NEW PERSPECTIVES IN SACRAL NERVE STIMULATION

FOR CONTROL OF LOWER URINARY TRACT DYSFUNCTION

Edited by **Udo Jonas & Volker Grünewald**

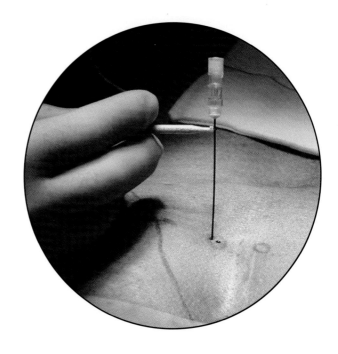

Includes full-colour atlas on surgical procedures

Kindly sponsored by
an unrestricted grant from Medtronic

MARTIN DUNITZ

© 2002 Martin Dunitz Ltd., a member of the Taylor & Francis group

First published in the United Kingdom in 2002 by
Martin Dunitz Ltd., The Livery House, 7–9 Pratt Street, London NW1 0AE
Tel: +44 (0) 20 74822202
Fax: +44 (0) 20 72670159
Email: info@dunitz.co.uk
Website: http://www.dunitz.co.uk

Although every effort has been made to ensure that all owners of copyright material have been acknowledged in this publication, we would be glad to acknowledge in subsequent reprints or editions any omissions brought to our attention.

The Authors have asserted their rights under the Copyright, Designs and Patents Act 1988 to be identified as the Authors of this Work.

Although every effort has been made to ensure that drug doses and other information are presented accurately in this publication, the ultimate responsibility rests with the prescribing physician. Neither the publishers nor the authors can be held responsible for errors or for any consequences arising from the use of information contained herein. For detailed prescribing information or instructions on the use of any product or procedure discussed herein, please consult the prescribing information or instructional material issued by the manufacturer.

A CIP record for this book is available from the British Library.
ISBN 1-84184-114-5

Distributed in the USA by
Fulfilment Center
Taylor & Francis
7625 Empire Drive
Florence, KY 41042, USA
Toll Free Tel: +1 800 634 7064
E-mail: cserve@routledge_ny.com

Distributed in Canada by
Taylor & Francis
74 Rolark Drive
Scarborough, Ontario M1R 4G2, Canada
Toll Free Tel: +1 877 226 2237
E-mail: tal_fran@istar.ca

Distributed in the rest of the world by
ITPS Limited
Cheriton House
North Way
Andover, Hampshire SP10 5BE, UK
Tel: +44 (0)1264 332424
E-mail: reception@itps.co.uk

Project management services by publish2day, Oxford
Indexed by Laurence Errington
Design and layout by InPerspective, London
Artwork by Peter Dolan, Medtronic Inc
Printed and bound in Singapore

Contents

List of contributors

Agnew, W.F., PhD, Director, Neural Engineering Laboratory, Huntington Medical Research Institutes, Pasadena, CA, USA

Arduini, A., MD, Field Engineer, Medtronic, Italy

Benson, J.T., MD, FACOG, Clinical Professor, Obstetrics and Gynaecology, University of Indiana, Indianapolis, IN, USA

Bertapelle, P., MD, Department of Urology, CTO-CRF-MA, Torino, Italy

den Boon, J., MD, Department of Gynaecology, Leiden University Medical Centre, The Netherlands

Bosch, J.L.H.R., MD, PhD, FEBU, Professor of Urology, Academic Hospital Rotterdam, The Netherlands

Braun, P.-M., MD, Department of Urology, University of Mannheim, Germany

Cappellano, F., MD, Department of Urology, Multimedica, Sesto S. Giovanni, Italy

Chai, T.C., MD, FACS, Assistant Professor of Urology, University of Maryland School of Medicine, Baltimore, MD, USA

Chancellor, M.B., MD, Professor of Urology and OBGYN, University of Pittsburgh School of Medicine, PA, USA

Chartier-Kastler, E. J., MD, PhD, Associate Professor of Urology, GH Pitié-Salpêtrière, Université Paris VI, Paris, France

Dahms, S., MD

Everaert, K., MD, Department of Urology, University Hospital Gent, Belgium

Fowler, C.J., MSc, FRCP, Department of Uro-Neurology, National Hospital for Neurology and Neurosurgery, London, UK

Ganio, E., MD, Department of Surgery, ORC, Colorectal Eporediensis Centre, Ivrea, Italy

Gerber, M., BSEE, MBA, Senior Product Development Manager, Medtronic, Minneapolis, MN, USA

Giardiello, G., Electronic Engineer, Clinical Manager, Medtronic, Italy

Groenendijk, P.M., MD, Department of Urology, Leiden University Medical Centre, The Netherlands

Grünewald, V., MD, Department of Urology, Medizinische Hochschule Hannover, Germany

Hampel, C., MD, Department of Urology, University of Mainz, Germany

Hassouna, M.M., MD, PhD, FRCSC, FACS, Associate Professor of Surgery, University of Toronto, Canada

Höfner, K., MD, PhD, Chairman, Department of Urology, Evangelisches Krankenhaus Oberhausen, Germany

Hohenfellner, M., MD, Associate Professor of Urology, University of Mainz, Germany

van den Hombergh, U., MD, Clinical Study Manager, Medtronic BRC, Maastricht, The Netherlands

Jonas, U., MD, Chairman, Department of Urology, Medizinische Hochschule Hannover, Germany

Jünemann, K.-P., MD, Department of Urology, University of Kiel, Germany

van Kerrebroeck, P.E.V., MD, PhD, FEBU, Chairman, Department of Urology, University of Maastricht, The Netherlands

Leng, W., MD, Assistant Professor of Urology, University of Pittsburgh School of Medicine, PA, USA

Lycklama à Nijeholt, A.A.B., MD, PhD, Department of Urology, Leiden University Medical Centre, The Netherlands

Mamo, G.A., MD, Clinical Instructor, University of Maryland Hospital, Baltimore, MA, USA

Matzel, K.E., MD, Department of Surgery, University of Erlangen-Nürenberg, Germany

McCreery, D.B., PhD, Senior Staff Scientist, Neural Engineering Laboratory, Huntington Medical Research Institutes, Pasadena, CA, USA

Molho, D., MD, Psychologist Neurourology and Spinal Unit Magenta Hospital (Milan), Italy

Morganti, C., MD, Psychiatrist, Niguarda Hospital (Milan), Italy

Oleson, K.A., BA, Director of Clinical and Regulatory Affairs, Medtronic EP Systems, Minneapolis, MN, USA

Peeren, F., MD

Ruiz-Cerdá, J.L., MD, PhD, FEBU, Department of Urology, Hospital de la Ribera, Alzira (Valencia), Spain

Scheepens, W.A., MD, Research Fellow, Department of Urology, University of Maastricht, The Netherlands

Schlote, N., MD, Department of Urology, Medizinische Hochschule Hannover, Germany

Schmidt, R.A., MD, HSC Division of Urology, University of Colorado, Denver, CO, USA

Schultz-Lampel, D., MD, Associate Professor of Urology, Kontinenzzentrum Südwest, Klinikum der Stadt Villingen-Schwenningen, Germany

Siegel, S.W., MD, Director, Center for Continence Care, Metropolitan Urologic Specialists, St. Paul, MN, USA

Spinelli, M., MD, Neurology and Spinal Unit, Magenta Hospital (Milan), Italy

Swoyer, J., BACHEM, Senior Principle Product Development Engineer, Medtronic, Minneapolis, MN, USA

Tanagho, E.A., MD, Professor of Urology, University of California, San Francisco, CA, USA

Thüroff, J.W., MD, Professor of Urology, Johannes Gutenberg University Medical School, Mainz, Germany

Tronnes, C., BSME, Senior Product Development Engineer, Medtronic, Minneapolis, MN, USA

Yuen, T.G.H., PhD, Experimental Pathologist, Neural Engineering Laboratory, Huntington Medical Research Institutes, Pasadena, CA, USA

Foreword

In 1971 B.S. Nashold and co-workers published a paper which incited great scientific interest*. They reported the successful implantation of a neural prosthesis on the sacral segment of the spinal cord, which was then used to activate detrusor contraction and micturition in spinal-cord-injured patients. In the same year, the newly-founded neural prosthesis programme within the National Institute of Neurological Communicative Diseases and Stroke (NINCDS), under the directorship of Dr. F. Terry Hambrecht, funded various neuroprosthesis programmes. These included helping the blind to see, the deaf to hear, the paraplegic to walk and the quadriplegic to use their hands, and constituted only a few of the efforts they supported. Control of bladder and bowel function in the spinal-cord-injured patient was also studied. However, when micturition could not be controlled through electrode implantation on the spinal cord, researchers moved towards the periphery, applying stimulation to the sacral roots in the hope of controlling the detrusor muscle and its sphincteric mechanism.

At the University of California, San Francisco, we were fortunate to be part of the team that initiated this work almost 30 years ago. We developed numerous experimental models to evaluate the feasibility of stimulation of various sacral roots or components, to thereby gain control of bladder function, restoring its storage and evacuative capabilities. From these experiments on both normal and paraplegic animals we learned a great deal. Work continued uninterrupted and, after the basic scientific foundation for sacral root stimulation had been established, clinical application was begun. The co-editor of this volume, Professor Udo Jonas, was one of the very first scientists to explore the possibilities of sacral nerve stimulation to control bladder function.

This book distinguishes itself in being concerned not only with reporting successful clinical application but also with discussing the basic research that led up to it. Chapters deal with the neurophysiology and mechanisms of neural control, the principles of safe stimulation, its effectiveness in refractory urge incontinence and chronic retention and the wider scope of other voiding dysfunctions. Emerging indications (pelvic pain, interstitial cystitis,

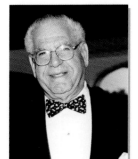

fecal incontinence and chronic constipation) are also explored by experts in the field.

Although this technology is still in its infancy, it offers successful treatment options to a core of unfortunate patients with intractable voiding dysfunction. We anticipate further refinement in neuromodulation as well as new frontiers for its application.

E. A. Tanagho, MD
University of California, San Francisco

*Nashold BS, Friedman H, Boyarsky S. Electrical activation of micturition by spinal cord stimulation. *J Surg Res* 1971; 11 (3): 144–70.

Introduction

This textbook, describing sacral nerve stimulation (SNS) and its aim of restoration of lower urinary tract function, is an important introduction to this specific branch of urological surgery. It should give the reader an insight into this new field and the state-of-the-art of a 'high-tech' surgical procedure. It is hoped that the reader will become familiar with the specific anatomy, with the principles of neurostimulation and neuromodulation, patient selection, and with the results obtained in the last two decades from using this intriguing technique. For a better understanding, the surgical atlas gives a visual demonstration of the 'tricks of the trade' — how to conduct preoperative screening as well as how to perform the implantation of the device itself.

The editors were delighted at their success in recruiting worldwide experts in this field to contribute to this book. Their impact in the development and clinical application of SNS has been pivotal in making this procedure a successful and a clinically accepted therapy. With regard to the role of SNS in the control of lower urinary tract dysfunction, the technique developed in cooperation with Medtronic is described here. With this in mind, the editors wish to thank the many members of the Medtronic InterStim investigators group worldwide — those with active participation in this volume as authors, as well as those who were co-investigators in the trials and co-authors in the publications cited herein. It is clear to all of us that SNS is not a first-line therapy: the indications for use are for those patients in whom conservative treatment has failed and in whom extensive and 'heroic' surgery might be necessary in order to solve their voiding and storage problems.

In order to validate a new therapy it is always important to look back in history, because research always builds on the successes and failures of the past. All the various techniques mentioned in Chapter 1, by Drs. Schlote and Tanagho, were the basis on which the practice of SNS was constructed and finally brought to clinical use. Because the sacral region is not necessarily familiar territory for urologists, Chapter 2 covers the anatomy of the sacrum, with special emphasis on localisation of the sacral foramina by the use of anatomical landmarks for electrode placement. Two chapters (Chapters 3 and 4) deal with neural control and the principles of safety and efficacy in nerve stimulation, in particular with the aim of avoiding nerve damage during stimulation and with a special focus on electrode design, stimulation characteristics, and long-term outcome. Chapters 5–7 are devoted to diagnosis and to clinical and urodynamic assessment. The correlation between clinical improvement following SNS, and the abolition of uninhibited bladder contractions, has been poor, and it has been shown that SNS may have a primary effect on urethral and pelvic-floor function. It is concluded that more studies on the interaction between urethra and bladder should be performed as soon as possible to increase our knowledge regarding the clinical applications of SNS (Chapters 4 and 5).

In Chapter 6, Dr. Hassouna discusses neuromodulation and growth factors in the lower urinary tract. He reports on the normal distribution of substance P and calcitonin-gene-related peptides in normal and pathological conditions, and the expression of c-*fos* and the distribution of nerve growth factor (again in both normal and pathological conditions). In Chapter 7, Drs. Grünewald and Höfner sum up pretreatment diagnostic evaluation, with special emphasis on the influence of drugs affecting lower urinary tract function. They describe the clinical examination and the general and specific tests, and focus on the peripheral nerve evaluation (PNE) test, which is mandatory prior to final implantation. In Chapter 8, Martin Gerber and co-workers describe the development and current design of the hardware. This information is important for the reader and the user in order to understand the principles and mechanism of SNS; it will enable appreciation of how this technique is applied and of why technical failures might occur.

In Chapters 9–11, Drs. van Kerrebroek, Siegel, and Benson discuss the indications for implantation as well as the predictive factors, again summarising the technique of PNE, which is (as a screening method) mandatory prior to each implantation. Furthermore, they introduce the principle of electrophysiological monitoring in SNS. Such monitoring can be helpful to validate the response during stimulation, especially because, at present, SNS is still in its infancy and future modifications and improvements are to be expected.

In Chapters 12 and 13, a sophisticated description of PNE and of the final implantation is given by the editors. This, again, helps the reader — and, certainly, also the surgeon — to understand the pre-implantation screening as well as the implantation itself. It enhances understanding of the surgical technique and can be used as a guideline for testing, as well as for implantation.

In Chapter 14, reprints of three publications (which all appeared in the *Journal of Urology*) describe the clinical results of SNS in patients with refractory urinary incontinence (R. Schmidt *et al.*) and in those with urinary retention (U. Jonas *et al.*), as well as the use of SNS in the treatment of urgency–frequency (M. Hassouna *et al.*). The data in these three papers represent the many years of intensive work of the Medtronic InterStim investigator group. In cooperation with Medtronic InterStim, they finally succeeded in obtaining FDA approval and in making this very intriguing and sophisticated work available for wide clinical use. To date, there have been more than 5000 implantations.

In Chapter 15, Dr. Spinelli and his group discuss patient selection and outcome evaluation in two groups of patients with symptoms of urgency–frequency or retention. It was concluded that psychological evaluation could be useful in the diagnosis of this very difficult patient population in order to determine eligibility for permanent electrode implantation. In the second half of Chapter 15, Dr. Cappellano and co-workers assessed the problem of quality of life (QoL) and concluded that SNS is an effective therapy that undoubtedly has a very positive effect on the patient's QoL.

There is no surgery without potential complications. Chapter 16 (U. Jonas and U. van den Hombergh) deals with this aspect and elucidates the safety data obtained in the investigational trial described in Chapter 14. These data showed clearly that no patient ultimately displayed permanent adverse effects after SNS. It was also noted that, in the 250 patients receiving an implant, no unanticipated event associated with the implanted system was reported. Overall, nearly 90% of 368 events in the study population were fully resolved at the time of database closure. However, the overall number of adverse events and the re-operation rate were significant enough to require further detailed analysis and efforts to improve this.

Chapters 17–19 look at the way ahead. In Chapter 17 the issue of bilateral stimulation is addressed by D. Schultz-Lampel, M. Hohenfellner, J.W. Thüroff, P.M. Braun and K.P. Jünemann. These authors present their experiences with bilateral SNS, using different surgical approaches for placement of the stimulating leads. Although the results in all studies are retrospectively obtained from a small number of treated patients without randomisation between unilateral and bilateral implants, all authors report improved results of bilateral compared with unilateral stimulation in their series. However, it remains unclear at this stage if this holds good for the long-term efficacy. Furthermore, it is not yet known whether the mere fact of bilateral stimulation alone might increase efficacy, or whether modifications of the surgical technique (in general, increasing the invasiveness of the procedure) also contribute to these improved results — and if so, to what extent.

In Chapter 18, M. Spinelli and co-workers introduce a new, minimally-invasive surgical technique (derived from PNE) for placement of the permanent lead. The percutaneous canal is dilated for final placement of a quadripolar lead inside the sacral foramen.

Under the lead-authorship of J.L.H.R. Bosch, Chapter 19 focuses on emerging new indications of SNS. The technique is not restricted to the treatment of other urological conditions, such as neurogenic refractory urge incontinence (J.L.H.R. Bosch) or interstitial cystitis (T.C. Chai), but may also be indicated for the treatment of disorders like faecal incontinence (K.E. Matzel), chronic faecal constipation (E. Ganio), and pelvic pain (K. Everaert and F. Peeren) as an isolated or associated symptom.

Finally, Chapter 20 (J.L. Ruiz Cerdá) focuses on the follow-up procedure and on the life expectancy of the system; trouble-shooting guidelines for outpatient follow-up are provided. It is concluded that those physicians who undertake implantation procedures must commit themselves to long-term follow-up assessments, because it is mandatory that these patients are seen regularly for their entire lifetime after surgery. Successful results can only be achieved if all aspects of patient care are covered; mere evaluation of technical aspects of the surgical and follow-up procedures would definitely be inappropriate.

In summary, this book is the first comprehensive, overall view of most aspects of sacral nerve stimulation. Any urologist with an interest in neurourology, and especially in the treatment of lower urinary tract dysfunction, should read this book and peruse the surgical atlas. Thus informed, urologists will gain a better insight into this new techique and the relevant aspects of the method. This will hopefully enable them to perform successful implants and to follow up satisfied patients.

U. Jonas, MD and
V. Grünewald, MD.
Hanover Medical School, Germany

1 Electrical stimulation of the lower urinary tract: historical overview

N. Schlote and E.A. Tanagho

Introduction

The discovery of electricity introduced enormous changes to human society: it not only improved daily life but also opened up new opportunities in scientific research. In the eighteenth century, the connection was made between nerves and electricity [1]. However, the observation that electricity could produce muscular contraction did not lead immediately to the conclusion that muscles and nerves produce and use electricity in order to function. Luigi Galvani was the first to suggest this possibility in his animal experiments [2]. He found that a device constructed from dissimilar metals, when applied to the nerve or muscle of a frog's leg, would induce muscular contraction. However, he thought that the metal provided a path to discharge the electricity inherent in the animal's muscle. Although it was impossible at that time for him to understand the relevant physical and chemical processes, his work formed the foundation for later discoveries of transmembrane potential and electrically-mediated nerve impulses.

Alessandro Volta, the inventor of the electrical battery (or voltaic pile) [3], was later able to induce a muscle contraction by producing a potential with his battery and conducting it to a muscle strip. He realised that the applied current in the metal, rather than 'animal electricity', was the source of the muscular contraction. He also showed that, if the metal conductors were eliminated and the end of the nerve was looped back to touch the muscle and then stimulated, contraction resulted; this phenomenon proved that the muscle contraction was caused by electricity transmitted by the nerve. The use of Volta's battery for stimulating nerves or muscles became known as galvanic stimulation.

Another basis for modern neural stimulators was the discovery of the connection between electricity and magnetism, demonstrated by Oersted in 1820; he described the effect of current passing through a wire on a magnetised needle. One year later, Faraday showed the converse — that a magnet could exert a force on a current-carrying wire. He continued to investigate magnetic induction by inducing current in a metal wire rotating in a magnetic field. This device was a forerunner of the electric motor and made it possible to build the magneto-electric and the induction coil stimulator. The latter, the first electric generator, was called the Faraday stimulator. Faradaic stimulation could produce sustained tetanic contractions of muscles, instead of a single muscle twitch as galvanic stimulation had done.

Key Points

- The connection between electricity and muscular contraction was made in the 18th century by Galvani and Volta.
- This led to development of the induction coil (Faraday) stimulator producing sustained, tetanic contractions.
- This facilitated study of the functional anatomy of individual muscles and of neuromuscular contraction.

Duchenne used an induction coil stimulator to study the anatomy, physiology and pathology of human muscles. Finally, he was able to study the functional anatomy of individual muscles [4,5]. This work is still valid for the investigation of functional neuromuscular stimulation.

In the early twentieth century, with the development of electric oscillators, stimulators, and amplifiers for neurophysiological studies, there was improved understanding of nerve impulses, synaptic transmission and functional areas within the nervous system. The German neurosurgeon Förster was the first to expose the human occipital pole under local anaesthesia and to stimulate this area electrically [6]. This stimulation caused the subject to see a spot of light, the location of this light being dependent on the location of the stimulated area. These findings formed the basis of efforts to develop visual prostheses for the blind.

Another basis for modern stimulator devices lay in the work of Chaffee and Light [7]. They examined the problem of stimulating neural structures deep in the body, while avoiding the risk of infection from percutaneous leads: they implanted a secondary coil underneath the skin and placed a primary coil outside the body, using magnetic induction for energy transfer and modulation. Further improvement was achieved by radio-frequency induction [8,9]. The group around Glenn developed a totally implanted heart pacemaker — one of the first commercially available stimulators. In the ensuing years, stimulators for different organ systems were developed, among them the above-mentioned heart pacemaker, a diaphragmatic pacemaker [8,9], and the cochlear implant [10].

Bladder stimulation

The concept of electrical stimulation of the bladder dates back to 1878. The Danish surgeon M.H. Saxtorph treated patients with urinary retention by inserting a special catheter with a metal electrode into the urinary bladder transurethrally and placing a neutral electrode suprapubically [11]. Katona *et al.* have described their technique of intraluminal electrotherapy; this method was initially designed to treat a paralytic gastrointestinal tract but was later used for neurogenic bladder dysfunction in patients with incomplete central or peripheral nerve lesions [12,13]. The activation of specific receptors in the bladder wall leads to small, local, muscular contractions, which further depolarise other receptor cells. Their stimuli create centrally induced, better coordinated, stronger detrusor contractions.

Further interest in the electrical control of bladder function began in the 1950s and 1960s. The most pressing question at that time was the appropriate location for stimulation. Several groups attempted to initiate or prevent voiding (in urinary retention and incontinence, respectively) by stimulation of the pelvic floor, the detrusor directly, the spinal cord, or the pelvic and sacral nerves or sacral roots. Even other parts of the body, such as the skin, were stimulated in an attempt to influence bladder function.

In 1954, McGuire performed a series of direct bladder stimulations in dogs [14] with a variety of electrodes, both single and multiple, in a variety of positions. These studies showed that a single pair of electrodes did not cause uniform spread of the stimulus to the entire detrusor but that multiple pairs of electrodes gave a more uniform increase in intravesical pressure. This research was continued by Boyce and associates [15]. Their experiments, also in a dog model, demonstrated the importance of the size of the electrode (which, at that time, was recommended not to exceed 1.0–1.5cm in diameter). Either a wire coil or a perforated plate was equally effective, although the coil could more easily be buried in the detrusor. With a single pair of electrodes, the maximal response was obtained when the electrodes were placed on both lateral bladder walls so that the points of stimulation encompassed a maximal amount of detrusor muscle. In human studies, the same group implanted an induction coil for direct bladder stimulation in three paraplegic men with complete paralysis of the detrusor muscle. The secondary coil was implanted in the subcutaneous tissue of the lower abdominal wall. In these three patients the results were an unqualified failure in one, a partial success in one, and highly successful in the third [15].

In 1963, Bradley and associates published their experience with an implantable stimulator [16]. They were able to achieve complete bladder evacuation in the chronic dog model over 14 months. However, when the stimulator was implanted in seven patients, detrusor contraction was produced but bladder evacuation resulted in only two. Further experiments were performed in the sheep, calf and monkey to seek to resolve species discrepancies. These animals were chosen because, in the sheep and calf, the bladder is approximately the same size as in the human, and this similarity could determine whether more power is needed for a bladder larger than that of the dog. In addition, the pelvis of monkeys and humans is similarly deep; thus, the influence (if any) of pelvic structure could be investigated. The results showed that a larger bladder needs more power and wider contact between the electrodes and that differences in structure do not necessitate different stimulation techniques [16].

Pelvic floor stimulation

In 1963, Caldwell described his clinical experience with the first implantable pelvic floor stimulator [17]. The electrodes were placed into the sphincter, with the secondary coil placed subcutaneously near the iliac spine. This device was primarily designed for the treatment of faecal incontinence; nonetheless, Caldwell also treated urinary incontinence successfully.

The development of a transrectal stimulator for electrical pelvic floor stimulation [18] later provided a relatively simple method for treating incontinence. Although this technique was used primarily for outlet incontinence, it was also shown to be effective in treating urinary incontinence due to detrusor instability [19], although Menu cited some restrictions in its benefit to patients with upper motor-neuron lesions [20].

In female patients, another approach to pelvic floor stimulation is intravaginal electrical stimulation, reported initially by Magnus Fall's group in 1977 [21]. They published numerous studies dealing

Key Points
- Animal experiments were conducted in the 1960s.
- Bladders of different sizes require different power levels and electrode spacing.
- Structural differences do not necessitate different stimulation techniques.
- Pelvic floor stimulation was used to treat outlet and detrusor instability.

with this subject in the ensuing years and found that intravaginal electrical stimulation also induces bladder inhibition in patients with detrusor instability. Lindström, a member of the same group, demonstrated that bladder inhibition is accomplished by reflexogenic activation of sympathetic hypogastric inhibitory neurons and by central inhibition of pelvic parasympathetic excitatory neurons to the bladder [22]. The afferent pathways for these effects could be shown to originate from the pudendal nerves.

Another interesting application of electrical stimulation for inhibition of detrusor activity is the transcutaneous stimulation of the posterior tibial or common peroneal nerve. This technique, drawn from traditional Chinese medicine, is based on the acupuncture points for inhibition of bladder activity and was reported by McGuire *et al.* in 1983 [23]. Although simple, it has never found widespread acceptance.

Pelvic nerve stimulation

In 1957, Ingersoll *et al.* reported the effects of unilateral pelvic nerve stimulation on the urinary bladder [24]. Unfortunately, pelvic nerves do not tolerate chronic stimulation and the pudendal nerves are activated, increasing outflow resistance. Additionally, in humans the fibres of the parasympathetic nervous system innervating the bladder split early in the pelvis, forming a broad plexus unsuitable for electrode application.

Detrusor stimulation

Direct detrusor stimulation offers high specificity to the target organ [25], but its disadvantages are electrode displacement and malfunction due to bladder movement during voiding, and fibrosis — even erosion — of the bladder wall. In 1967, Hald *et al.* [26] reported their experience of direct detrusor stimulation with a radio-linked stimulator in four patients, three with upper motor-neuron lesions and one with a lower motor-neuron lesion. The receiver was placed in a paraumbilical subcutaneous pocket. Two wires from the receiver were passed subcutaneously to the ventral bladder wall, where they were implanted. A small portable external transmitter generated the necessary energy. The procedure worked in three patients; in one it failed because of technical problems.

Spinal cord stimulation

Nashold, Friedman and associates were the first to attempt to achieve micturition via spinal cord stimulation [27]. They explored the possibility of direct electrical activation of the micturition centre in the sacral segments of the conus medullaris and reported that the region for optimal stimulation is S1–S3. Effectiveness was determined not only by location but also by frequency. In subsequent experiments, the same group compared the stimulation of the dorsal surface of the spinal cord at L5, S1 and S2 with depth stimulation (2–3mm) at S1 and S2 in acute and chronic settings [28]. It was only through the latter, the depth stimulation, that voiding was produced: high bladder pressures were achieved by surface stimulation but external sphincter relaxation did not occur, and was noted only after direct application of the stimulus to the micturition centre in the spinal cord. Stimulation between L5 and S1 produced pressure without voiding, even with depth stimulation.

Jonas *et al.* continued the investigation of direct spinal-cord stimulation to achieve voiding [29–31]. They compared 12 different types of electrodes — three surface (bipolar surface electrode, dorsal column electrode, and wrap-around electrode) and nine depth electrodes. These differed in many parameters (e.g. bipolar–tripolar, horizontal–vertical–transverse). Regardless of the type of electrode, the detrusor response to stimulation was similar. Interestingly, the wrap-around surface electrode with the most extended current spread provoked the same results as the coaxial depth electrode with the least current spread, prompting those authors to theorise that current does not cross the midline of the spinal cord. Unfortunately, no real voiding was achieved. It was found that the stimulation of the spinal cord motor centres stimulates the urethral smooth and striated sphincteric elements simultaneously: the expected detrusor contraction resulted, but sphincteric contraction was associated. The sphincteric resistance was too high to allow voiding — it allowed only minimal voiding at the end of the stimulation, so-called poststimulus voiding. These results contrasted with the earlier work of Nashold and Friedman [27,28].

The next attempt was to locate and differentiate the principal neuronal cells in the spinal cord to overcome the problem of simultaneous contraction of striated sphincter and detrusor. In retrograde tracer studies with horseradish peroxidase injected into various locations in the autonomic and somatic systems of the lower urinary tract, Thürhoff *et al.* determined the existence of two nuclei, a parasympathetic and a pudendal nucleus [32]. The parasympathetic nucleus could be shown within the pudendal nucleus; thus, at the level of the spinal cord, stimulation of the bladder separate to that of the sphincter is difficult.

Sacral root stimulation

For these reasons the feasibility of sacral rootlet stimulation was investigated, based on the hypothesis that different roots would carry different neuronal axons to different locations. The University of California, San Francisco (UCSF) group performed numerous experiments on a canine model [33], as the anatomy of bladder innervation of the dog is similar to that of the human. After laminectomy, the spinal roots were explored and stimulated, either intradurally or extradurally, but within the spinal canal, in the following modes: (1) unilateral stimulation of the intact sacral root at various levels; (2) simultaneous bilateral stimulation of the intact sacral root at various levels; (3) stimulation of the intact ventral and dorsal root separately; (4) stimulation of the proximal and distal ends of the divided sacral root; (5) stimulation of the proximal and distal ends of the divided dorsal and ventral roots. From these studies it became clear that stimulating the intact root is least effective and stimulating the ventral component is most effective and that no difference exists between right- and left-root stimulation [33]. Besides detrusor contraction, stimulation caused some sphincteric

Key Points
- Sacral root stimulation has been investigated extensively in dogs.
- Stimulation of the ventral sacral root is more effective than intact root stimulation.

Key Points

- Detrusor and sphincter contraction can be activated separately.
- Sphincter contraction can be sustained without detrusor reaction.
- Stimulation of human sacral roots is effective in neurogenic bladder dysfunction.
- Long-term treatment uses a permanently implanted electrode in contact with deafferented S3 nerve roots.

contraction, owing to the presence of both autonomic and somatic fibres in the ventral root, and the studies were continued with the addition of neurotomy to eliminate the afferent fibres. The dorsal fibres were separated and cut, and only the ventral component was stimulated. In this model the stimulated sacral roots became the carriers of autonomic efferent fibres. These experiments showed that, to achieve maximally specific detrusor stimulation, the dorsal component must be separated from the ventral component and the somatic fibres of the root must be isolated and selectively cut [34]. The experiments also demonstrated that stimulation with low frequency and low voltage can maintain adequate sphincteric activity, but that stimulation with high frequency and low voltage will fatigue the external sphincter and block its activity. When high-frequency/low-voltage stimulation is followed by high-voltage stimulation, bladder contraction will be induced and voiding achieved.

The finding that detrusor contraction can be activated separately from sphincteric activity and that adequate sphincteric contraction can be sustained without exciting a detrusor reaction made it seem possible that a true bladder pacemaker could be achieved. In addition, in histological and electron-microscopic examination of the stimulated sacral roots, no damage was found when they were compared with the contralateral non-stimulated roots. Neither the operation nor the chronic stimulation damaged the ventral root, and the responses remained reliable and stable.

For further development of this technique in humans, Tanagho's group later performed detailed anatomical studies on human cadavers. The aim was to establish the exact anatomical distribution of the entire sacral plexus, following it from the sacral roots in the spinal cord through the sacral foramen inside the pelvic cavity. Emphasis was placed on the autonomic pelvic plexus as well as the somatic fibres. With this anatomical knowledge, the stimulation of human sacral roots in neurogenic bladder dysfunction was developed and made clinically applicable as a long-term treatment [35]. Direct electrical stimulation was performed through a permanently implanted electrode, placed mostly in contact with S3 nerve roots in the sacral foramen, after deafferentation.

As noted above, studies had shown the existence of separate parasympathetic and pudendal nuclei. The ventral sacral roots emerge as numerous separate rootlets. The spatial orientation of these rootlets implies that each carries the axons of the closest neuronal cell group in the spinal cord, meaning that the axons emerging from the parasympathetic nucleus and those emerging from the pudendal nucleus are separate. These rootlets group into rootlet bundles that later constitute the ventral root, in which form they exit the dura. Dissection of these rootlets throughout their entire course in the dura showed that they maintain their identity. This could mean that stimulation of specific rootlets might be equivalent in specificity and selectivity to microstimulation of specific neuron groupings in the spinal cord. The fibres that carry autonomic fibres to the detrusor muscle could be isolated by stimulating these rootlets. If this could be done intradurally, they could be cut and electrodes placed extradurally at the entire ventral root.

This was successfully shown in the dog model [36]. The stimulation of sacral rootlet bundles isolated from the rest of the sacral root gave the same increase of bladder pressure when stimulated close to the exit from the dura, in the mid-segment, or close to the origin in the spinal cord. This could make the stimulation more selective, eliminating detrusor–sphincter dyssynergia.

In additional work, taking advantage of the knowledge that high-frequency current can block large somatic fibres, electrical blockade of undesired responses was tested to replace selective somatic neurotomies. High-frequency sinusoidal stimulation was effective in blocking external sphincter activity. However, the sinusoidal waveform is not efficient. Alternate-phase, rectangular wave is more efficient and induces the same blockade: alternating pulses of high frequency and low amplitude followed by pulses of low frequency and high amplitude were effective in inducing low-pressure voiding without the need for somatic neurotomies. This approach has not yet been tried clinically, but it might prove to be the answer to the problem of detrusor–sphincter dyssynergia in electrically stimulated voiding.

Key Points

- Increased selectivity of stimulation by isolated root bundles eliminates detrusor–sphincter dyssynergia.
- Electrical blockade of undesired responses may replace selective somatic neurotomies.
- Clinically, this would solve the problem of detrusor–sphincter dyssynergia in electrically stimulated voiding.

Conclusions

Thus, neurostimulation of the bladder has had a long and arduous history. Neurogenic bladder dysfunction can now be treated; however, many groups continue to carry out pioneering work in this field. With increasing anatomical and physiological knowledge and greater technical improvements, artificial means may no longer be required.

References

1. Brazier MAB. *A History of Neurophysiology in the 17th and 18th Centuries*. New York: Raven Press, 1984.
2. Galvani L. *De viribus electricitatis in motu musculari, commentarius*. De Bononiensi Scientarium et Artium Instituto Atque Academia 1791; 7: 363–418.
3. Volta A. Letter to Sir Joseph Banks, March 20, 1800. On electricity excited by the mere contact of conducting substances of different kinds. *Philos Trans R Soc Lon* [Biol] 1800; 90: 403–31.
4. Duchenne GBA. *De l'électrisation localisée et de son application à la physiologie, à la pathologie et à la therapeutique*. Paris, 1855.
5. Duchenne GBA. *Physiologie des mouvements demonstrée à l'aide de l'experimentation electrique et de l'observation clinique, et applicable à l'étude des paralysies et des deformations*. Paris, 1867.
6. Förster O. Beiträge zur pathophysiologie der sehbalin und der sehsphaere. *J Psychol Neurol Lpz* 1929; 39: 463–85.
7. Chaffee EL, Light RE. A method for remote control of electrical stimulation of the nervous system. *Yale J Biol Med* 1934; 7: 83.
8. Glenn WWL, Phelps MŁ. Diaphragm pacing by electrical stimulation of the phrenic nerve. *Neurosurgery* 1985; 17: 974–84.
9. Glenn WWL, Mauro A, Longo E et al. Remote stimulation of the heart by radiofrequency transmission. *N Engl J Med* 1959; 261: 948.
10. House WF. Cochlear implants. *Ann Otol Rhinol Laryngol* 1976; 85(27): 1–93.
11. Saxtorph MH. *Strictura urethrae — Fistula perinei — Retentio urinae*. Clinisk Chirurgi. Copenhagen: Gyldendalske Forlag, 1878.
12. Katona F, Benyo L, Lang J. Uber intraluminare elektrotherapie vor verschiedenen paralytischen zuständen des gastrointestinalen tractes mit quadrangularstrom. *Zentralbl Chir* 1959; 84: 929.

13. Katona F. Stages of vegetative afferentation in reorganization of bladder control during electrotherapy. *Urol Int* 1975; 30: 192–203.

14. McGuire WE. Response of the neurogenic bladder to various electrical stimuli. Research Thesis, Department of Surgery, Bowman Gray School of Medicine, Jan. 1955.

15. Boyce WH, Lathem JE, Hunt LD. Research related to the development of an artificial electrical stimulator for the paralyzed human bladder: a review. *J Urol* 1964; 91: 41–51.

16. Bradley WE, Chou SN, French LA. Further experience with the radio transmitter receiver unit for the neurogenic bladder. *J Neurosurg* 1963; 20: 953–60.

17. Caldwell KPS. The electrical control of sphincter incompetence. *Lancet* 1963; 2: 174.

18. Glen ES. Guard for intra-anal-plug electrode. *Lancet* 1969; 2: 325–6.

19. Kock NG, Pompeius R. Inhibition of vesical motor activity induced by anal stimulation. *Acta Clin Scand* 1963; 126: 244.

20. Menu DC. The treatment of detrusor incontinence by electrical stimulation. *J Urol* 1979; 122: 515.

21. Fall M, Erlandson BE, Carlsson CA, Lindström S. The effect of intravaginal electrical stimulation on the feline urethra and urinary bladder. *Scand J Urol Nephrol* (Suppl) 1977; 44: 19–30.

22. Lindström S, Fall M, Carlsson CA, Erlandson BE. The neurophysiological basis of bladder inhibition in response to intravaginal electrical stimulation. *J Urol* 1983; 129: 405–10.

23. McGuire EL, Zlang SC, Horwinski ER, Lytton B. Treatment of motor and sensory detrusor instability by electrical stimulation. *J Urol* 1983; 129: 78–9.

24. Ingersoll EH, Jones LL, Hegre ES. Effect on urinary bladder of unilateral stimulation of pelvic nerves in the dog. *Am J Physiol* 1957; 189: 167.

25. Hald T, Agrawal O, Kantrowitz A. Studies in stimulation of the bladder and its motor nerves. *Surgery* 1966; 60: 848–56.

26. Hald T, Meier W, Khalili A *et al*. Clinical experience with a radio-linked bladder stimulator. *J Urol* 1967; 97: 73–78.

27. Nashold BS, Friedman H, Boyarsky S. Electrical activation of micturition by spinal cord stimulation. *J Surg Res* 1971; 11: 144–7.

28. Friedman H, Nashold BS, Senechal P. Spinal cord stimulation and bladder function in normal and paraplegic animals. *J Neurosurg* 1972; 36: 430–7.

29. Jonas U, Heine JP, Tanagho EA. Studies on the feasibility of urinary bladder evacuation by direct spinal cord stimulation. I. Parameters of most effective stimulation. *Invest Urol* 1975; 13: 142–50.

30. Jonas U, James LW, Tanagho EA. Spinal cord stimulation versus detrusor stimulation. A comparative study in six acute dogs. *Invest Urol* 1975; 13: 171–4.

31. Jonas U, Tanagho EA. Studies on the feasibility of urinary bladder evacuation by direct spinal cord stimulation. II. Poststimulus voiding: a way to overcome outflow resistance. *Invest Urol* 1975; 13: 151–3.

32. Thürhoff JW, Bazeed MA, Schmidt RA *et al*. Regional topography of spinal cord neurons innervating pelvic floor muscles and bladder neck in the dog: a study by combined horseradish peroxidase histochemistry and autoradiography. *Urol Int* 1982; 37: 110–20.

33. Tanagho EA, Schmidt RA. Bladder pacemaker: scientific basis and clinical future. *Urology* 1982; 20: 614–9.

34. Schmidt RA, Bruschini H, Tanagho EA. Sacral root stimulation in controlled micturition: peripheral somatic neurotomy and stimulated voiding. *Invest Urol* 1979; 17: 130–4.

35. Probst M, Piechota HJ, Hohenfellner M *et al*. Neurostimulation for bladder evacuation: is sacral root stimulation a substitute for microstimulation? *Br J Urol* 1997; 79: 554–66.

36. Tanagho EA, Schmidt RA. Electrical stimulation in the clinical management of the neurogenic bladder. *J Urol* 1988; 140: 1331–9.

2 Anatomy of the sacral region

G.A. Mamo

Introduction

Urologists and gynaecologists are generally unfamiliar with the surgical anatomy of the sacral region. Surgical techniques used to localise the foramina and nerves during sacral neuromodulation are often challenging and time consuming, even with radiological assistance. The clinical response to the therapy is often dependent on precise positioning of the lead within the foramen; placing the lead at the wrong angle or even a few millimetres away from the nerve can alter the clinical outcome. With full understanding of the anatomy of this area, such difficulties can be avoided and better clinical results obtained. This chapter provides a detailed description of the anatomy involved in sacral neuromodulation.

ilium. the haunch bone a wide bone forming the upper part of each side of the hip bone

The sacrum

→ houses all sacral nerves.

The sacrum is a triangular bone extending from the inferior aspect of the vertebral column. It consists of five, fused, false vertebrae and houses all the sacral and coccygeal nerves. The sacrum articulates with the last lumbar vertebra at its base, with the ilium on either side laterally and with the coccyx at its apex. On its inferolateral aspect the sacrum is attached to the ischium by the sacro-sciatic ligament complex.

The ventral surface is concave in the vertical plane, and slightly so in the transverse plane. On the surface are four transverse lines, which represent the original division of the bone into five, separate vertebral bodies (Fig. 2.1). At the extremities of these lines are the anterior foramina, lateral to which is the 'lateral mass', formed by the coalesced transverse processes of the sacral vertebrae, and in which there are four shallow grooves containing the anterior sacral nerves.

The dorsal surface of the sacrum is convex but irregular, consisting of many ridges and grooves (Fig. 2.2). In the middle line is the median sacral crest, consisting of three or four tubercles, of which the first is usually very prominent and completely separate from the rest; these tubercles represent the rudimentary spinous processes. This crest ends inferiorly beneath the lowest tubercle, where there is a gap in the sacral canal termed the sacral hiatus; this defect is due to the failure of the fusion of

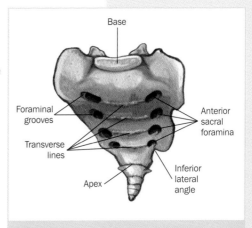

Figure 2.1 View of ventral surface of sacrum.

(Labels: Base; Foraminal grooves; Transverse lines; Apex; Anterior sacral foramina; Inferior lateral angle)

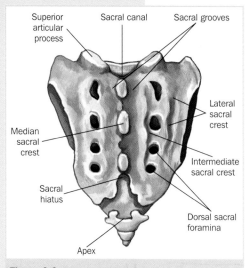

Figure 2.2 *View of dorsal surface of sacrum.*

the laminae of the fifth sacral vertebra (S5). On either side of the crest are the sacral grooves, with the intermediate sacral crest just lateral to them. This crest comprises a row of four small tubercles representing the fusion of the articular processes, forms the medial aspect of the posterior foramina. The lateral sacral crest, found just lateral to the foramina, is a ridge that is formed by the fusion of the transverse processes and is the site of insertion of the gluteus maximus muscle. Just beneath S4 the inferior lateral angle can be identified by the point at which the lateral sacral surface narrows abruptly and curves medially (Fig. 2.1).

The sacral canal runs throughout the greater part of the bone (Fig. 2.2). It is large and triangular superiorly, but shallow and flat inferiorly. It houses the sacral nerves, and is perforated by the anterior and posterior sacral foramina.

The sacrum can vary in shape and structure among different individuals and genders [1]. In females, it is wider than in males and less curved; the upper half tends to be straighter than the lower half. The sacrovertebral angle is greater in females than in males, which increases the size of the pelvic cavity. In males, the curvature is more evenly distributed over the whole length of the bone, and is altogether greater than that in females. Some individuals can have five sacral foramina if the dorsal laminae of the fifth vertebra fuse completely; in others, the sacral canal can be open for the entire lower half of the bone.

Sacral foramina

Each sacral foramen is a Y-shaped complex of canals, with the anterior foramen forming the stem and the posterior and intervertebral foramina forming the two limbs. The anterior foramina, which are analogous to the intervertebral foramina, are found approximately 2cm lateral to the midline on either side. They are trumpet shaped and widen laterally into broad, shallow grooves where the ventral rami of the upper four sacral nerves exit into the pelvis.

The posterior foramina are somewhat smaller; they diminish in size from above downwards and are covered by a fibrous membrane, which is probably analogous to the ligamentum flavum of the vertebral column [2]. The small dorsal branches of the corresponding sacral nerves traverse these foramina to innervate the multifidus muscle over the sacrum and the integument over the posterior part of the coccyx and gluteal region.

The posterior foramina appear to be equidistant in the vertical plane (Fig. 2.3). In a detailed anatomical study of cadaveric foramina, Hasan *et al.* [3] found that the mean interforaminal distances between each of the S2, S3 and S4 foramina was 4cm in both males and females: the mean distances between the S1 and S2 foramina was 3cm; that between S2 and S3 was 3cm in males and 2cm in females; and that between S3 and S4 was 3cm in males and 2cm in females. The upper sacrum tends to curve more than its lower part, especially in males [4]; this causes S1 and S2 to face away from S3 and S4. Thus, skin markings may not be equidistant between S1–2 and S3–4.

During test stimulation, needles can be inserted into the foramina at a wide range of angles in both the vertical and horizontal planes. Hasan *et al.* [3] found that the angulation in the vertical plane ranged from 25 to 80 degrees in S2 (mean of 47 degrees in males and 53 degrees in females), from 45 to 95 degrees in S3 (mean of 69 degrees in both males and females), and from 40 to 98 degrees in S4 (mean of 69 degrees in males and 70 degrees in females). In the transverse plane the range of angulation was 85–115 degrees for S2, 72–118 degrees for S3, and 85–105 degrees for S4.

Needle insertion into the foramina can result in damage to nerve roots and vessels. Because these structures are more likely to be found on the medial aspect of the foramen, injury can be minimised by using a more lateral foramen entry [3]. Investigators have also found that increasing the angle of needle entry in the vertical plane can increase the risk of injury to the vessels [3]. The S2 foramen is nearly half filled by its nerve root and ganglion [2], which increases the likelihood of penetration during needle placement; the S3 and S4 foramina, on the other hand, are filled mostly with fat, their nerve roots occupying a relatively smaller portion of the foramen. The fat provides added protection to the nerve by allowing it to be pushed aside during the procedure.

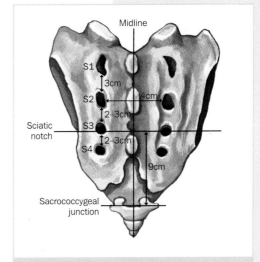

Figure 2.3 Dorsal view of the sacrum depicting the relative distances between the foramina and the relationship between the sciatic notch, sacrococcygeal junction and the S3 foramina.

Key Points

- Needle injury to nerve roots and vessels is minimised by a more lateral entry.
- Structures in the S2 foramen are at more risk than those in the S3 and S4 foramina.

Sacral nerves

The spinal nerves emerge from the dorsal root ganglia, course a few millimetres, and then split into ventral and dorsal spinal rami. The ventral sacral rami emerge from the anterior sacral foramina (Fig. 2.4) and the dorsal rami exit through the dorsal foramina. All five sacral nerves descend from the conus medullaris, then traverse the central sacral canal; the first four then exit through the foramina, whereas the fifth exits between the sacrum and the coccyx. All sacral nerves communicate with the sacral sympathetic ganglia as they exit from their foramina.

Sacral nerve root width decreases in size from above downwards: Hasan *et al.* [3] found that the width of the S1 nerve was between 6 and 8mm,

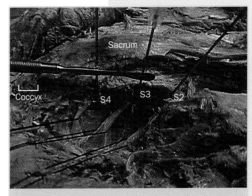

Figure 2.4 A lateral view cadaveric dissection showing the S2, S3 and S4 nerves exiting the sacrum, and needles placed through the exposed anterior and posterior foramina.

Key Points

- Electrical stimulation of each sacral nerve elicits specific sensorimotor responses.
- Individual variations in sacral spinal cord structure may cause mixed/inconsistent responses.

that of S2 was between 5 and 6mm, that of S3 was between 3 and 4mm, and that of S4 was between 2 and 3mm.

After the nerve roots exit anteriorly they pass in the superior portion of the foramen and groove, then proceed in an inferolateral direction to meet the other nerves to form the sacral plexus. These sacral nerves proceed in different directions: S1 and S2 pass obliquely outwards, S3 and S4 exit nearly horizontally [1]. The sacral plexus is triangular: its base corresponds to the exit of the nerves from the sacrum; its apex corresponds to the lower part of the great sacrosciatic foramen. The plexus rests upon the anterior surface of the piriformis muscle and divides into four principal peripheral nerves: these are the sciatic nerve (L4, 5, S1–3) — which divides into the common peroneal (L4, 5, S1, 2) and tibial nerves (L4, 5, S1–3) — the superior gluteal nerve (L4, 5, S1), the inferior gluteal nerve (L5, S1, 2), and the posterior femoral cutaneous nerve (S1–3).

The sacral nerves provide many branches to the pelvis and lower extremities: S1 and S2 ventral rami give their major contribution to the sciatic nerve; the S3 contribution is minor; S4 and S5 never contribute to the sciatic nerve. Sacral nerves S2, S3, and S4 contribute to the pudendal nerve, which is the main sensory and motor nerve of the pelvic floor. The ventral branches of S5, together with the coccygeal nerve, emerge between the sacrum and the coccyx to form the coccygeal plexus, which innervates the skin of the anococcygeal region.

Electrical stimulation of the sacral nerves elicits specific sensory and motor responses: stimulating the S2 nerve results in contraction of the gluteus maximus muscle through the inferior gluteal nerve, together with stimulation of the superficial perineal musculature, which causes anteroposterior (AP) contraction of the anal sphincter and perineum ('clamp' response) [5, 6]. Stimulation of the S2 nerve also causes contraction of the calf and plantar flexion of the foot through the tibial nerve, and eversion of the foot through the superficial peroneal branch of the common peroneal nerve. Patients also feel a sensation in the upper posterior thigh and buttocks through the inferior clunial nerve (gluteal branches of posterior cutaneous nerve of thigh) and posterior femoral cutaneous nerve.

Stimulation of nerves S3 and S4 causes a contraction of the levator ani ('bellows' response), coccygeus, and external anal sphincter muscles through the pudendal nerve. This also results in (a) a sensation in the labia majora, urethra, penis, and scrotum through the perineal branch of the pudendal nerve and posterior femoral cutaneous nerve, and (b) rectal sensation through the inferior rectal nerve. Stimulation of S3 also results in flexion of the toes through the tibial branch of the sciatic nerve.

Many investigators have found numerous variations and interconnections within the sacral spinal cord, particularly between the S2 and S3 ventral rami [7, 8]. They also found inconsistencies in the innervation of the S3 nerve; occasionally, the sacral ventral roots were completely missing. This probably explains the mixed and inconsistent nerve-root responses that are sometimes encountered during nerve stimulation.

Vascular supply

The lateral sacral artery, a branch of the internal iliac artery, provides branches to each of the foramina. The venous plexuses, which are found in about two-thirds of the foramina [2], communicate with the presacral venous plexuses formed by the medial and lateral sacral veins. Bleeding encountered during needle insertion is usually the result of injury to these veins.

Superficial soft tissues of the sacral region

The soft tissues found dorsal to the sacrum consist of muscle, fat, and fascia (Fig. 2.5). Under the skin lies fat followed by the superficial fascia, which is a layer of condensed connective tissue. Beneath, more fatty tissue is encountered, followed by the lumbodorsal (thoracolumbar) fascia and sacrospinalis muscle. The amount of fat found on either side of the superficial fascia varies significantly among individuals. This fascial layer is often confused with the lumbodorsal fascia during surgical dissection; the latter fascia can easily be identified by its glistening appearance and the occasional presence of muscle fibres from the gluteus maximus on its surface. The lumbodorsal fascia is extremely strong and relatively immobile. In our institution, we have been able to fix our permanent lead to this fascia, and found no evidence of lead movement after long-term follow-up.

The lumbodorsal fascia encloses the sacrospinalis (which is the sacral portion of the erector spinae) and the multifidus muscles, the latter inserting directly on the posterior surface of the sacrum. Laterally, the gluteus maximus originates on the inferiolateral edge of the sacrum, below the level of the third sacral foramen. Sometimes, fibres from this muscle insert more medially and need to be retracted or cut in order to expose the lumbodorsal fascia.

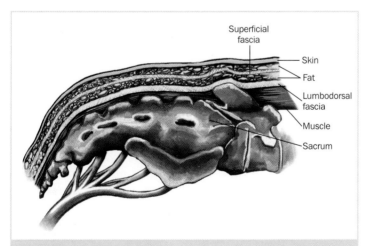

Superficial fascia

Skin

Fat

Lumbodorsal fascia

Muscle

Sacrum

Figure 2.5 *Lateral view illustration of the sacral region. The various soft tissue layers dorsal to the sacrum can be seen.*

13

Key Points

- Sacral foramina can be identified by bony landmarks.
- S3 foramina are also located in relation to the sacrococcygeal junction.
- Radiological localisation of foramina is also useful, especially in obese patients.

Anatomical landmarks for localising the foramina

There are many ways in which to identify the sacral foramina by using bony landmarks, such as the sciatic notch, midline sacral spinous processes, iliac crest and sacral hiatus [6, 9–11]. The sciatic notch landmark is that most commonly used (Fig. 2.3). The S3 foramen is found by palpating the upper edge of the greater sciatic notch, just lateral to the sacrum; this usually corresponds to the level of S3. The notches are sometimes difficult to palpate, especially in obese patients.

We have devised another method of localising the S3 foramen, based on cadaveric dissections and experience with over 200 neurostimulation procedures. This technique estimates the location of the S3 foramina at approximately 9cm above the sacrococcygeal junction (Fig. 2.3). The latter is identified by a knuckle-like protuberance at the apex of the sacrum. However, sometimes this cannot be palpated in obese patients; instead, it is identified by a sudden drop at the tip of the sacrum. Occasionally, this technique underestimates the location of the foramen, especially in obese patients whose sacra are larger; in such patients the foramen can be estimated as 2–3cm higher than expected.

Radiological landmarks for localising the foramina

Radiological localisation of the foramina can also be valuable, particularly in obese patients whose bony landmarks cannot be palpated. Fluoroscopy is especially helpful in those patients in whom the midline cannot be discerned by the skin markings. In obese patients the skin often shifts to one side, causing erroneous placement of the midline mark; this is probably one of the most common causes of frustration during foramen localisation. It is possible to locate S3 radiographically by placing a needle horizontally on the skin and adjusting it so that it coincides with the lowest radiographic aspect of the sacroiliac joint (Fig. 2.6). The S3 foramen can also be located just below an imaginary midpoint between the base of the sacrum and the tip of the coccyx on a lateral view radiograph (Fig. 2.7).

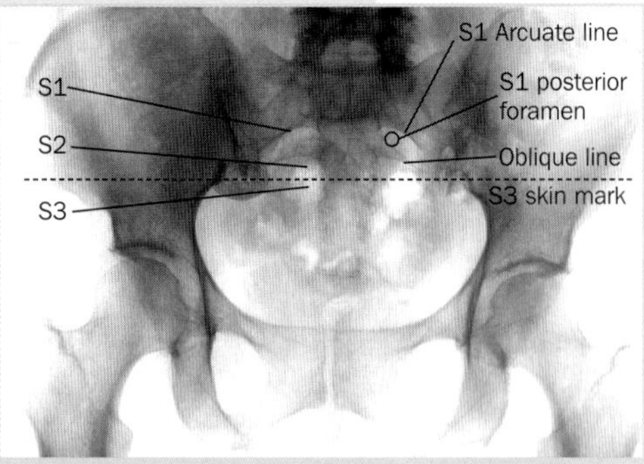

***Figure 2.6** Anteroposterior radiograph of the pelvis. The arcuate lines and some of the oblique lines of the first 3 foramina are seen. The interrupted line across the inferior aspect of the sacroiliac joint corresponds with the S3 foramina and can be used as a skin landmark.*

The shape and relative position of the anterior and posterior foramina vary with different projections. The outlet projection provides the best view of the posterior foramina on plain radiograph [12]: they are partially visible as elliptical radiolucencies on an AP 15–20-degree craniad tilt radiograph [13]. At this angle, the opening of the foramina are visualised as the anterior and posterior foramina overlap (Fig. 2.8).

The roofs of the anterior foramina project on AP radiograph as the 'arcuate lines' (Fig. 2.6), which are seen only in S1, S2 and S3; the fourth sacral foramen has no arcuate line. In the AP radiograph an oblique line, starting near the

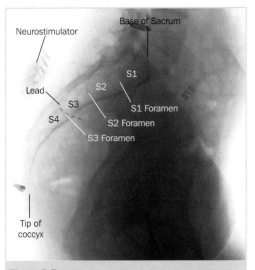

Figure 2.7 *Lateral view radiograph showing the location of the S3 foramen just below the imaginary midpoint between the base of the sacrum and the tip of the coccyx.*

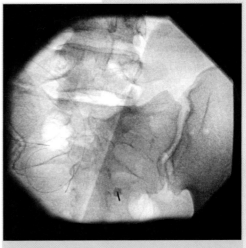

Figure 2.8 *Outlet view of the pelvis. The overlapping anterior and posterior foramina expose the posterior foramen. A test wire on the right and a needle on the left are seen inside the corresponding S3 posterior foramina.*

lateral end of the arcuate line and extending superomedially, represents the lateral wall of the anterior foramen. Anatomically, and in some radiographs, this line continues into the lateral wall of the posterior foramen above and therefore can be used as a guide in localising it (Fig. 2.6); however, this lateral wall is less often seen than the arcuate line [13].

References

1. Gray H. *Anatomy, descriptive and surgical*; *Osteology*. London: J. W. Parker and Son, 1858; 1–720: 12–16.
2. Liguoro D, Viejo-Fuertes D, Midy D *et al*. The posterior sacral foramina: an anatomical study. *J Anat* 1999; 195: 301–4.
3. Hasan ST, Shanahan DA, Pridie AK *et al*. Surface localization of sacral foramina for neuromodulation of bladder function. *Eur Urol* 1996; 29: 90–8.
4. Abitbol MM. Sacral curvature and spinal posture. *Am J Physiol Anthropol* 1989; 80: 379–89.
5. Schmidt RA. Applications of neurostimulation in urology. *Neurourol Urodyn* 1988; 7: 585–92.
6. Siegel SW. Management of voiding dysfunction with an implantable neuroprosthesis. *Urol Clin North Am* 1992; 19: 163–70.
7. Marani E, Pijl ME, Kraan MC *et al*. Interconnections of the upper ventral rami of the human sacral plexus: a reappraisal for dorsal rhizotomy in neurostimulation operations. *Neurourol Urodyn* 1993; 12: 585–98.
8. Mersdorf A, Schmidt RA, Tanagho EA. Topographic–anatomical basis of sacral neuromodulation: neuroanatomical variations. *J Urol* 1993; 149: 345–9.
9. Essenhigh DM, Ryan DW. An appraisal of S3 blocks in the management of incontinence. *J Urol* 1982; 54: 697–9.
10. Hassouna MM, Elhilali MM. Role of the sacral root stimulator in voiding dysfunction. *World J Urol* 1991; 9: 145–8.
11. Thon WF, Baskin LS, Jonas U *et al*. Neuromodulation of voiding dysfunction and pelvic pain. *World J Urol* 1991; 9: 138–41.
12. Xu R, Ebraheim NA, Robke J *et al*. Radiologic and anatomic evaluation of the anterior sacral foramens and nerve grooves. *Spine* 1996; 21: 407–10.
13. Jackson H, Burke JT. The sacral foramina. *Skeletal Radiol* 1984; 11: 282–8.

3 The mechanism of action of sacral nerve stimulation in the treatment of detrusor overactivity and urinary retention

M.B. Chancellor and W. Leng

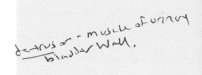

Introduction

The overactive bladder represents one of the most challenging problems in urology. Current treatments for the uninhibited bladder include pharmacotherapy, surgical denervation and surgical augmentation procedures. However, these forms of treatment have significant adverse effects [1]. Functional electrical stimulation appears to be a favourable non-surgical treatment for many patients with detrusor instability. Stimulation techniques have utilised surface electrodes, anal and vaginal plug electrodes [2–4], and dorsal penile nerve electrodes [5,6]. The recently FDA-approved sacral nerve stimulation (SNS) techniques represent a major advance in neuromodulation.

The purpose of this chapter is to discuss how SNS can treat both urinary urge incontinence and dysfunctional voiding, including idiopathic urinary retention [7–10]. The implantable system comprises a neurostimulator, an extension cable, and a lead with quadripolar electrodes. The electrode is implanted in one of the sacral foramina, most commonly the S3 foramen. The pulse generator is implanted subcutaneously in a lower quadrant of the abdomen. The urologist uses an electronic programmer to adjust the stimulation parameters non-invasively [11–14]. We will first discuss the pertinent neuroanatomy and neurophysiology relating to SNS. Following this background discussion, hypotheses on how SNS can resolve lower urinary tract dysfunction are presented.

Pelvic afferent pathways

Efferent outflow to the lower urinary tract can be reflexly activated by spinal afferent pathways as well as by input from the brain. Afferent input from the pelvic visceral organs, and also somatic afferent pathways from the perineal muscle and skin, are very important. Somatic afferent pathways in the pudendal nerves that transmit noxious and innocuous stimuli from the genital organs, urethra, prostate, vagina, anal canal and skin can modulate voiding function [15–17].

afferent. sensory nerve.

axon- nerve fiber

Bladder afferent nerves are critical for sending signals of bladder fullness and discomfort to the brain and initiating the micturition reflex. The bladder afferent pathways are composed of two types of axons: these are small, myelinated A_δ fibres and unmyelinated C fibres. The former transmit signals mainly from mechanoreceptors that detect bladder fullness or wall tension; on the other hand, C fibres mainly detect noxious signals and initiate painful sensations. The bladder C-fibre nociceptors perform a similar function and send signals to the central nervous system (CNS) when an infection or irritative condition exists in the bladder. C-fibre bladder afferents also have reflex functions to facilitate or trigger voiding [18–20]: this can be viewed as a defence mechanism to eliminate irritants or bacteria. The C-fibre bladder afferents have been implicated in the triggering of reflex bladder hyperactivity associated with neurological disorders such as spinal cord injury and multiple sclerosis. Capsaicin, and its ultrapotent analogue, resiniferatoxin, are specific C-fibre afferent neurotoxins; these are currently undergoing clinical trials for the treatment of lower urinary tract dysfunction relating to C-fibre alterations [15].

Bladder hyperactivity and urinary incontinence are assumed to be mediated by the loss of voluntary control of voiding and the appearance of primitive voiding reflex circuitry. This can occur as a result of the re-emergence of neonatal reflex patterns that were suppressed during postnatal development or the formation of new reflex circuits mediated by C-fibre afferents [21]. Under normal conditions, the latter are thought to be mechano-insensitive and unresponsive to bladder distension (hence the term 'silent' C fibres); however, as a consequence of neurological and inflammatory diseases (or possibly during ageing), the silent C fibres become sensitive to bladder distension and can trigger micturition reflexes [18–20]. This type of bladder hyperactivity may be suppressed by blocking C-fibre afferent activity or by interrupting reflex pathways in the spinal cord by SNS.

Micturition reflexes

Normal micturition is completely dependent on neural pathways in the central nervous system. These pathways perform three major functions — namely, amplification, coordination, and timing [16]. The nervous control of the lower urinary tract must be able to amplify weak smooth-muscle activity to provide sustained increases in intravesical pressures sufficient to empty the bladder. The bladder and urethral sphincter function must be coordinated to allow the sphincter to open during micturition but to be closed at all other times. Timing represents the voluntary control of voiding in the normal adult and the ability to initiate voiding over a wide range of bladder volumes (Fig. 3.1). In this regard, the bladder is a unique visceral organ which exhibits predominately voluntary rather than involuntary (autonomic) neural regulation. A number of important reflex mechanisms contribute to the storage and elimination of urine and modulate the voluntary control of micturition [17].

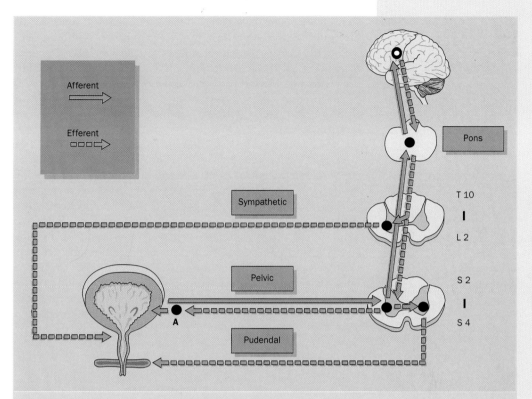

Figure 3.1 *Micturition requires positive feedback to ensure complete bladder emptying. As the bladder fills, myelinated A$_\delta$ tension receptors are (A) activated. This afferent signal must reach the pontine micturition centre with subsequent activation of parasympathetic efferent outflow.*

The bladder is also an unusual organ because it is functionally 'turned off' most of the time and then turned on in an 'all-or-nothing' manner to eliminate urine. It therefore differs from many other visceral organs such as the heart, blood vessels and gastrointestinal tract, which receive tonic autonomic regulation. The ability to turn on micturition in a switch-like fashion is facilitated by positive feedback loops in the micturition reflex pathway. Thus, bladder afferent activity can activate efferent excitatory input to the bladder that can initiate a bladder contraction. This positive loop can activate more afferent firing and more intense reflex efferent activity. This positive feedback, mediated in part by supraspinal parasympathetic pathways to the pontine micturition centre, is a very effective mechanism for promoting efficient bladder emptying and for minimising residual urine. However, the positive feedback mechanism is a potential liability because, in the presence of pathological conditions, it can contribute to the emergence of bladder hyperactivity and incontinence. Because of positive feedback, loss of central inhibitory controls or sensitisation of bladder afferent input can easily lead to the unmasking of involuntary voiding. Thus, nature has provided other mechanisms for inhibitory modulation of the micturition reflex. These mechanisms, which reside in the spinal cord and can be activated by various somatic and visceral afferent nerves, might be viewed as a counterbalance for the bladder reflex pathways [22–24]. The spinal organisation of these inhibitory mechanisms has been elucidated by electrophysiological studies in animals [25,26]. We here hypothesise that these modulatory mechanisms can be activated by SNS in the treatment of overactive bladders.

Guarding reflexes (guarding against stress urinary incontinence)

There is an important bladder–urethra reflex that is mediated by sympathetic efferent pathways to the urethra: this excitatory reflex contracts the urethral smooth muscle and is thus termed a 'guarding' reflex [27,28]. The positive reflex is not activated during micturition but when bladder pressure is increased; for example when the subject coughs or exercises. A second guarding reflex is triggered by the bladder afferents that synapse with sacral interneurons which, in turn, activate urethral external sphincter efferent neurons that send axons into the pudendal nerve [8]. The activation of pudendal urethral efferent pathways contracts the external urinary sphincter and prevents stress urinary incontinence (Fig. 3.2). The brain inhibits the guarding reflexes during micturition.

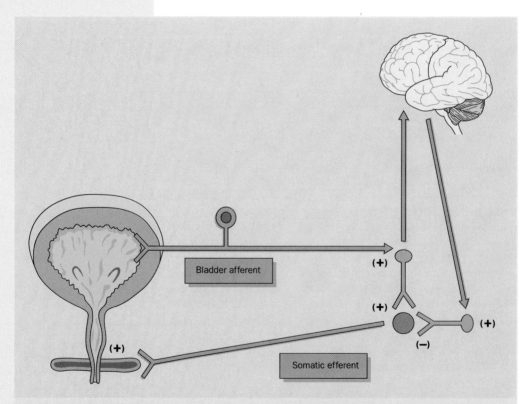

Figure 3.2 *The guarding reflex prevents urinary incontinence. When there is a sudden increase in intravesical pressure, such as during a cough, the urinary sphincter contracts via the spinal guarding reflex to prevent urinary incontinence. The spinal guarding reflex is turned off by the brain to allow urination.*

Bladder–bladder and bladder–urethral reflexes (promoting micturition)

The bladder afferent (A_δ or C-fibre) nerves connect with interneurons in the sacral spinal cord. Interneurons synapse with bladder preganglionic (efferent) parasympathetic neurons to form the bladder–bladder reflex [27–30]. Interneurons activated by bladder afferents also synapse with urethral parasympathetic efferent neurons to form a bladder–urethra reflex. The bladder–bladder reflex is a positive reflex that activates the full bladder. Once this reflex is 'turned on' it remains *on* to empty the bladder completely. The bladder–urethra parasympathetic reflex is an inhibitory reflex that induces the smooth muscle of the proximal urethra to relax and the urethral outlet to open reflexively during a bladder contraction (Fig. 3.3).

Sacral afferent input modifying micturition reflexes

The guarding and voiding reflexes discussed above are activated at different times under completely different clinical scenarios. However, anatomically, they are located in close proximity in the

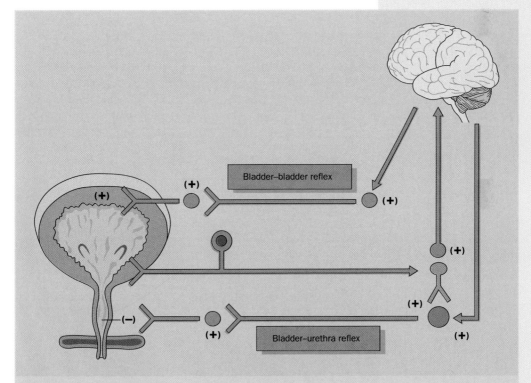

Figure 3.3 *The voiding reflex with supraspinal bladder facilitation and spinal pathway urethral relaxation. Afferents from the bladder project on spinal tract neurons that ascend to the brain. Descending pathways connect to parasympathetic efferent nerves to contract the bladder (bladder–bladder reflex). A spinal bladder–urethra reflex is activated via a similar bladder afferent innervation.*

Key Points

- SNS activates somatic afferent axons modulating both sensory processing and micturition reflex pathways in the spinal cord.

S2–S4 levels of the human spinal cord. Both sets of reflexes are modulated by a number of centres in the brain. Thus, these reflexes can be altered by a variety of neurological diseases, some of which can unmask involuntary bladder activity mediated by C fibres (Fig. 3.4). It is possible to modulate these reflexes by SNS and to restore voluntary micturition.

Experimental data from animals indicate that somatic afferent input to the sacral spinal cord can modulate the guarding and bladder–bladder reflexes: de Groat [29] has shown that sacral preganglionic outflow to the urinary bladder receives inhibitory inputs from various somatic and visceral afferents, as well as from a recurrent inhibitory pathway [22–24]. The experiments have also provided information about the organisation of these inhibitory mechanisms [25,26]. Electrical stimulation of somatic afferents in the pudendal nerve elicits inhibitory mechanisms [21]. This is supported by the finding that interneurons in the sacral autonomic nucleus exhibit firing correlated with bladder activity and are inhibited by activation of somatic afferent pathways. This electrical stimulation of somatic efferent nerves in the sacral spinal roots could inhibit reflex bladder hyperactivity mediated by spinal or supraspinal pathways. In neonatal kittens and rats, micturition as well as defecation are elicited when the mother cat licks the perineal region [21]. This reflex appears to be the primary stimulus for micturition, as urinary retention occurs when the young kittens and rat pups are separated from their mother.

To induce micturition, the perineal afferents must activate the parasympathetic excitatory input to the bladder but also suppress the urethral sympathetic and sphincter somatic guarding reflexes. Suppression of guarding reflexes by SNS contributes to the enhancement of voiding in patients with urinary retention.

The perineum-to-bladder reflex is very prominent during the first four postnatal weeks and then becomes less effective and usually disappears in kittens by the age of 7–8 weeks (which is

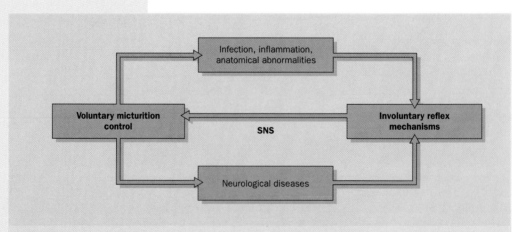

Figure 3.4 *The concept of SNS is to modulate the abnormal involuntary reflexes of the lower urinary tract and restore voluntary control.*

the approximate age of weaning). In adult animals and humans, perineal stimulation or mechanical stimulation of the sex organs (vagina or penis) inhibits the micturition reflex [17,23,27,28].

As well as convincing data from the animal research work that identified somatic afferent modulation of bladder and urethral reflexes, there are also data from clinical physiological studies supporting the view that stimulation of sacral afferents can modify bladder and urethral sphincter reflexes. Functional electrical stimulation appears to be a favourable non-surgical treatment for many patients with detrusor instability. Stimulation techniques have utilised surface electrodes, anal and vaginal plug electrodes [2–4], and dorsal penile nerve electrodes [5,6].

The success of pelvic floor electrical stimulation relies on convergence in the CNS of visceral and somatic sensory innervation [31]. By stimulating somatic afferent pathways, it is possible to block the processing of visceral afferent signals impinging upon the same region of the spinal cord. An example of this is posterior tibial nerve stimulation: by electrical stimulation of this nerve (or its dermatome) it is possible to block sensory afferents from the bladder [32,33]. Ohlsson and associates [4] report encouraging success using electrical somatic nerve stimulation with transvaginal probes in women and transrectal probes in men. Despite a documented average 45% increase in bladder capacity, however, only half of their patients reported a 30% decrease in the frequency of micturition. Fall [2] also reported favourable long-term results of vaginal electrical stimulation in the treatment of refractory detrusor instability and stress urinary incontinence. Of those women with detrusor instability studied, 73% became asymptomatic during treatment, and 45% remained free from symptoms despite discontinuation of therapy. Many patients, however, required up to 6 months of therapy before benefit was apparent.

Hypotheses of SNS mechanisms

SNS activates somatic afferent axons that modulate sensory processing and micturition reflex pathways in the spinal cord. Urinary retention and dysfunctional voiding can be resolved by inhibition of the guarding reflexes. Detrusor hyperreflexia can be suppressed by direct inhibition of bladder preganglionic neurons as well as inhibition of interneuronal transmission in the afferent limb of the micturition reflex.

We hypothesise that the effects of SNS depend on electrical stimulation of afferent axons in the spinal roots which, in turn, modulate voiding and continence reflex pathways in the CNS. The afferent system is the most likely target because beneficial effects can be elicited at intensities of stimulation that do not activate movements of striated muscles [34–36].

How do sacral somatic afferents alter lower urinary tract reflexes to promote voiding? To understand this mechanism it should be recognised that, in adults, brain pathways are necessary to turn

Key Points
- Both urinary retention and dysfunctional voiding can be resolved by inhibition of guarding reflexes.

off sphincter and urethral guarding reflexes to allow efficient bladder emptying. Thus spinal cord injury produces bladder–sphincter dyssynergia and inefficient bladder emptying by disrupting the brain mechanisms (Figs. 3.2 and 3.5). This may also occur after more subtle neurological lesions in patients with idiopathic urinary retention, such as after a bout of prostatitis or urinary tract infection. Before the development of brain control of micturition, at least in animals, stimulation of somatic afferent pathways passing through the pudendal nerve to the perineum can initiate efficient voiding by activating bladder efferent pathways and turning off the excitatory pathways to the urethral outlet [15,16,18]. Tactile stimulation of the perineum in the cat also inhibits the bladder–sympathetic reflex component of the guarding reflex mechanism. We hypothesise that SNS can elicit similar responses in patients with urinary retention and turn off excitatory outflow to the urethral outlet, thus promoting bladder emptying. Because sphincter activity can generate afferent input to the spinal cord that can, in turn, inhibit reflex bladder activity, an indirect benefit of suppressing sphincter reflexes would be facilitation of bladder activity; this may also be useful in the patient population with idiopathic urinary retention.

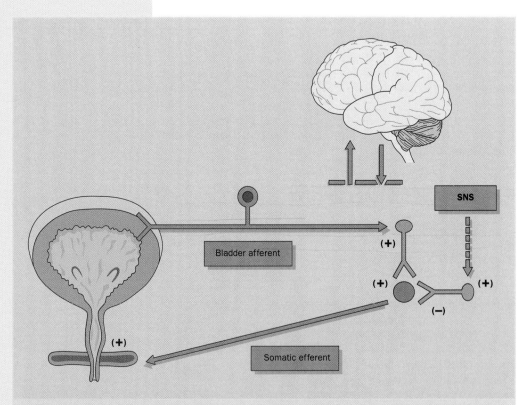

Figure 3.5 *The spinal guarding reflexes (Fig. 3.2) can be turned off by the brain for urination to take place. In cases of neurological diseases, the brain cannot turn off the guarding reflex and retention can occur. SNS restores voluntary micturition in cases of voiding dysfunction and urinary retention by inhibiting the guarding reflex.*

How do sacral afferents inhibit the overactive bladder? Several reflex mechanisms may be involved in the SNS suppression of bladder hyperactivity. Afferent pathways projecting to the sacral cord can inhibit bladder reflexes in animals and humans. The source of afferent input may be from sphincter muscles, distal colon, rectum, anal canal, vagina, uterine cervix, and cutaneous afferents from the perineum (Figs 3.3 and 3.6). As mentioned previously, two mechanisms have been identified in animals for somatic and visceral afferent inhibition of bladder reflexes. The most common mechanism is suppression of interneuronal transmission in the bladder reflex pathway [18,37,38]. It is assumed that this inhibition occurs in part on the ascending limb of the micturition reflex and therefore blocks the transfer of information from the bladder to the pontine micturition centre. This action would prevent involuntary (reflex) micturition but would not necessarily suppress voluntary voiding that would be mediated by descending excitatory efferent pathways from the brain to the sacral parasympathetic preganglionic neurons. A second inhibitory mechanism is mediated by a direct inhibitory input to the bladder preganglionic neurons. This can be induced by electrical stimulation of the pudendal nerve or by mechanical stimulation of the anal canal and distal bowel; it is not elicited by tactile stimulation of

Key Points
- Detrusor hyperreflexia is counteracted in two ways: 1. Direct inhibition of bladder preganglionic neurons suppresses detrusor hyperreflexia. 2. Inhibition of interneuronal transmission in the afferent limb of the micturition reflex.

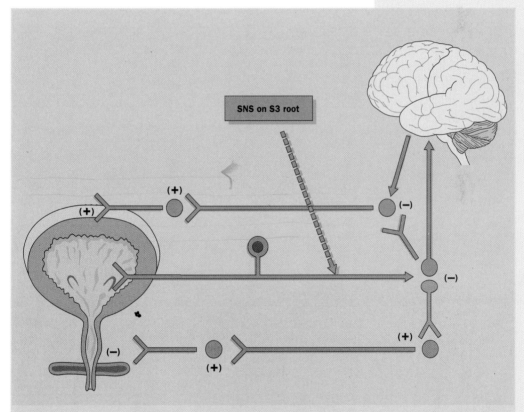

Figure 3.6 *In cases of supraspinal dysfunction overactive micturition bladder reflexes occur (Fig. 3.3). SNS inhibits urinary urgency, frequency, and urge incontinence by inhibiting the bladder–bladder and bladder–urethra reflexes.*

penile or perineal afferents. The latter mechanism would be much more effective in turning off bladder reflexes because it would directly suppress firing in the motor outflow from the spinal cord. It would also be expected to block non-selectively both voluntary and involuntary voiding. Thus, this inhibitory response may be less important clinically in the responses to SNS because patients usually retain normal voiding mechanisms (Table 3.1).

Table 3.1 SNS: mechanisms

1	Inhibits spinal tract neurons involved in the micturition reflex
2	Inhibits interneurons involved in spinal segmental reflexes,
3	Inhibits postganglionic neurons directly
4	May inhibit primary afferent pathway
5	May indirectly suppress guarding reflexes by turning off bladder afferent input to internal sphincter sympathetic or external urethral sphincter interneurons
6	Postganglionic stimulation can directly activate postganglionic neurons and induce bladder activity, but at the same time can turn off bladder–bladder reflex by inhibiting afferent–interneuronal transmission. This explains how SNS can induce voiding but turn off hyperactive voiding mediated by spinal micturition reflex

Conclusions

The principles behind SNS can be summarised as somatic afferent inhibition of sensory processing in the spinal cord. Pudendal afferent input can also trigger voiding reflexes by suppressing the guarding reflex pathways. Pudendal afferent input to the sacral spinal cord can turn off supraspinally mediated hyperactive voiding by blocking ascending sensory systems. SNS, a minimally-invasive urological technique, holds great promise for a large number of patients who suffer from a spectrum of lower urinary tract disorders.

References

1. Schmidt RA. Treatment of unstable bladder. *Urology* 1991; 37: 28–32.
2. Fall M. Electrical pelvic floor stimulation for the control of detrusor instability. *Neurourol Urodyn* 1985; 4: 329.
3. Janez J, Plevnik S, Suhet P. Urethral and bladder responses to anal electrical stimulation. *J Urol* 1979; 122: 192–4.
4. Ohlsson BL, Fall M, Frankenbers-Sommar S. Effects of external and direct pudendal nerve maximal electrical stimulation in the treatment of the uninhibited overactive bladder. *Br J Urol* 1989; 64: 374–80.
5. Walter JS, Wheeler JS, Robinson CJ, Wurster RD. Inhibiting the hyperreflexic bladder with electrical stimulation in a spinal animal model. *Neurourol Urodyn* 1993; 12: 241–52.

6. Wheeler JS, Walter JS. Bladder inhibition by dorsal penile nerve stimulation in spinal cord injured patients. *J Urol* 1992; 147: 100–3.
7. Bosch JLHR, Groen J. Sacral (S3) segmental nerve stimulation as a treatment for urge incontinence in patients with detrusor instability: results of chronic electrical stimulation using an implantable prosthesis. *J Urol* 1995; 154: 504–7.
8. Shaker HS, Hassouna M. Sacral nerve root neuromodulation: an effective treatment for refractory urge incontinence. *J Urol* 1998; 159: 1516–19.
9. Shaker HS, Hassouna M. Sacral root neuromodulation in idiopathic nonobstructive chronic urinary retention. *J Urol* 1998; 159: 1476–8.
10. Vapnek JM, Schmidt RA. Restoration of voiding in chronic urinary retention using neuroprosthesis. *World J Urol* 1991; 9: 142.
11. Jünemann KP, Lue TF, Schmidt RA, Tanagho EA. Clinical significance of sacral and pudendal nerve anatomy. *J Urol* 1988; 139: 74–80.
12. Schmidt RA, Tanagho EA. Feasibility of controlled micturition through electric stimulation. *Urol Int* 1979; 34: 199–230.
13. Schmidt RA, Senn E, Tanagho EA. Functional evaluation of sacral nerve root integrity. Report of a technique. *Urology* 1990; 35: 388–92.
14. Tanagho EA, Schmidt RA. Electrical stimulation in the clinical management of the neurogenic bladder. *J Urol* 1988; 140: 1331–9.
15. Yoshimura N, de Groat WC. Neural control of the lower urinary tract. *Int J Urol* 1997; 4: 111–25.
16. de Groat WC. Central nervous system control of micturition. In PD O'Donnell (ed) *Urinary Incontinence*. St. Louis: Mosby, 1997; 33–47.
17. de Groat WC, Araki I, Vizzard MA et al. Developmental and injury induced plasticity in the micturition reflex pathway. *Behav Brain Res* 1997; 92: 127–40.
18. Kruse MN, de Groat WC. Spinal pathways mediate coordinated bladder/urethral sphincter activity during reflex micturition in normal and spinal cord injured neonatal rats. *Neurosci Lett* 1993; 152: 141–4.
19. Cheng CI, Ma CP, de Groat WC. Effect of capsaicin on micturition and associated reflexes in rats. *Am J Physiol* 1993; 265 (1–2): R132–8.
20. Cheng CI, Ma CP, de Groat WC. Effect of capsaicin on micturition and associated reflexes in chronic spinal rats. *Brain Res* 1995; 678 (1–2): 40–8.
21. de Groat WC. Changes in the organization of the micturition reflex pathway of the cat after transection of the spinal cord. In: RP Verra, B Grafstein (eds). *Cellular mechanisms for recovery from nervous systems injury: a conference report. Exp Neurol* 1981; 71: 22.
22. de Groat WC, Ryall RW. The identification and antidromic responses of sacral preganglionic parasympathetic neurons. *J Physiol (Lond)* 1968; 196: 533.
23. de Groat WC, Ryall RW. Recurrent inhibition in sacral parasympathetic pathways to the bladder. *J Physiol (Lond)* 1968; 196: 579.
24. de Groat WC. Nervous control of the urinary bladder of the cat. *Brain Res* 1975; 87: 201–11.
25. de Groat WC. Excitation and inhibition of sacral parasympathetic neurons by visceral and cutaneous stimuli in the cat. *Brain Res* 1971; 33: 499.
26. de Groat WC. Mechanisms underlying recurrent inhibition in the sacral parasympathetic outflow to the urinary bladder. *J Physiol* 1976; 257: 503–13.
27. de Groat WC, Vizzard MA, Araki I, Roppolo JR. Spinal interneurons and preganglionic neurons in sacral autonomic reflex pathways. In: G Holstege, R Bandler, C Saper (eds). *The emotional motor system. Prog Brain Res* The Netherlands: Elsevier, 1996; 107: 97.
28. de Groat WC, Nadelhaft I, Milne RJ et al. Organization of the sacral parasympathetic reflex pathways to the urinary bladder and large intestine. *J Auton Nerv Syst* 1981; 3: 135–60.
29. de Groat WC. Inhibitory mechanisms in the sacral reflex pathways to the urinary bladder. In: Ryall RW, Kelly JS (eds). *Iontophoresis and Transmitter Mechanisms in the Mammalian Central Nervous System*. The Netherlands: Elsevier, 1978; 366–368.
30. de Groat WC. Mechanisms underlying the recovery of lower urinary tract function following spinal cord injury. *Paraplegia* 1995; 33: 493–505.
31. Morrison JFB. Neural connections between the lower urinary tract and the spinal cord. In: M Torrens, JFB Morrison (eds). *The Physiology of the Lower Urinary Tract*. London: Springer Verlag, 1987: 53–85.
32. McGuire EJ, Shi-Chun Z, Horwinski R, Lytton B. Treatment of motor and sensory detrusor instability by electrical stimulation. *J Urol* 1983; 129: 78–9.
33. Crocker M, Doleys DM, Dolce JJ. Transcutaneous electrical nerve stimulation in urinary retention. *South Med J* 1985; 78: 1515–6.

34. Thon WF, Baskin LS, Jonas U et al. Surgical principles of sacral foramen electrode implantation. *World J Urol* 1991; 9: 133.
35. Vadušek DB, Light JK, Liddy JM. Detrusor inhibition induced by stimulation of pudendal nerve afferents. *Neurourol Urodyn* 1986; 5: 381.
36. de Groat WC, Kruse MN, Vizzard MA et al. Modification of urinary bladder function after neural injury. In: F Seil (ed) *Adv Neurol Vol. 72: Neuronal Regeneration, Reorganization, and Repair*. New York: Lippincott-Raven, 1997; 33: 347–64.
37. Kruse MN, Noto H, Roppolo JR, de Groat WC. Pontine control of the urinary bladder and external urethral sphincter in the rat. *Brain Res* 1990; 532: 182–90.
38. de Groat WC, Theobald RJ. Reflex activation of sympathetic pathways to vesical smooth muscle and parasympathetic ganglia by electrical stimulation of vesical afferents. *J Physiol* 1976; 259: 223–37.

4 Principles for safe and effective nerve stimulation

W.F. Agnew, D.B. McCreery

and T.G.H. Yuen

Introduction

This chapter reviews various designs of nerve electrodes and stimulation protocols from the perspectives of safety and effectiveness. We focus primarily on work carried out at Huntington Medical Research Institutes (HMRI), Pasadena, California, USA, using cat peroneal and sciatic nerve models. This work, performed over a 15-year period (1984–99), helped to elucidate the mechanisms underlying mechanically- and electrically-induced injury and to define the range of stimulus parameters within which nerves can be safely and effectively stimulated. These studies led to the development of a nerve electrode array which was used in sacral nerve for micturition and is also being used for vagal nerve stimulation (VNS) for epilepsy. Preliminary results of histological studies of post-mortem nerve taken from human vagal nerve implants are also presented.

The potential for mechanically-induced neural injury in long-term implants of electrodes on cranial and peripheral nerves

The mechanical configuration of the electrode and its relation to neural injury

There have been several recent reviews of the use of nerve electrodes for both experimental and clinical applications [1–5]. Naples *et al.* [2] reviewed nerve electrode configurations and their propensity to produce or avoid neural injury. They described the evolution of nerve arrays from the standpoints of materials biocompatibility, and mechanically-induced neural damage. Although these authors acknowledged that the mechanisms of electrode-induced neural damage are not fully understood, they concluded that the electrode configuration itself (incorrect fit to the nerve), surgical trauma, pressure caused by postsurgical oedema, excessive scar formation (which could bind the nerve to surrounding tissue) and tension on the electrode cables, were all potential contributors to neural damage.

Of concern in the installation of any type of nerve electrode is the degree of interference with the nerve's regional blood supply and to what extent this may contribute to the, 'mechanically-induced' neural changes. The relative importance of the longitudinal (versus the regional) vascular supply of nerves has been

Key Points

- Nerve constriction and compression is injurious.
- Nerve stretching by lead implantation is not a significant risk.

reviewed [3, 6]. These workers agree that ligation of vessels subserving the nerve's regional blood supply has no pronounced effect on the nerve. Although ligation of a regional source of supply produces a temporary local diminution of blood flow, the effect is most probably transient since the longitudinal pathway is capable of dilation and thus compensating for the local loss. Thus, the necessary mobilisation, or 'freeing-up', of segments of nerve for implantation of circumneural arrays appears to be of little consequence. Using intravital microscope techniques on the rabbit sciatic–tibial nerve, no changes in microcirculation were observed at the mid-level of a 15cm mobilised segment of the nerve [7]. In the cat peroneal–sciatic model developed in our laboratory at HMRI, we frequently ligated the inferior gluteal artery and vein in order to facilitate installation of bipolar helical electrodes. No neural damage attributable to these ligations was noted, and we have not observed evidence of damage that might be attributed to partial loss of regional blood supply, such as patchy areas of necrosis or an infarcted fascicle alongside normal fascicles [8].

However, there is no doubt that peripheral nerves can be affected adversely by chronic constriction and compression. Closed cuff electrodes (sutured closed) may compromise the structural integrity of nerve. Larsen *et al.* [9] implanted recording cuff electrodes 3cm in length on the tibial nerve of rabbits for up to 16 months: a 27% loss of myelinated axons (all sizes except the smallest) was found beneath and distal to the cuff 2 weeks after implantation. However, by 16 months after implantation the number of myelinated axons had been restored to control values, demonstrating the remarkable regenerative capacity of peripheral nerve. Since the cuff was sutured closed, the authors postulated entrapment, secondary to postsurgical oedema, as one explanation for the fibre loss. Another possible source of the injury could be local compression of the nerve at the ends of this exceptionally long and closed cuff. On the other hand, open (unsealed) cuffs, chronically implanted on the dog sacral nerve, had a propensity to extrude the nerve, resulting in mechanically induced damage in the form of axonal loss due to compression [10]. Mackinnon *et al.* [11] reported on the consequences of chronic nerve compression by circumneural silastic bands placed on the multifascicular median nerve of the cynomolgus monkey. The fascicles near the periphery of those nerves compressed for 12 months demonstrated perineurial thickening and a loss of axons, and marked thinning of the myelin of surviving axons.

Mild stretching of a nerve does not appear to be a significant risk in nerve electrode array implantation. Nerve trunks, fascicles and their constituent axons are arranged in an undulating, interwoven configuration so that stretching of the whole nerve causes little strain on the axons [12]. Lundborg and Rydevik [7] found that rabbit tibial nerves stretched to their 'upper stretch limit' (mean value of 15% elongation) for 30 minutes, were subjected to total ischaemia which, however, was reversible when the tension was relaxed. At the 'lower stretching limit' of 8% elongation, circulation through the arterioles and capillaries was maintained. This is well in excess of the degree of nerve stretch required for elevation and implantation of the HMRI helical electrode lead being used at present for vagal and other clinical nerve stimulations.

In our experience with nerve implants at HMRI, the most common type of mechanically-induced injury is manifested as subperineurial crescents of endoneurial connective tissue. These areas of increased connective tissue were most frequently situated at the periphery of the fascicles and occasionally were accompanied by degenerating axons, localised axonal loss, and remyelinating axon profiles [8]. The subperineurial crescents may be adaptive to some degree since they closely resemble 'Renaut bodies' (hyaline-appearing, loosely-textured, whorled, cell-sparse structures found in the subperineurial space) [13]. Weis *et al.* [14] reported an association between the development of Renaut bodies and nerve entrapment, and proposed that these structures may serve as a pressure-absorbing cushion for entrapped nerve.

> **Key Points**
> - Renaut bodies may cushion entrapped nerve.
> - Cable routing and electrode stability reduce electrode tension.

Routing of cables and positional stability of electrode arrays

In our early studies using a seven-coil, helical, electrode array, subperineurial crescents were observed in at least one fascicle of 40% of the nerves. Subsequently, we minimised the incidence of subperineurial crescents by several methods of reducing the tension exerted on the electrodes by the cable. In a series of 12 cats (24 nerves), Huntington Helix electrodes were implanted on the sciatic nerves for periods of 1–6 months, and the arrays were sutured to the superficial epineurium at three points. A second measure was to route the cable so that minimal tension was exerted on the array, by forming a loop in the cable immediately adjacent to the electrode array. Although a few perineurial crescents were still observed in this series, only one of 78 fascicles (1.3%) showed significant neural damage in the form of axonal loss and remyelinating profiles. This routing technique is being used in clinical applications of the NeuroCybernetic Systems lead for vagus nerve stimulation for epilepsy [15, 16]. In our studies it was helpful to monitor the postsurgical positional stability of electrode arrays and cables by the use of radiographs (Fig. 4.1).

Intraneural electrode arrays

A few attempts have been made to stimulate nerves by endoneurial (penetrating) electrodes. At a symposium held at Case Western Reserve University, the feasibility of selective activation of muscles by conventional (extraneural) and intraneural (intrafascicular) electrode arrays was discussed [4]. Conclusions from this symposium were that intraneural electrodes offer the advantages of greater selectivity and lower power requirements, but these may be offset by the difficulty of introducing very fine wire or silicon-substrate electrodes through the collagenous epineurium and perineurium. It was also concluded that cuff electrodes may provide more

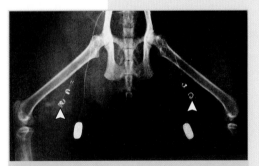

Figure 4.1 Radiograph through pelvic region of the cat taken immediately after implantation, to show bilateral electrode implants on sciatic nerves. A marker coil (of platinum in silastic) was sutured to the nerve just distal to the distal electrode (arrowheads). Rectangular platinum indifferent electrodes are visible in the subcutaneous tissue just dorsal to the arrays. Subsequent radiographs and examination at autopsy showed no movement between markers and arrays. Note the coil in the cable (arrow) which prevents tension on the electrode array.

Key Points
• Intraneural electrodes may
increase trauma risk.

stable recruitment patterns over time, and are easier to remove or replace should the need arise. Grill and Mortimer [17] subsequently demonstrated the feasibility of using chronically implanted multiple-contact spiral cuff electrodes to effect selective activation of individual nerve fascicles.

A major concern with intraneural electrodes is the danger of breaching the perineurium, particularly with large wire microelectrodes (in excess of 75μm in diameter). The perineurium acts as a diffusion barrier between the epineurium and the endoneurium. Trauma to the perineurium can result in endoneurial oedema, leading to an increase of endoneurial pressure and creating a 'miniature compartment syndrome' in the nerve fascicle [3]. Bowman and Erickson [18] histologically evaluated sites beneath pulsed and unpulsed electrodes implanted intraneurally in the posterior tibial nerve of rabbits for 4 years. The electrodes were of stainless-steel wire, 51μm in diameter but wound into helical coils (280–300μm in diameter). The nerve showed little axonal loss, although 40% of the specimens exhibited a 'bulbous formation' associated with endoneurial oedema, suggesting injury to the perineurial membrane. Lefurge *et al.* [19] obtained chronic intrafascicular recordings from the radial nerve of cats. Although the nerve appeared physiologically normal during the course of the experiment, micrographs of the nerves showed redundant myelin, marked axonal loss, and endoneurial oedema, suggesting perineurial injury as a result of insertion or residence of the intrafascicular recording electrodes. These studies indicate that excitation of nerves by intraneural rather than epineurial electrodes carries a greater risk of trauma, at least at this stage of their development.

Post-mortem studies

Our laboratory has recently begun to evaluate tissue taken post mortem from VNS patients. To date, we have studied seven patients who were implanted and stimulated with the NeuroCybernetic prosthesis for periods of 9 months to 3 years. Their deaths were not associated with malfunction of the device. The implanted nerve site on the left vagus was studied, as well as the unimplanted right vagus. At autopsy, electrode arrays of all patients were found to be well positioned and well invested with connective tissue without distortion of the nerves. Histological studies revealed that cellular changes were remarkably similar in both pulsed and unpulsed nerves and were limited to the types of morphological alterations (including degenerating myelinated fibres) that can be attributed to post-mortem preservation artefacts. That the degenerating myelinated fibres in both stimulated and control nerves was due to changes post mortem is supported by the fact that no macrophages or any other inflammatory cells were present, as would be the case if the ongoing damage had occurred when the patient was alive. In addition, morphometric analysis of the nerves of one of the specimens was carried out by image analysis on a personal computer, as described previously [20]. This study demonstrated that the distribution of fibre diameters in stimulated and unstimulated vagal nerves was very similar (unpublished studies). Important conclusions from these post-mortem studies are that the arrays and tethers were properly placed and there was no evidence of mechanically-induced injury (distortion of the nerve, subepineurial crescents) or of electrically-induced injury.

These post-mortem human studies, carried out on VNS patients who had used clinically-effective stimulus protocols and in which the arrays had been implanted for longer periods than most animal studies, are highly relevant to the objectives of this volume and should be conducted in any clinical application at every opportunity.

The role of connective tissue in chronic implants on nerve

The presence of a connective tissue sheath around the implanted nerve can be both beneficial and detrimental. For the most part, connective tissue ensheathment appears to aid in binding the electrode to the nerve and allows the electrode and nerve to move as a unit, which is desirable. A disadvantage would be reduced or restricted mobilisation of the nerve due to a build-up of excess connective tissue, which could bind the array to neighbouring muscle tissue.

Connective tissue ensheathment also presents a problem in explantation of chronic implants, whether in experimental or clinical studies. We have found the removal of connective tissue, preparatory to processing the nerve for histology, to be a laborious process. One of our group (T.G.H. Yuen) used the erbium laser by which the connective tissue sheath can be rapidly and effectively removed in increments of a few micrometres without damaging the underlying fixed nerve or the electrode array.

Protocols for safe stimulation of peripheral and cranial nerves

Characteristics of electrically-induced injury

In addition to minimising mechanically-induced injury during implantation and residence of the electrode on the nerve, it is vital that the nerve is not injured by the electrical stimulation itself. A number of animal studies have demonstrated that prolonged electrical stimulation may, under certain circumstances, cause injury to the axons in peripheral and cranial nerves. Injury may occur even when the principles of prudent, functional electrical stimulation are adhered to, including the use of controlled-current stimuli that inject no net charge, the use of noble metal electrodes, and use of a stimulus charge density that does not tax the electrode's charge-injection capacity [1, 8, 20–26].

After several hours of stimulation of a nerve at a damaging amplitude and frequency, some of the myelinated axons begin, within a few days, to undergo early axonal degeneration (EAD). The myelin surrounding the axons collapses into the axonal space, forming redundant myelin and myelin ovoid bodies [1, 8, 20–25]; non-myelinated fibres are not damaged. The histological manifestations of EAD are very conspicuous by 7 days after the damaging stimulation. The damaged axons are distributed quite uniformly throughout a fascicle, and are interspersed with others (usually the majority) that appear essentially normal (Fig. 4.2). There is a major

Key Points

- Post-mortem studies on VNS patients show no mechanically/electrically-induced neural injury, given correct protocols.
- In animal studies, prolonged/excessive stimulation may cause early axonal degeneration (EAD).

Key Points

- Electrical stimulation may injure axons in several ways.
- Some injuries follow electrochemical reactions at the electrode/fluid interface.
- Others involve neural activity or changes in polarisation.

difference between this type of injury and that which may be caused by a poorly-fitting cuff or helical electrode, wherein the histological changes are usually confined to crescentic inclusions at the periphery of the fascicle.

The fate of electrically-induced EAD was recently evaluated in a chronic study following 8 hours of continuous stimulation of the sciatic nerve using charge-balanced wave forms at high intensities, 50Hz and 2100–4500μA [27]. Degenerating axonal profiles were present for up to 60 days following the stimulation. Computer-assisted morphometric and ultrastructural studies indicated that a few of the damaged fibres had not regenerated within as long as 125 days following stimulation. Functional deficits were not observed in any of the animals. These findings indicated that there is relatively little late-onset injury associated with the stimulation. However, the slow, possibly incomplete, recovery of the damaged axons emphasised the importance of using stimulus protocols with adequate margins of safety.

Mechanisms of electrically-induced injury

There are several mechanisms by which electrical stimulation might injure axons. These fall into two broad categories: those related to the passage of the stimulus current across the interface between the electrode and the physiological fluid and those associated with the flow of the current through the tissue. The first category includes tissue toxicity from the products of electrode dissolution as well as other products arising from electrochemical reactions at the interface [26]. The second category encompasses those processes that are not linked specifically to the electrochemistry at the tissue interface but, rather, are associated with the induced neural activity or with the depolarisation and hyperpolarisation of the axonal membranes by the stimulus current. Several studies support the premise that the

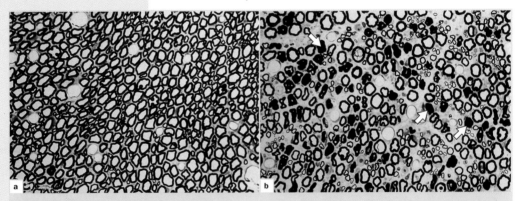

Figure 4.2a *Normal-appearing, 1μm cross-section of a cat sciatic nerve subjected to continuous stimulation at 20Hz and 3000μA (3 × full α component) for 8 hours. Note lack of early axonal degeneration (EAD) or other abnormalities (a safe and effective stimulation). Bar = 20μm.*

Figure 4.2b *Plastic section 1μm from the contralateral sciatic nerve of the same cat as in Figure 4.2a pulsed with 100Hz, 1700μA (3 × full α component) for 8 hours. Note numerous profiles of EAD (arrows). Larger and smaller axons are spared. Bar = 20μm.*

axonal injury is related to the neuronal activity induced by the prolonged high-rate electrical stimulation — a type of activity-related
injury. For example, blocking the action potentials in a peripheral
nerve with a local anaesthetic will protect the nerve from stimulation-induced injury [21]. Other workers have described activity-
associated ultrastructural changes in the nodes of Ranvier, including
extra-axonal vacuoles separating the myelin terminal lamella of the
perinodal apparatus [28]. There is very good evidence that excessive
neuronal activity can injure neurons in the brain [29–31]. However,
the current required to induce axonal injury in a peripheral nerve is
greater than the amplitude that is required to excite the axons, and
this poses a difficulty for the hypothesis that the axonal injury is
related to the induced neural (hyper)activity. If the injury is activity-
related, the process cannot be simply that a particular axon is injured
by its own activity. Were this the case, it would not be possible safely
to activate the fibres in a peripheral nerve, at the stimulus frequency
that exceeds a critical value [24, 25]. However, the results from our
'local anaesthetic' study strongly implicate neuronal activity as a
factor in the damage. These findings can be reconciled by the
premise that the damage is due to a 'mass action' phenomenon in
which the vulnerable axons are injured when a sufficient number of
fibres are recruited by the stimulus [24]. Possibly, the injury might be
precipitated by mass activity-related changes in the extra-axonal
environment, such as accumulation of potassium [32].

An alternative hypothesis is that the axonal injury is due to electroporation of the axonal membranes by the applied electric field,
rather than to the induced neuronal activity *per se*. In electroporation, the electric field generated by the stimulus current moment-
arily opens pores in the cellular membrane, thereby disturbing
intracellular homoeostasis by allowing ions such as calcium to enter
the axon [33, 34]. This is consistent with the observation that the
damage threshold to electrical stimulation in a peripheral nerve is
much higher than the excitation threshold. Indeed, there is good
evidence that membrane permeabilisation by electroporation is a
major cause of the damage to nerve and muscle after severe electric shock [35, 36]. However, the electroporation hypothesis is difficult to reconcile with the findings from our study of local
anaesthesia. Another difficulty is that the myelinated axons of intermediate size (those with axonal diameter of 3–9μm) are more
vulnerable to stimulation-induced injury than are the largest or the
smallest myelinated fibres [20] (Fig. 4.2). Experimental measurements
and mathematical modelling have shown that the largest axons
would experience the greatest depolarisation and repolarisation [37,
38]. Therefore, if membrane electroporation were primarily responsible for the stimulation-induced damage, the largest fibres should
be most vulnerable to the injury, which is not the case. It is unclear
why the intermediate-sized fibres would be more vulnerable to
injury from a change in the composition of the extracellular environment. However, the 'mass-action' hypothesis of axonal injury seems
to best fit the experimental observations, at least for the moderate
levels of current that were tested in the animal models, and which
are likely to be generated by clinical stimulators.

> **Key Points**
> - EAD may be related to induced neuronal activity, rather than tissue toxicity.
> - Electroporation is probably not culpable.

The premise that the axonal injury is activity related has a number of implications for the design of protocols for safe and effective nerve stimulation. One corollary, which is supported by experimental data, is that for there to be a high correlation between the neural injury and the stimulus, the latter must be specified in terms of units that are related to the stimulation-induced neuronal activity. Indeed, the correlation between the neural damage and the stimulus amplitude is very poor when the latter is expressed as electrical units such as current, charge density or charge per phase [24]. We have used as a normalising factor the stimulus current that is required to recruit fully the earliest (α) component of the compound action potential (CAP) induced by the stimulation. The α component of the CAP is composed of the action potentials from group I and group II efferent fibres as well as the afferent fibres that have overall diameters of approximately 5–22μm [39].

The results from peripheral nerves stand in contrast with those from a study in which the stimulus was applied through disc-shaped platinum electrodes implanted directly on the surface of the cerebral cortex, and where the threshold of neural damage was correlated strongly with both charge density and charge per phase [40]. The difference may be due to the rather complex relation between the stimulus current and the neural activity induced in the nerve. Our recent studies of peripheral nerve stimulation have utilised the Huntington Helical circumneural electrode, in which the stimulus current is injected via a pair of helical platinum bands which are spaced 10mm apart and completely encircle the nerve. The portion of the stimulus current which actually enters the nerve is affected strongly by the snugness of the fit between the electrode and the nerve and, subsequently, it appears to be affected by the growth of connective tissue around the implant site. Furthermore, the relation between the stimulus current field within the nerve, the longitudinal component of the intraneural electric field induced by the current, and the depolarisation (and subsequent excitation) of the individual axons may be quite complex [37, 38, 41, 42].

In the cat sciatic nerve the threshold for axonal damage is determined by a synergistic interaction of the stimulus amplitude (in α units) and frequency. Figure 4.3 shows data from 33 feline sciatic nerves implanted chronically with helical circumneural electrodes. Several weeks after implantation, the nerves were stimulated for 8 hours with charge-balanced, controlled-current pulse pairs. Each phase (the first and second pulses) was separated by an interphase delay of 400μs. This waveform excites myelinated axons over a wide range of sizes [43]. The stimulus frequency was either 20, 50, or 100Hz. The abscissa of Figure 4.3 is the percentage of myelinated axons undergoing early axonal degeneration at 7 days after the stimulation [25]. It should be interpreted as a relative, rather than an absolute, scale of axonal injury since, during EAD, a particular myelinated fibre may appear quite normal at one point along the nerve (i.e. in a particular histological cross-section) but will appear markedly degenerated at another level [20]. When the stimulus frequency was 20Hz, there was virtually no axonal injury that could be attributed to the stimulation, even when the stimulus amplitude was eight times greater than that necessary to recruit fully the α component of the compound action potential; when the stimulus frequency was 50Hz, axonal damage occurred when the stimulus amplitude exceeded approximately one α unit; when the stimulus frequency was 100Hz, the threshold for the neural injury was nearly unchanged, but the slope of the regression line increased markedly.

Figure 4.3 shows that there are two thresholds for stimulation-induced axonal injury — one related to stimulus amplitude and a second related to stimulus frequency. In the cat sciatic nerve implanted with the helical electrodes, and with a pulse duration of 100μs per phase, the amplitude threshold for EAD is approximately one α unit, and the frequency threshold is between 20 and 50Hz. Below these thresholds, there was no histologically detectable axonal injury that could be attributed to the stimulation.

The first-order correlation coefficients of the regression analysis of the data shown in Figure 4.3 are of some interest. At a pulse rate of 50 or 100Hz, the coefficients (*R*) are 0.87 and 0.85, respectively. Thus, by specifying the stimulus amplitude in terms of α units, we can predict the amount of EAD with an accuracy of R^2 (75% or 72%), for a pulse rate of 50 or 100Hz, respectively. The remaining variance in the amount of EAD must be due to factors that were not controlled in our study.

The neural damage threshold is also determined by the particulars of the stimulus waveform. When the stimulus frequency is 50Hz and the stimulus pulse duration is 100μs per phase with a 400μs interphase delay, the damage threshold is approximately one α unit, as shown in Figure 4.3. However, when the pulse duration is reduced to 50μs per phase and the interphase delay is eliminated, the damage threshold increases, to approximately two α units [24]. This also lends credence to the premise that the axonal injury is linked to the excitation of a large number of axons, since the short-duration stimulus pulses will tend to excite the large axons [43] whose action potentials contribute to the component of the compound action potential. Therefore, when the stimulus is one α unit, fewer small axons (and hence fewer axons in total) are excited than would be the case with the long-duration pulses. Thus, the short-pulse waveform may afford some additional margin of safety, but only when the objective is to excite the axons that are represented in the α component of the CAP (the group I and the group II efferent fibres and the larger afferent fibres). If the objective is to excite small axons, the mass-action hypothesis

Key Points
- Thresholds of stimulus amplitude/frequency affect axonal injury.
- Stimulus waveform is also important.

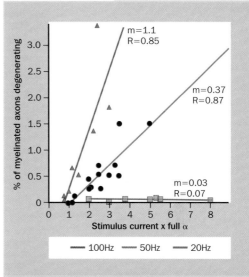

Figure 4.3 *Plots of the percentage of myelinated axons in a cat sciatic nerve undergoing EAD, 7 days after 8 hours of continuous stimulation. The abscissa is the amplitude of the stimulus current pulses, expressed as multiples of the current required to fully recruit the α component of the compound action potential recorded over the spinal cord. Data from nerves stimulated at 20, 50 and 100Hz are plotted as different symbols. The first-order regression coefficients for each stimulus frequency are also listed: R is the correlation coefficient and m is the slope of the regression line in units of percentage axons degenerating per α unit. (From ref. 25 with permission.)*

implies that the margin of safety will be larger for a stimulus waveform that preferentially recruits the smaller axons [44]. Even the inclusion of an interphase delay will at least reduce the tendency to recruit the larger fibres before the smaller ones [43].

The risk of injury is also affected by the duration of continuous stimulation. The amount of EAD in the cat peroneal nerve increased markedly as the length of the session of continuous stimulation was increased from 4 to 8 hours, and then to 16 hours [23].

In addition to the protective effects of low frequency and decreasing the total duration of stimulation, additional safety is provided by intermittent stimulation of nerve. The feline peroneal nerve sustained no injury during 8 hours of intermittent stimulation using a 50% duty cycle (5 seconds of stimulation, then 5 seconds without stimulation) whereas continuous stimulation at 50Hz caused considerable EAD [8]. Thus, the propensity for stimulation-induced axonal injury appears to be related to the average pulse frequency, rather than to the instantaneous frequency.

Recommendations

We can now consider how the data from these animal studies might be used to aid in the design of protocols for safe, long-term stimulation in human patients. We should note that there is no evidence that the electrode arrays or protocols that have been used for sacral or vagal nerve stimulation are injurious to the nerve, and our emphasis here is how to ensure the greatest margin of safety.

It may be concluded, from the review of mechanical factors involved in neural injury, that the ideal nerve electrode array should (a) be fabricated from soft pliable material, (b) be self-sizing to accommodate a reasonable range of nerve sizes for the particular application, in order to avoid constricting the nerve, and (c) be able to survive indefinitely in the environment of tissue fluids. It should also (d) have features that prevent it from being dislodged from the nerve, and (e) be equipped with a strong, yet flexible, cable.

Certainly, Figure 4.3 should not be considered a 'quantitative recipe' for specifying protocols for safe stimulation of the human vagus nerve. Indeed, that figure was derived from data using a helical electrode, but the electrode was implanted on the cat sciatic nerve, and the nerve was stimulated continuously during a single 8-hour session rather than intermittently over a period of many months or years. We have no data from the animal studies as to whether the propensity for the stimulus to cause axonal injury is cumulative over many days or data relating to the differences in the neural damage threshold for different nerves or for different species. However, the fact that the current protocols for clinical stimulation of the vagus entail stimulating the nerve for no more than about 2–3 hours each day is surely advantageous from the standpoint of safety [15]. Protocols that require prolonged stimulation may carry greater risk; furhermore, other factors, such as the stimulus pulse duration, can affect the damage threshold. However, Figure 4.3 can still provide some valuable (albeit qualitative) guidelines. First, there appears to be a threshold frequency below which there is no axonal damage at all, even when the stimulus amplitude is quite high; therefore, in a clinical nerve stimulator, the average stimulus frequency should not be in excess of that required to obtain the desired effect. Secondly, the stimulus amplitude should not be greater than that required to obtain the desired clinical effect, since if the stimulus frequency does happen to exceed the threshold for inflicting axonal injury, the propensity to cause the injury will increase with the stimulus amplitude.

The hypothesis that the damage is due to the composite induced neuronal activity suggests that some additional margin of safety may be derived from the use of a stimulus waveform that affords some degree of selective excitation of the relevant fibre population. At present there is some uncertainty as to which fibre populations are primarily responsible for the anti-epileptic activity of vagal nerve stimulation. Resolution of this issue may permit the design of stimulation protocols that further enhance the safety of this treatment modality, as well as further improving the electrical efficiency of the stimulator [45].

> **Key Points**
> - Stimulus frequency/amplitude should not exceed that clinically required.
> - A waveform that excites relevant nerve fibres may confer extra safety.

Acknowledgements

We thank Cheryl Long for secretarial assistance. This work was supported in part by Contract Nos. NO1-NS-2-2323, NO1-NS-5-2324 and NO1-NS-8-2388 from the NINDS of the NIH.

References

1. Agnew WF, McCreery DB, Yuen TGH, Bullara LA. Local anesthetic block protects against electrically-induced damage in peripheral nerve. *J Biomed Eng* 1990; 12: 301–8.
2. Naples GG, Mortimer JT, Yuen TGH. Overview of peripheral nerve electrode design and implantation. In: Agnew WF, McCreery DB (eds) *Neural Prostheses: Fundamental Studies*. Englewood Cliffs: Prentice Hall, 1990; 107–45.
3. Rydevik BL, Danielson N, Dahlin LB, Lundborg G. Pathophysiology of peripheral nerve injury with special reference to electrode implantation. In: Agnew WF, McCreery DB (eds) *Neural Prostheses: Fundamental Studies*. Englewood Cliffs: Prentice Hall, 1990; 85–105.
4. Mortimer JT, Agnew WF, Horch K *et al.* Perspectives on new electrode technology for stimulating peripheral nerves with implantable motor prostheses. *IEEE Trans Rehabil Eng* 1995; 3: 145–54.
5. Bhadra N, Peckham PH. Peripheral nerve stimulation for restoration of motor function. *J Clin Neurophysiol* 1997; 14: 378–93.
6. Adams WE. The blood supply of nerves: the effects of exclusion of its regional sources of supply of the sciatic nerve of the rabbit. *J Anat* 1942; 77: 243–50.
7. Lundborg G, Rydevik B. Effects of stretching the tibial nerve of the rabbit: a preliminary study of the intraneural circulation and the barrier function of the perineurium. *J Bone Joint Surg* 1973; 55: 390.
8. Agnew WF, McCreery DB, Yuen TGH, Bullara LA. Histologic and physiologic evaluation of electrically stimulated peripheral nerve: considerations for the selection of parameters. *Ann Biomed Eng* 1989; 17: 39–60.
9. Larsen JO, Thomsen M, Haughland M, Sinkjaer T. Degeneration and regeneration in rabbit peripheral nerve with long-term nerve cuff electrode implant: a stereological study of myelinated and unmyelinated axons. *Acta Neuropathol* 1998; 96: 365–78.

10. Yuen TGH, Agnew WF, Bullara LA. Histopathological evaluation of dog sacral nerve after chronic electrical stimulation for micturition. *Neurosurgery* 1984; 14: 449–55.
11. Mackinnon SE, Dellon AL, Hudson AR, Hunter DA. A primate model for chronic nerve compression. *J Reconstr Microsurg* 1985; 3: 185–94.
12. Sunderland S. *Nerves and Nerve Injuries*. 2nd edition. Edinburgh: Churchill Livingstone, 1978.
13. Asbury AK. Renaut bodies. A forgotten endoneurial structure. *J Neuropathol Exp Neurol* 1973; 22: 334–43.
14. Weis J, Alexianu ME, Heide G, Schroeder JM. Renaut bodies contain elastic fiber components. *J Neuropathol Exp Neurol* 1993; 52: 445–451.
15. Uthman BM, Wilder BJ, Hammond EJ, Reid SA. Efficacy and safety of vagus nerve stimulation in patients with complex partial seizure. *Epilepsia* 1990; 31(Suppl 2): S44–S50.
16. Landy HJ, Ramsey RE, Slater J et al. Vagus nerve stimulation for complex partial seizures: surgical technique, safety and efficacy. *J Neurosurg* 1993; 78: 26–31.
17. Grill WM, Mortimer JT. Stability of the input–output properties of chronically implanted multiple contact nerve cuff stimulating electrodes. *IEEE Trans Rehabi Eng* 1998; 6: 364–73.
18. Bowman BR, Erickson RC. Acute and chronic implantation of coiled wire intraneural electrodes during cyclical electrical stimulation. *Ann Biomed Eng* 1985; 13: 75–93.
19. Lefurge T, Goodall E, Horch K et al. Chronically implanted intrafascicular recording electrodes. *Ann Biomed Eng* 1991; 19: 197–207.
20. McCreery DB, Yuen TGH, Agnew WF, Bullara LA. A quantitative computer-assisted morphometric analysis of stimulation-induced injury to myelinated fibers in a peripheral nerve. *J Neurosci Methods* 1997; 73: 159–68.
21. Agnew WF, McCreery DB (eds). *Neural Prostheses: Fundamental Studies*. Englewood Cliffs: Prentice Hall, 1990.
22. Agnew WF, McCreery DB, Bullara LA, Yuen TGH. Effects of prolonged electrical stimulation of peripheral nerve. In: Agnew WF, McCreery DB (eds) *Neural Prostheses: Fundamental Studies*. Englewood Cliffs: Prentice Hall, 1990: 147–67.
23. Agnew WF, McCreery DB. Considerations for safety with chronically implanted nerve electrodes. *Epilepsia* 1990; 31(Suppl 2): S27–S32.
24. McCreery DB, Agnew WF, Yuen TGH, Bullara LA. Damage in peripheral nerve from continuous electrical stimulation: comparison of two stimulus waveforms. *Med Biol Eng Comput* 1992; 30: 109–14.
25. McCreery DB, Agnew WF, Yuen TGH, Bullara LA. Relation between stimulus amplitude, stimulus frequency, and neural damage during electrical stimulation of the sciatic nerve of the cat. *Med Biol Eng Comput* 1995; 33: 426–29.
26. Robblee LS, Rose TL. Electrochemical guidelines for selection of protocols and electrode materials for neural stimulation. In: Agnew WF, McCreery DB (eds) *Neural Prostheses: Fundamental Studies*. Englewood Cliffs: Prentice Hall, 1990. 25–66.
27. Agnew WF, McCreery DB, Yuen TGH, Bullara LA. Evolution and resolution of stimulation-induced axonal injury in peripheral nerve. *Muscled Nerve* 1999; 22: 1393–402.
28. Wurtz CC, Ellisman MH. Alterations in the ultrastructure of peripheral nodes of Ranvier associated with repetitive action potential propagation. *J Neurosci* 1986; 6: 3133–43.
29. Ben-Ari Y, Tremblay E, Ottersen OP, Meldrum BS. The role of epileptic activity in hippocampal and remote cerebral lesions induced by Kainic Acid. *Brain Res* 1980; 191: 79–97.
30. Olney JW, de Gubareff T, Sloviter RS. "Epileptic" brain damage in rats induced by sustained electrical stimulation of the perforant path: ultrastructural analysis of acute hippocampal pathology. *Brain Res Bull* 1983; 10: 699–712.
31. Seisjo BK, Abdul-Rahman A. A metabolic basis for the relative vulnerability of neurons in status epilepticus. *Acta Physiol*. 1979; 106: 377–78.
32. McCreery DB, Agnew WF. Changes in extracellular potassium and calcium concentration and neural activity during prolonged electrical stimulation of the cat cerebral cortex at defined charge densities. *Exp Neurol* 1983; 79: 371–96.
33. Weaver JC. Electroporation: a general phenomenon for manipulating cells and tissues. *J Cell Biochem* 1993; 51: 426–35.
34. Tsong TY. Electroporation of cell membranes. *Biophys J* 1991; 60: 297–306.
35. Lee RC, River LP, Pan FS et al. Surfactant-induced sealing of electropermeabilized skeletal muscle membranes *in vivo*. *Proc Nat Acad Sci USA* 1992; 89: 4524–28.
36. Chen W, Lee RC. Altered ion channel conductance and ionic selectivity induced by large imposed membrane potential pulses. *Biophys J* 1994; 67: 603–12.

37. Rattay F. Analysis of models for extracellular fiber stimulation. *IEEE Trans Biomed Eng* 1989; 36: 676–82.
38. Rubenstein JT. Analytical theory for extracellular stimulation of nerve with focal electrodes II: passive myelinated axon. *Biophysical J* 1991; 60: 538–55.
39. Ruch TC, Fulton JF. *Medical Physiology and Biophysics*. Philadelphia: W.B. Saunders Co., 1960.
40. McCreery DB, Agnew WF, Yuen TGH, Bullara LA. Charge density and charge per phase as cofactors in neural injury induced by electrical stimulation. *IEEE Trans Biomed Eng* 1990; 37: 996–1001.
41. McNeal DR. Analysis of a model for excitation of myelinated nerve. *IEEE Trans Biomed Eng* 1976; 23: 329–37.
42. Rijkhoff NJM, Holshimer J, Debruyne FMJ, Wijkstra H. Modeling selective activation of small myelinated nerve fibers using a monopolar point electrode. *Med Biol Eng Comput* 1995; 33: 762–68.
43. Gorman PH, Mortimer JT. The effect of stimulus parameters on the recruitment characteristics of direct nerve stimulation. *IEEE Trans Biomed Eng* 1983; 30: 407–14.
44. Fang ZP, Mortimer JT. Selective activation of small motor axons by quasi-trapezoidal current pulses. *IEEE Trans Biomed Eng* 1991; 38: 168–74.
45. McCreery DB, Agnew WF. A comparison of stimulation modes for electrical excitation of fibers in the cat tibial nerve, with reference to anti-epileptic stimulation of the human vagus nerve. In: *American Epilepsy Society Meeting*, Boston, Mass., 1997; Vol. 38, Suppl. 8: 18–19.

5 Clinical and urodynamic assessments of the mode of action of sacral nerve stimulation

A.A.B. Lycklama à Nijeholt,

P.M. Groenendijk and J. den Boon

Introduction

Sacral nerve stimulation (SNS) can be very effective in the treatment of refractory urge incontinence, urgency–frequency, and voiding difficulty. The clinical results of this treatment, published in recent years, are promising: the reported cure rate varies from 41 to 100%, with an average of 70% [1].

Explanation of the neurophysiological mode of action of this treatment is based on human electrophysiological studies and on animal experiments. In SNS treatment, both afferent and efferent sacral nerve fibres (constituting the pelvic plexus) and pudendal nerve fibres (innervating the external sphincter and pelvic floor) are stimulated. The thicker myelinated somatic fibres are affected more than the thinner parasympathic fibres, resulting in a primary effect on urethral and pelvic floor activity; because the threshold for a motor effect on bladder activity is higher, a direct simultaneous motor effect on the bladder is avoided. According to some investigators [2, 3, 4, 5], the modulating effect of the enhanced urethral sphincter and pelvic floor tone inhibits detrusor instability. If this is true, the effect of neuromodulation on voiding difficulty can also be explained: neuromodulation reduces the spastic behaviour of the pelvic floor, which is permanently inhibiting bladder activity. By reducing this inhibitory effect, neuromodulation restores normal bladder contractility. However, according to another concept [6], neuromodulation primarily affects the bladder via the afferent sacral nerve fibres.

In this chapter we present both clinical and urodynamic data which underline the effect of SNS treatment on urethral and pelvic floor function.

Patients and methods

Three clinical and urodynamic observations are presented here. First, the clinical and urodynamic results of 22 patients, undergoing surgery in Leiden during the international multicentre SNS study, were analysed. As part of this study, 6 months postoperatively, a urodynamic investigation was performed, during which the Itrel* stimulator was switched off and on. The efficacy of SNS treatment

Key Points
- SNS affects thicker, myelinated, somatic fibres more than thinner, parasympathetic fibres.
- Urethral/pelvic floor activity is affected more than bladder activity.

*A predecessor of the current InterStim device.

and the effect of switching the stimulator on and off on both ure-thral and bladder instability were studied.

Five female patients, in whom bladder stability had been achieved by neuromodulation, were selected for a pudendal block with lignocaine (lidocaine). For the pudendal block we used a trumpet-needle, isolated by a glove, except for the tip, which was connected to a neurostimulator. On vaginal examination the ischial spine was palpated and the pudendal nerve was located by apply-ing electrical stimulation via the tip of the trumpet-needle. After this nerve had been identified, 15ml 0.5% lignocaine was injected through the sacrospinous ligament. A bilateral block was applied. Some 20 minutes after injection, the effect of the pudendal block was assessed by testing the bulbocavernous reflex and by testing the vulvar and perineal sensitivity with a needle and clamp. A urodynamic study was performed before injection and was repeated during the pudendal block.

The final clinical and urodynamic observation was in a female patient with recurrent urge incontinence after a bladder substitution operation. This patient (JV, born in 1963), had presented originally with severe, refractory urgency–frequency (diurnal frequency, 25; nocturnal frequency, 3) and severe urge incontinence. At that time urodynamic investigation had revealed severe bladder and urethral instability. Interstitial cystitis was excluded by bladder biopsies. Because the bladder had a functional capacity of 150ml, a supra-trigonal cystectomy was performed, in combination with a bladder substitution according to the Mainz technique. Three years later, this patient presented again with recurrent, severe urge incontinence. Urodynamic investigation showed that the urge incontinence was due to severe urethral instability and minor 'bladder' instability. The functional 'bladder' capacity was 600ml. A peripheral nerve evalua-tion (PNE) test was performed on S3, on the left side. Both the clini-cal and urodynamic effects of the subchronic PNE test, which was carried out over a period of 2 weeks, were documented.

Results

At our institution, 22 patients underwent surgery in the course of the multicentre SNS study. These patients were selected as candi-dates for implantation because of symptomatic improvement of at least 50% during the subchronic PNE test. Of these patients, 15 were in the urge incontinence group, five were in the urgency–frequency group (including one male patient) and two underwent surgery because of chronic voiding dysfunction. In the majority of these patients, especially in the incontinence group and in the urgency–frequency group, urethral and bladder instability was noted. In a considerable number of patients, SNS treatment resulted in marked improvement in both urethral and bladder stability.

Figure 5.1 refers to patient JB, born in 1952, who had suffered from severe, refractory urge incontinence and urgency–frequency (diurnal frequency, 30; nocturnal frequency, 4) for 7 years. Urodynamic studies demonstrated urethral and bladder instability

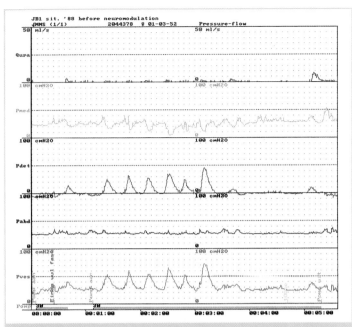

Figure 5.1 *Patient JB, with severe refractory urge incontinence and urgency–frequency: urodynamics before neuromodulation operation: urethral and bladder instability with concomitant incontinence.*

    Q_{ura} = urinary flow (ml/s); scale 0–50ml/s

    P_{med} = urethral pressure (cmH$_2$O; scale 0–100cmH$_2$O)

    P_{det} = detrusor pressure (cmH$_2$O; scale 0–100cmH$_2$O)

    P_{abd} = abdominal pressure (cmH$_2$O; scale 0–100cmH$_2$O)

    P_{ves} = vesical pressure (cmH$_2$O; scale 0–100cmH$_2$O)

with concomitant incontinence. She was selected for a PNE test and, because of an impressive improvement, for a SNS implant. At interim analysis at 6 months postoperatively (S3 left), urodynamic investigation (Fig. 5.2) showed, in accordance with an excellent clinical response, stable bladder and urethral function. During this urodynamic study the Itrel stimulator was switched off (Fig. 5 3): this brought about an instant recurrence of urethral and bladder instability, with concomitant incontinence. According to the time-scale, in the second half of the filling phase the decrease in urethral pressure precedes a rise in bladder pressure.

    Five patients, in whom neuromodulation had brought about stability, were selected for bilateral pudendal block with ligno-caine. The efficacy of the pudendal block was assessed by disappearance of the bulbocavernous reflex and absence (or marked decrease) of perineal and vulvar sensitivity. In two patients, these clinical parameters indicated a satisfactory pudendal nerve block; however, in three patients the block was inadequate. The application of the pudendal block, performed by an experienced gynaecologist, appeared to be rather uncomfortable for the patient,

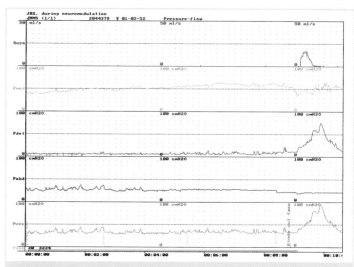

Figure 5.2 *Patient JB during SNS: interim analysis 6 months postoperatively (S3 left).In accordance with an excellent clinical response there is stable bladder and urethral function during filling, followed by normal voiding.*

    Q_{ura} = *urinary flow (ml/s); scale 0–50ml/s*
    P_{med} = *urethral pressure (cmH$_2$O; scale 0–100cmH$_2$O)*
    P_{det} = *detrusor pressure (cmH$_2$O; scale 0–100cmH$_2$O)*
    P_{abd} = *abdominal pressure (cmH$_2$O; scale 0–100cmH$_2$O)*
    P_{ves} = *vesical pressure (cmH$_2$O; scale 0–100cmH$_2$O)*

and identification of the pudendal nerve appeared to be more diffi-cult than in patients in labour, which explains the failure of the pudendal nerve block in three patients. In two patients the successful pudendal block was followed by a urodynamic inves-tigation. Figure 5.4 again refers to patient JB, after pudendal block: the bulbocavernous reflex was absent; perineal and vulvar sensi-tivity was absent on the left and markedly decreased on the right. Urodynamic studies showed recurrent severe bladder and urethral instability with severe incontinence during filling. This is in sharp contrast to the urodynamic investigation performed before the pudendal nerve block. The results of this investigation were simi-lar to those depicted in Figure 5.2 in that they showed a stability of bladder and urethral function as a result SNS treatment.

In patient JV who underwent a bladder substitution operation, it was possible to compare preoperative clinical and urodynamic data with such data 3 years later, when she complained of recur-rent urinary incontinence, and with data during the subsequent chronic PNE test. Before the bladder-substitution operation, JV complained of severe urgency–frequency and severe urge incon-tinence. At that time, a urodynamic investigation revealed severe bladder and urethral instability (Fig. 5.5). This investigation illus-trates very clearly the initial decrease in urethral pressure, followed by the rise in bladder pressure. The clinical result of the bladder

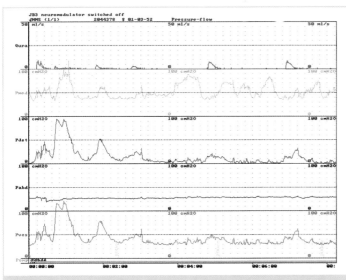

Figure 5.3 *Patient JB interim analysis 6 months postoperatively: when the Itrel stimulator is switched off there is an instant recurrence of urethral and bladder instability with concomitant incontinence. According to the timescale, in the second half of the filling phase the decrease in urethral pressure precedes a rise in bladder pressure.*

Q_{ura} = *urinary flow (ml/s); scale 0–50ml/s*

P_{med} = *urethral pressure (cmH$_2$O; scale 0–100cmH$_2$O)*

P_{det} = *detrusor pressure (cmH$_2$O; scale 0–100cmH$_2$O)*

P_{abd} = *abdominal pressure (cmH$_2$O; scale 0–100cmH$_2$O)*

P_{ves} = *vesical pressure (cmH$_2$O; scale 0–100cmH$_2$O)*

substitution operation was initially satisfactory — a normal functional 'bladder' capacity, spontaneous voiding and continence. However, 3 years later, JV presented again with severe urge incontinence. Urodynamic studies of the neobladder showed urge incontinence due to severe urethral instability and minor 'bladder' instability (Fig. 5.6). The pattern of urethral instability, characterised by major fluctuations in urethral pressure, was the same as before: the most significant decreases in urethral pressure resulted, in combination with minor increases in 'bladder' pressure (perhaps as a result of contractions of the original trigone), in incontinence.

Because of the marked urethral instability, a PNE test was discussed and performed. During the subchronic PNE phase (which lasted for 2 weeks), JV had no complaints at all of urge incontinence; this was documented in a voiding diary. A urodynamic investigation (Fig. 5.7), performed halfway through this subchronic PNE test, showed disappearance of the previous severe urethral and minor 'bladder' instability. According to the patient's diaries, the average bladder capacity increased from 286 to 348ml. After removal of the temporary wire electrode, the urge incontinence recurred; the patient was, therefore, selected for permanent SNS implantation.

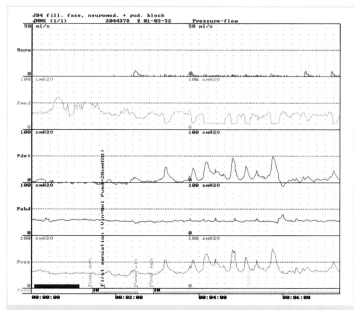

Figure 5.4 Patient JB during SNS after bilateral pudendal block with lignocaine. Recurrence of severe bladder and urethral instability due to the pudendal block, with severe incontinence during filling. (This is in sharp contrast to Figure 5.2.)

Q_{ura} = urinary flow (ml/s); scale 0–50ml/s

P_{med} = urethral pressure (cmH$_2$O; scale 0–100cmH$_2$O)

P_{det} = detrusor pressure (cmH$_2$O; scale 0–100cmH$_2$O)

P_{abd} = abdominal pressure (cmH$_2$O; scale 0–100cmH$_2$O)

P_{ves} = vesical pressure (cmH$_2$O; scale 0–100cmH$_2$O)

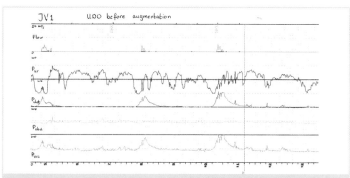

Figure 5.5 Patient JV with severe, refractory urgency–frequency and urge incontinence. Urodynamic investigation before bladder substitution operation: severe bladder and urethral instability with concomitant incontinence. This investigation illustrates clearly the initial decrease in urethral pressure, followed by the rise in bladder pressure.

Q_{ura} = urinary flow (ml/s); scale 0–50ml/s

P_{med} = urethral pressure (cmH$_2$O; scale 0–100cmH$_2$O)

P_{det} = detrusor pressure (cmH$_2$O; scale 0–100cmH$_2$O)

P_{abd} = abdominal pressure (cmH$_2$O; scale 0–100cmH$_2$O)

P_{ves} = vesical pressure (cmH$_2$O; scale 0–100cmH$_2$O)

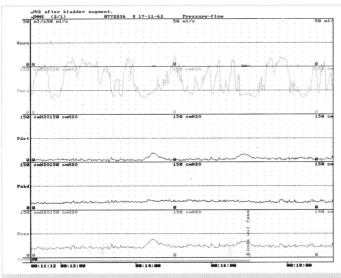

Figure 5.6 *Patient JV 3 years after bladder substitution. After a good clinical result initially, there is a recurrence of severe urge incontinence. Urodynamic study of the neobladder with urge incontinence due to severe urethral and minor 'bladder' instability. The pattern of the urethral instability, characterised by major urethral pressure fluctuations, is as before. The most significant falls in urethral pressure result (in combination with concomitant minor increases in 'bladder' pressure — perhaps as result of contractions of the original trigone) in incontinence.*

Q_{ura} = *urinary flow (ml/s); scale 0–50ml/s*
P_{med} = *urethral pressure (cmH$_2$O; scale 0–100cmH$_2$O)*
P_{det} = *detrusor pressure (cmH$_2$O; scale 0–100cmH$_2$O)*
P_{abd} = *abdominal pressure (cmH$_2$O; scale 0–100cmH$_2$O)*
P_{ves} = *vesical pressure (cmH$_2$O; scale 0–100cmH$_2$O)*

Discussion

SNS has proved to be effective for symptoms such as urinary urgency, frequency, incontinence, pelvic pain and voiding difficulty refractory to conservative treatment. The technique was first introduced in 1981 by Tanagho and Schmidt after animal studies and an extensive laboratory programme. The mode of action is discussed in several publications [4, 7].

Anatomically, the nerve fibres originating from S2 to S4 are autonomic fibres (comprising the pelvic plexus which innervates the bladder and the smooth muscle wall of the urethra) and somatic nerve fibres (forming the pudendal nerve). The pudendal nerve divides into the dorsal nerve of the penis or clitoris, the rectal branches, the transversus perinei branch and the scrotal or labial branches; it consists of both motor and sensory fibres [8].

According to Hohenfellner *et al.* [4] neuromodulation primarily affects the somatic A_α and A_γ fibres of the pudendal nerve. Depolarisation of these thicker myelinated A_α and A_γ somatomotor

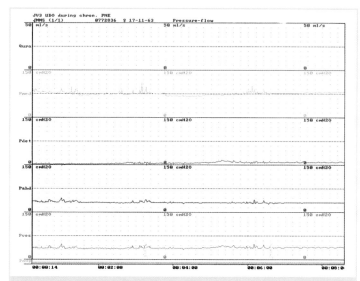

Figure 5.7 *Patient JV during subchronic PNE. Urodynamic studies, performed halfway through the subchronic PNE test (which lasted for 2 weeks), showing complete disappearance of the previous severe urethral and minor 'bladder' instability. As documented by a diary, the patient was continent during the subchronic PNE test.*

Q_{ura} = urinary flow (ml/s); scale 0–50ml/s
P_{med} = urethral pressure (cmH$_2$O; scale 0–100cmH$_2$O)
P_{det} = detrusor pressure (cmH$_2$O; scale 0–100cmH$_2$O)
P_{abd} = abdominal pressure (cmH$_2$O; scale 0–100cmH$_2$O)
P_{ves} = vesical pressure (cmH$_2$O; scale 0–100cmH$_2$O)

pudendal nerve fibres affects the external sphincter and pelvic floor and may inhibit detrusor activity. This stimulation does not result in depolarisation of the thin, unmyelinated B and C parasympathetic bladder fibres because of their higher threshold. This is probably due to the greater membrane capacitance of these small, unmyelinated fibres in comparison with the thicker, myelinated A$_\alpha$ fibres and skeletal muscle fibres [9]. According to Hohenfellner, the stimulator has to be switched off to initiate micturition; this is not, however, consistent with current daily practice in SNS, where usually a full 24 hours' stimulation is applied [4].

Thon *et al.* [3] discussed the concept of neural modulation by stimulation of A$_\delta$ myelinated fibres, typically sacral roots S3 and S4, resulting in a decreased spasticity of the pelvic floor and enhanced urethral sphincter tone. In the opinion of these authors, voiding dysfunction is often initiated by unstable urethral activity which activates voiding reflexes, leading to detrusor instability and associated symptoms. They conclude that detrusor instability is suppressed by the inhibitory effect of the enhanced urethral sphincter tone, stabilising detrusor activity.

Elabbady *et al.* [5] state that the most important benefit of neural modulation is rediscovery by the patient of pelvic floor muscles, because failure to feel the pelvic floor prevents the initiation of voiding. Neuromodulation suppresses spastic neuronal activity and modulates the behaviour of the pelvic muscles; this must result in recovery of voluntary control of pelvic floor muscles and, subsequently, in better control of voiding. In our opinion, however, this hypothesis cannot explain the fairly abrupt effect of SNS on urethral and bladder instability that we often see in urodynamic investigations in operated patients when the stimulator is switched off and on. More recently, Shaker *et al.* have concluded that sacral root stimulation exerts its effect by inhibiting the activity of the reflex arc conveyed by the C-afferent fibres [10]. This finding suggests that blockade of C-fibre activity is one of the mechanisms of action of sacral root neuromodulation.

According to Thon, Hohenfellner and Elabbady [3–5], the primary or most relevant effect of neuromodulation is motor, on urethral and pelvic floor function. According to Bosch and Groen [6,11], however, the clinical effect of neuromodulation is not related to an effect on urethral and pelvic floor function but, rather, to a stimulating effect on afferent anorectal branches of the pelvic nerve, to afferent sensory fibres in the pudendal nerve and to muscle afferents from the limbs, resulting in an inhibitory effect on detrusor contractility via the spinal inhibitory system. According to those authors, this concept is supported by the observation that the urethral pressure profile parameters such as maximum urethral closure pressure (MUCP) and functional urethral length (FUL) did not show a significant increase with stimulation switched on [9]. In general, the importance of a centrally regulated effect is supported by a recent study by Fowler *et al.* indicating that the motor pelvic floor contraction, observed during PNE is mediated by afferent input and is not the result of direct efferent stimulation [12]. This centrally-mediated effect is supported by the clinical observation that pelvic floor contraction in SNS is bilateral, with unilateral stimulation.

If it is true that the primary mode of action of SNS is through afferents, it is still a matter of debate whether the resulting efferent effect is focused mainly on bladder activity or on urethral and pelvic floor activity. We believe that the impact of urethral/pelvic floor function is important, as we discuss further in this chapter.

The main indications for SNS treatment are urge incontinence and urgency–frequency, which occur during the filling phase of the bladder. In these conditions, bladder instability can often be documented during urodynamic studies. However, urethral function can be assessed urodynamically only when, during filling, urethral pressure is measured throughout the study. In most published SNS studies this has not been the case. Only those investigators who have included integral urethral pressure measurement in the urodynamic set-up can study the distinct relation between (unstable) urethral and bladder contractions [13], as well as the distinct effect of neuromodulation treatment on both forms of instability. We have studied extensively the importance of urethral instability and its susceptibility to SNS; our results will be published separately (P.Groenendijk, A.A.B. Lycklama à Nijeholt). By taking the timescale during urodynamic studies into account, it can be

Key Points
- Blockade of C-afferent fibre activity may be a mechanism of action of SNS.
- Motor pelvic floor contraction may be mediated by afferent, not efferent, input.
- Integral urethral pressure measurement relates unstable urethral/bladder contractions.
- It also reveals the effect of SNS on both forms of instability.

blocks C-fibres. result SNS.

recorded that, both during normal voiding and in the presence of concomitant urethral and bladder instability, the fall in urethral pressure frequently precedes bladder contraction. This fall in urethral pressure can be experienced by the patient as an 'urge to void'. When this pressure drop is followed by a bladder contraction, as is often the case, voiding starts or an unstable bladder contraction is noted.

In the urodynamic literature, it is often argued that urethral instability is a problem in that it cannot easily be expressed in hard numbers in relation to fluctuations in urethral pressure. However, this should not deter us from referring to urethral instability when a distinct pattern of urethral pressure fluctuations can be seen during the filling phase. The relationship with some clinical conditions underlines the relevance of the phenomenon of urethral instability: for instance, we note quite often that, at filling, urethral instability starts at the first sensation of voiding. Frequently, we note urethral instability in a patient with sensory urge, in the absence of bladder instability.

Figures 5.1–5.3 illustrate the effect of SNS not only on bladder instability but also on urethral instability. As illustrated in Figure 5.4, a bilateral pudendal nerve block with lignocaine instantly undermines the stabilising effect of neuromodulation: both urethral and bladder instability recur, resulting in urge incontinence. Whether this effect is due to blockage of the motor pudendal effect on urethral and pelvic floor function or is due to blockage of the pudendal afferents towards the sacral nerves, is unclear. This observation, however, underlines the importance of the pudendal nerve in SNS treatment.

The urodynamic studies performed in patient JV clearly illustrates the presence of concomitant urethral and bladder instability in combination with urge incontinence (Fig. 5.5) In this patient, because of recurrent urge incontinence after the bladder substitution operation, the urodynamic investigation also illustrates the distinct fluctuations in urethral pressure and the concomitant minor unstable 'bladder' contractions following a significant drop in urethral pressure (Fig. 5.6). The most obvious event during the urodynamic investigation, performed in the subchronic PNE phase (Fig. 5.7), is the complete disappearance of urethral instability. This, and the stabilised 'bladder' function, result clinically in abolition of urge incontinence. With only the trigone left in this patient, this emphasises the possible role of this small portion of the bladder and the role of urethral/pelvic floor function in (in)continence and its susceptibility to SNS.

The above foregoing clinical and urodynamical data stress the importance of urethral and pelvic floor function in bladder function. They support the hypothesis regarding the impact of SNS via depolarisation of myelinated somatic (pudendal) nerve fibres resulting in stabilised urethral function and, subsequently, in stabilisation of bladder function.

The data presented are not in accordance with the hypothesis published by Bosch and Groen [6]. The urodynamic investigations that they performed in patients with SNS lack a permanent urethral pressure measurement in the filling phase. Instead of taking a stabilising effect of neuromodulation on urethral function into account, they anticipate enhanced urethral pressure if neuromodulation acts directly on urethral/pelvic floor function. In their opinion, the finding of only an insignificant increase in urethral pressure profile parameters (MUCP and FUL) indicates the absence of a beneficial effect of neuromodulation on urethral and pelvic floor muscles. Instead, the finding of greater bladder contractility 6 months postoperatively supports (in their opinion) the hypothesis that the mode of action of neuromodulation is via stimulation of afferent nerve fibres, resulting in a directly inhibitory effect on detrusor contractility via a spinal inhibitory system. They consider that animal experiments support this hypothesis because (at least in the cat) afferents from the pelvic floor muscles have no inhibitory effect on the bladder.

The relationship between the clinical outcome of SNS and the initial presence of bladder instability is unclear. A poor correlation between clinical improvement and disappearance of uninhibited bladder contractions has been reported [6]. This unsatisfactory correlation upholds the idea that other factors, such as urethral relaxation, play a part in the occurrence of urge incontinence [14].

It is becoming increasingly clear that neuromodulation, for the most successfully treated conditions — such as urge incontinence and urinary retention — probably relies on a combination of mechanisms that affect function at many levels in the neuroaxis [1].

> **Key Points**
> - Correlation between clinical improvement after SNS and abolition of uninhibited bladder contractions is poor.
> - Other factors are probably involved in successful neuromodulation.
> - SNS may have a primary effect on urethral and pelvic floor function.
> - It may also have a secondary effect on bladder function.

Conclusions

An increasing body of clinical data support the importance of SNS in refractory urge incontinence, urge–frequency complaints, and chronic voiding difficulties. In the main, in a number of publications, two concepts have been put forward to explain the physiological mode of action of SNS: a primary motor effect on urethral activity and pelvic floor muscles with a secondary effect on bladder function is postulated, as well as a primary motor effect, via the afferent sacral nerve fibres, on the bladder itself. In this respect, taking those urodynamic data that includes permanent urethral pressure measurements into account in several clinical conditions, an important (or even primary) effect of neuromodulation on urethral and pelvic floor function is endorsed.

The mode of action of SNS, based on our clinical and urodynamic observations, appears to be a primary afferent effect via pelvic and pudendal nerve fibres, resulting in a motor effect through the spinal system, mainly on urethral and pelvic floor function and perhaps (to a lesser degree), on bladder function. The main effect on urethral and pelvic floor function may subsequently, because of an inhibitory effect, affect bladder function.

In the near future, more studies on the (now well-illustrated) interaction between urethral and bladder instability and its susceptibility to SNS, may further enrich our knowledge regarding treatment by sacral neuromodulation.

References

1. Bemelmans BLH, Mundy AR, Craggs MD. Neuromodulation by implant for treating lower urinary tract symptoms and dysfunction. *Eur Urol* 1999; 36: 81–91.
2. Schmidt RA. Advances in genitourinary neurostimulation. *Neurosurgery* 1986; 19: 1041–4.
3. Thon WF, Baskin LS, Jonas U et al. Neuromodulation of voiding dysfunction and pelvic pain. *World J Urol* 1991; 9: 138–41.
4. Hohenfellner M, Thüroff JW, Schultz-Lampel D et al. Sakrale Neuromodulation zur therapie von Miktionsstörungen. *Aktuel Urol* 1992; 23: I–X.
5. Elabbady AA, Hassouna MM, Elhilali MM. Neural stimulation for chronic voiding dysfunctions. *J Urol* 1994; 152: 2076–80.
6. Bosch JHLR, Groen J. Sacral (S3) segmental nerve stimulation as a treatment for urge incontinence in patients with detrusor instability: results of chronic electrical stimulation using an implantable neural prothesis. *J Urol* 1995; 154: 504–7.
7. Tanagho EA, Schmidt RA. Electrical stimulation in the clinical management of the neurogenic bladder. *J Urol* 1988; 140: 1331–9.
8. McFarlane JP, Foley SJ, de Winter P et al. Acute suppression of idiopathic detrusor instability with magnetic stimulation of the sacral nerve roots. *Br J Urol* 1997; 80: 734–41.
9. Bosch JLHR, Groen J. Effects of sacral nerve stimulation on urethral resistance and bladder contractility: how does neuromodulation work in urge incontinence patients? [abstract 62]. *Neurourol Urodyn* 1995; 14: 502–4.
10. Shaker HS, Wang Y, Loung D et al. Role of C-afferent fibres in the mechanism of action of sacral nerve root neuromodulation in chronic spinal cord injury. *Br J Urol* 2000; 85: 905–10.
11. Bosch JLHR. Sacral neuromodulation in the treatment of the unstable bladder. *Curr Opin Urol* 1998; 8: 287–91.
12. Fowler CJ, Swinn MJ, Goodwin RJ et al. Studies of the latency of the pelvic floor contraction during peripheral nerve evaluation show that the muscle response is reflexly mediated. *J Urol* 2000; 163: 881–3.
13. Park JM, Bloom DA, McGuire EJ. The guarding reflex revisited. *Br J Urol* 1997; 80: 940–5.
14. Shaker HS, Hassouna MM. Sacral nerve root neuromodulation: an effective treatment for refractory urge incontinence. *J Urol* 1998; 159: 1516–19.

6 Neuromodulation and growth factors in the lower urinary tract

M.M. Hassouna

Introduction

Until the early 1980s, little information was available about the transmitter content of bladder sensory nerves and about their pharmacological modulation, although sensory nerves of the bladder and urethra have been extensively studied with neurophysiological techniques [1]. Over the past 20 years, much information has been amassed regarding the distribution, function and transmitter content of sensory nerves in the mammalian lower urinary tract. Anatomical and immunohistochemical techniques have provided evidence that neuropeptides, including substance P (SP), and calcitonin gene-related peptides (CGRP), are synthesised and stored in primary sensory neurons. It appears that these neuropeptides have a transmitter role in signalling events generated in the periphery to second-order sensory neurons engaged in micturition pathways in the spinal cord [2–4].

Afferent innervation of the bladder is carried out by two sets of nerve fibres — the A_α myelinated and the C unmyelinated fibres [5–7]. The A_α fibres are fast conducting (30m/s) and provide afferent input to the normal micturition reflex, whereas the C fibres are slow conducting (0.3m/s). These C fibres are involved in the pathogenesis of detrusor hyperreflexia, bladder instability, and chemical cystitis [8, 9]. Neuropeptides, including SP and CGRP, are synthesised in the neurons of dorsal root ganglia, and stored and released through C fibres [10–12]. These neuropeptides mediate epithelial permeability, smooth muscle relaxation, and neurotransmitter release from adjacent nerves [4]. Desensitisation of the C fibres by capsaicin can abolish the bladder hyperreflexia in both animals and humans [13–15].

The proto-oncogene c-*fos* encodes the synthesis of fos-protein in the central nervous system. This gene is devoid of basal expression in the spinal cord under physiological conditions, and is activated only when the sensory cells are exposed to transmembrane stimulation conveyed mainly by afferent C fibres [16]. The study of the expression of the c-*fos* gene is an excellent tool for evaluation of the spinal processing of afferent C-fibre input.

Nerve growth factor (NGF) is a trophic protein that acts as a retrograde messenger between peripheral effector tissue and innervating neurons. NGF in peripheral neurons is synthesised in the innervating target tissues including smooth muscle cells, fibroblasts and astrocytes [17–19]. Following *de novo* synthesis, NGF is not stored in the musculature but is rapidly secreted. Sympathetic and

Key Points

- Neuropeptides (NPs) e.g. substance P and calcitonin gene-related peptides (SP, CGRP) are synthesised/stored in primary sensory neurons.
- They signal peripheral events to sensory spinal neurons in micturition pathways.
- Bladder afferent nerve-fibre types are A (myelinated) and C (unmyelinated).
- Fast (A) fibres give afferent input to the normal micturition reflex.
- Detrusor hyperreflexia, bladder instability, chemical cystitis, involve slow (C) fibres.
- C fibres store/release NPs.
- NPs mediate epithelial permeability, smooth muscle relaxation, neurotransmitter release.
- Capsaicin desensitises C fibres and abolishes bladder hyperreflexia.
- C-fibre input is evaluated by study of c-fos expression.

(some) sensory neurons require NGF for survival, growth and to regulate neurotransmitter synthesis during development and in adulthood [20]. The distribution of neuropeptides SP and CGRP, as well as c-*fos* gene expression and NGF under physiological and pathological conditions, are reviewed.

Normal distribution of SP and CGRP

Nerve fibres immunoreactive to SP and CGRP can be detected in rats at the age of 2 weeks [21, 22]. There is then a sharp increase in both the total amount and concentration of SP and CGRP until the rats reach the age of 3–4 weeks. Following a peak at 3–8 weeks, the concentration of SP decreases with age, whereas that of CGRP remains unchanged [22]. In the rat or guinea-pig urinary bladder, a plexus of SP- and CGRP-positive fibres is present in the submucosal layer, more evident in the bladder neck than in the bladder dome. From this plexus some fibres enter the epithelium and terminate at this level [23, 24]. In the bladder there is a rich plexus of nerve fibres displaying CGRP in association with blood vessels and muscle layers. The nerve supply of the trigone is greater than that of other areas of the bladder [24, 25]. CGRP-positive fibres also enter the urethral epithelium [24]. As in the bladder, SP and CGRP are present mainly in nerve fibres, but are rarely found in ganglion cells in the bladder neck and urethra in a variety of species. The fibres within the smooth muscle layers and in the subepithelium represent sensory afferents because systemic capsaicin pretreatment depletes bladder SP [26–28]. In the guinea-pig, 2% of nerve cells in ganglia situated within the smooth muscle layer and near the mucosa at the base of the bladder are positive for SP [27]. In rats, the distribution of CGRP fibres is similar to that of SP, although the former are more numerous [24, 25]. In addition, SP and CGRP are present in dorsal root ganglion cells supplying the bladder and urethra; SP is almost invariably colocalised with CGRP, whereas some populations of sensory nerve cells contain CGRP without SP [28].

In humans, the overall innervation of a fetus can be visualised using protein gene product (PGP) 9.5, a general nerve marker. At 17 weeks gestation a rich plexus of PGP is present throughout the detrusor muscle coat. As gestational age increases, SP- and CGRP-containing nerves are observed with increasing frequency, although SP and CGRP are mainly confined to perivascular nerve plexuses. With increasing fetal age, small clusters of intramural neurons are observed in the urinary bladder. A delicate plexus of branching varicose nerves is observed in the fetal paraganglia; these nerves increase in density with increasing gestational age and some are SP- and CGRP-immunoreactive. Late fetal and early postnatal paraganglia contain Timofeew's sensory corpuscles, the central nerve fibres of which display immunoreactivity for SP and CGRP [29]. Nerves containing SP and CGRP are typically present within the subepithelial region, encircling intramural ganglia and around blood vessels; these are sparsely distributed, and only rarely projected to the smooth muscle bundles of the detrusor in humans. Approximately 26% of CGRP-immunoreactive nerves contain SP; conversely, all SP-immunoreactive fibres contain CGRP [30]. Varicose nerve fibres are in close proximity to some of the intramural neurons, the majority of such varicosities showing immunoreactivity to CGRP. Less common are pericellular varicosities immunoreactive to SP. No correlation is found between the peptide contents of the ganglion cells and that of the associated pericellular terminals. Neurochemical heterogeneity of intramural neurons is present in the human bladder neck, providing evidence for the complexity of the peripheral innervation of the bladder [31, 32].

In the human prostate, the greatest density of nerves is found in the proximal central prostate, followed by the anterior capsule and distal central prostate, with the least density in the peripheral prostate [33, 34]. In the ureterovesical junction, SP- and CGRP-containing nerves are rarely observed in association with the intramural ureter and none are detected in the human ureteric submucosa. Nerves containing SP and CGRP are not observed within the intermediate layer. Similarly, SP- and CGRP-positive nerve fibres are rarely encountered in detrusor muscle [35].

The SP and CGRP receptors can be visualised using emulsion autoradiography in the human bladder. The SP receptors are found over the endothelium of arterial blood vessels within the detrusor muscle, lamina propria and small vessels in the subepithelium, whereas CGRP receptors are expressed densely over the smooth muscle layer of arteries and arterioles, and weakly over collecting venules; they are not present over the detrusor muscle. Although the afferent nerves contain SP and CGRP, not all cell types express receptors for these peptides. The general distribution of receptors is in good agreement with the location of nerves, and with the known actions of SP and CGRP as vasodilator agents [36].

In studies *in vitro*, capsaicin produces a transient large contraction of guinea-pig muscle strips excised from the bladder dome but only a weak contraction followed by relaxation of strips from the bladder neck. Both effects undergo full desensitisation, indicating a specific and indirect origin, via activation of transmitter release from sensory nerves [37]. On application of capsaicin, SP and CGRP are simultaneously released from the guinea-pig bladder. SP is a more potent contractile agent in the bladder dome than in the bladder neck, whereas CGRP is a more potent relaxant agent in the neck than in the dome. In addition, the coupling between CGRP receptors and cyclic adenosine monophosphate generation occurs more efficiently in the neck than in the dome. Therefore, the full expression of the contractile activity of SP in the neck of guinea-pig bladder is prevented by the concomitant powerful relaxant activity of CGRP [38].

SP and CGRP are simultaneously released from sensory nerves in the bladder and their overall effect on a given target depends upon several variables: these are the relative amounts of peptides stored and released from sensory nerves, the type of receptors present on target cells, the efficacy of the coupling between receptors and second-messenger systems and the difference in the inactivation rate of released peptides [37]. Density of innervation is important in regulating the biological response produced by

Key Points

- Distribution of SP/CGRP receptors reflects nerve location.
- It also accords with the vasodilatory role of SP/CGRP.
- SP contracts guinea-pig bladder muscle; CGRP relaxes it.
- SP is more potent in guinea-pig bladder dome than neck muscle.
- CGRP is more potent in guinea-pig bladder neck than dome muscle.

endogenous peptides in the bladder. There is a direct correlation between the bladder tissue content of SP and the amplitude of contraction produced by application of capsaicin [39]. The local effects of peptides released from the peripheral endings of afferent C fibres are collectively known as neurogenic inflammation [40, 41].

SP is a potent and direct stimulant of bladder motility in various species including humans [4]. In rat and guinea-pig, plasma protein extravasation induced by SP is more intense in the urethra than in the bladder; at bladder level, it is more intense in the neck than in the dome [42]. Plasma protein extravasation produced by exogenous SP in the rat bladder is unaffected by chronic extrinsic denervation (removal of pelvic ganglia) which, by contrast, abolished plasma protein extravasation produced by the administration of capsaicin [42]. Although CGRP exerts a relaxant effect on the detrusor muscle of some species (guinea-pig, dog), it does not in others (rat, human) [4]. In the urethra of rat, CGRP exerts a relaxant effect and is responsible for the relaxation following application of capsaicin [43]. It is a potent vasodilator that increases blood flow and decreases vascular resistance in the urinary bladder [44]; in humans it relaxes the bladder neck and prostate, but not the bladder body. Thus, lower urinary tract tissues are responsive to certain bioactive peptides in an inhomogeneous fashion. These studies indicate that selective modulation of peptide function may be an approach to therapy of urogenital disorders [45].

Distribution of SP and CGRP in pathological conditions

The SP and CGRP content of the rat or guinea-pig urinary bladder can be completely depleted by capsaicin pretreatment, as well as by chronic extrinsic denervation [39, 46]. The SP and CGRP nerve fibres present in the subepithelium of the bladder represent the terminal endings of the bladder sensory afferents. The presence of afferent C fibres within bladder and urethral subepithelium is of particular interest because many chemicals that are normally present in the urine, or that are produced during cystitis, stimulate these sensory nerves. The location of sensory nerve terminals in the bladder and urethral epithelium, and the peculiar chemosensitivity of C fibres make them candidates to detect any eventual backflow of urine [38].

In rats with cystitis, micturition reflexes become hyperexcitable. Instillation of mustard oil into the bladder causes a massive leucocyte infiltration of the bladder tissues, partial damage of the mucosal layer, and marked hyperreflexia of the detrusor muscle. Primary sensory neurons in the dorsal root ganglia L1–L2 and L6–S1, and postganglionic efferent neurons in the major pelvic ganglia that innervate the rat urinary bladder, are labelled with retrogradely transported Fast Blue. Two days after induction of the cystitis, the proportion of Fast Blue-labelled bladder afferent neurons that express SP and CGRP are significantly increased in both the rostral lumbar dorsal root ganglia (L1, L2) and the lumbosacral dorsal root ganglia (L6, S1). These results indicate that upregulation of SP and CGRP synthesis in sensory and efferent neurons is involved in the response to acute cystitis [47]. Whereas SP stimulates the release of histamine, prostaglandin E2, prostaglandin F2α and leukotriene B4 in guinea-pig urinary bladder, CGRP suppresses their release. SP induces an immediate and transient release of histamine and activation of cyclooxygenase and delayed activation of 5-lipoxygenase; these actions may directly regulate the participation of these peptides in the pathogenesis of cystitis [48]. The regulation of the sympathetic efferent outflow to the urinary bladder differs from that of the parasympathetic efferent outflow because of the differences in the segmental pattern and degree of upregulation of these substances in bladder afferents that project to the rostral lumbar and lumbosacral spinal cord [47].

In rats with spinal cord injury, bladder hyperreflexia develops, correlated with an increase in SP and CGRP levels in the bladder and L6 dorsal root ganglia. Capsaicin treatment or neuromodulation of the sacral nerve roots can abolish bladder hyperreflexia, which corresponds to a decrease in SP and CGRP content in the dorsal root ganglia [49, 50]. However, no change is found in the detrusor contractility and neurokinin receptor pharmacology as shown by responses to KCl, electric field stimulation and neurokinin receptor-selective agonists in a study *in vitro* [49].

The density of SP- and CGRP-immunoreactive nerves within the subepithelium of women with urodynamically-proven idiopathic detrusor instability is increased by 82% and 94%, respectively. This effect is not due to an increase in overall nerve density, because immunoreactivity for PGP (a general nerve marker) does not differ significantly between these patients and controls. Patients with detrusor instability demonstrate an increase in SP- and CGRP-containing nerve fibres [30].

In the rat urinary bladder following X-ray irradiation, there is a significant increase in the density of SP- but not of CGRP-immunoreactive nerves. There are regional differences within the bladder, that is, there is an increase in SP-immunoreactive nerves around and within the urothelium. The increase in the density of SP-immunoreactive nerves in the irradiated bladders may be due to axonal sprouting which contributes to the symptoms of radiation injury [51].

In rats pretreated with capsaicin or vehicle, no difference in binding site for SP in smooth muscle and submucosal blood vessels is apparent between the two treated groups. Specific CGRP-binding sites are located over the epithelium and weakly over submucosal arterioles. The density of CGRP-binding sites on the epithelium, but not blood vessels, is increased by 22% after chronic capsaicin pretreatment, indicating receptor upregulation. Although SP and CGRP are colocalised in primary afferent sensory fibres in rat urinary bladder, the receptors for these neuropeptides are located on different cell types and may be subject to different neural influences [52].

In diabetic rats, SP produces hypotension and increased plasma extravasation in the urinary bladder, respiratory tissues and skin, whereas CGRP has no effect on blood pressure or vascular

> **Key Points**
> - SP/CGRP levels change in pathological states.
> - SP/CGRP-containing nerve-fibre density increases in patients with detrusor instability.

permeability in these rats. The simultaneous administration of CGRP and SP results in modest potentiation of the vascular permeability actions of SP in both normal and diabetic rats. Defective neurogenic inflammatory responses in diabetic rats may result from decreased responses in their effector tissues to the neuropeptides released from sensory nerves [53].

In the human bladder with outlet obstruction, the density of innervation of the bladder detrusor by nerves containing SP and CGRP is assessed in bladder tissue taken from the lateral wall below the peritoneal reflection. A reduction in the density of innervation by SP- and CGRP-immunoreactive nerve fibres is found in the bladder with outlet obstruction. These findings, combined with the significant reduction in SP content of the obstructed bladder and, in particular, of the bladder with acute urinary retention, indicate that there is an afferent nerve dysfunction resulting from bladder outflow obstruction [54]. In the prostate gland of patients with benign prostatic hyperplasia, there is a reduction in the density of SP-containing nerves and an increase in CGRP-containing nerves in patients with urinary retention [34].

Normal expression of c-*fos*

As previously mentioned, c-*fos* is a proto-oncogene that encodes the synthesis of fos-protein in the central nervous system. Fos-protein-positive neurons were detected in fewer than two cells per section in the spinal cord of a normal rat [17]. The level of c-*fos* gene expression can be quantified by counting the number of fos-protein-positive neurons in spinal cord sections. After nociceptive and non-nociceptive stimulation of the urinary bladder, c-*fos* gene expression is increased as detected by immunocytochemical methods; this increase occurs within 30–60 minutes [55, 56]. The c-*fos* gene is devoid of basal expression in the spinal cord under physiological conditions, and is activated only when the sensory cells are exposed to transmembrane stimulation conveyed mainly by afferent C fibres. Its expression is mediated by the spinal pathway, because spinal cord transection does not alter the c-*fos* gene expression induced by chemical irritation [17]. A c-*fos* gene expression study is an excellent tool by which to evaluate the spinal processing of afferent C-fibre input.

Expression of c-*fos* in pathological conditions

In rats, fos-protein-positive neurons can be detected following chemical irritation or overdistension of the bladder in the L6 and S1 spinal segments, but mainly in the former [17]. The maximum expression of the c-*fos* gene is 2 hours after such irritation of the bladder; c-*fos* expression reverts to the baseline level 24 hours after chemical irritation. No fos-protein-positive neurons are found in the spinal cord of rats with chronic cystitis [55, 57]. Fos-protein-positive cells are mainly located in four areas in the spinal cord — namely, medial dorsal horn, lateral dorsal horn, dorsal commissure and lateral laminae V–VII near the sacral parasympathetic nucleus [58].

Many factors, including the vehicle [59], anaesthesia [60], catheterisation and bladder distension [17], can affect c-*fos* expression. Acute electrical stimulation of the pelvic nerve for 1.5 hours can induce c-*fos* expression in L6–S1 spinal cord segments and the number of fos-protein-positive cells increases with increased intensity of stimulation [61]; however, chronic neuromodulation of the sacral nerve roots can inhibit c-*fos* expression [62], possibly because of desensitisation. The effect of sacral nerve root neuromodulation is very similar to that of capsaicin, a neurotoxin specific to C fibres. Intravesical capsaicin instillation initially increases c-*fos* expression but, after 24 hours, the c-*fos* immunoreaction in the spinal cord disappears [17]. Furthermore, capsaicin pretreatment can inhibit a nociceptive stimulus to the bladder, as demonstrated by the marked reduction (83.6%) of c-*fos* response to chemical irritation [17]. Electroacupuncture at the Sanyinjiao acupoints on the hind legs of rats also inhibits c-*fos* expression in rat spinal cord after chemical irritation of the rat bladder. The effect of electroacupuncture at acupoints is through nociceptive modulation after circulating enkephalin combines with its receptors in the spinal micturition centre [63].

Placement of a urethral catheter alone elicits c-*fos* expression in a similar number of neurons (mainly in the medial dorsal horn and dorsal commissure in the segments L1–2 and L5–S1) in rats with spinal cord injury and control rats. Distension-induced bladder contractions markedly increase c-*fos* expression, primarily in the spinal segments L5–S1 in the control rats, where the majority of bladder and urethral afferent fibres terminate. Compared with controls, c-*fos* expression after spinal cord injury occurs in a significantly greater number of neurons throughout the segments L3–S1 following induction of bladder distension. The greatest proportional increase in the number of fos-positive cells occurred in L3–5, which normally receive only little afferent input from the urinary bladder. Cell numbers predominantly increase in the lateral dorsal horn and lateral lamina V–VII. This indicates a neuroplastic reorganisation of spinal pathways after spinal cord injury. The unmasking of silent synapses or formation of new connections by afferent axonal sprouting caudal to the lesion, as evident from the increased numbers of cells expressing c-*fos* after bladder distension, could be factors underlying the emergence of reflexogenic micturition in rats with chronic spinal cord injury [64]. Pretreatment with capsaicin significantly reduces the number of fos-immunoreactive cells induced by bladder distension after spinal cord injury. Spinal cord injury reveals an altered c-*fos* expression pattern in response to an innocuous bladder stimulus [65].

Previous instillation of lignocaine (lidocaine) markedly reduces the number of fos-immunoreactive cells in the spinal cord responding to capsaicin-induced bladder afferent excitation. The number of fos-immunoreactive cells induced by acetic acid instillation in a bladder desensitised by capsaicin administered 24 hours previously is not changed by lignocaine application prior to capsaicin. The local anaesthetic pretreatment of the bladder with lignocaine reduces the

Key Points

- c-*fos* expression varies with pathological state, *inter alia*.
- Lignocaine pretreatment blocks capsaicin-induced excitation of rat bladder afferents.

capsaicin-induced noxious excitation of the sensory fibres without decreasing the subsequent desensitisation by capsaicin [66].

Although c-*fos* gene expression is inhibited in all four regions of the L6 spinal cord after chronic neuromodulation, a significant reduction in the number of fos-protein-positive neurons is found only in the dorsal commissure area [62]. Cruz *et al.* [67] have reported that the highest number of fos-protein-positive cells was found in the dorsal commissure and the intermediolateral grey matter in the L5–S1 spinal cord segment in rats. The reduction of fos-protein-positive cells was more pronounced in the dorsal commissure and intermediolateral grey matter (95%) in capsaicin-treated rats [67]. The dorsal commissure is more important than other regions in the control of the micturition reflex because more fos-protein-positive neurons are present in this area than in other regions [67]. In addition, Al-Chaer *et al.* [68, 69] have compared the role of the dorsal column and the spinothalamic tract in the processing of visceral nociceptive information transmitted to the ventral posterolateral nucleus of the thalamus: the dorsal column has a more important role than that of the spinothalamic tract in visceral nociception, and the pelvic visceral stimulus depends on activity in the dorsal column–medial lemniscus system. Furthermore, both anatomical and physiological studies of the grey matter in the spinal cord of rats show that neurons around the central canal, including the dorsal commissure, may contribute strongly to long ascending spinal cord projections. These neurons are reminiscent of the noxious-specific cells in the outermost layers of the dorsal horn [70].

Normal distribution of NGF

Nerve growth factor (NGF) is a trophic protein that acts as a retrograde messenger between peripheral effector tissue and innervating neurons. The source of NGF for peripheral neurons is the innervating target tissue. Smooth muscle cells [18], fibroblasts [19] and astrocytes [20] can all synthesise NGF, which is not stored in the musculature but is secreted rapidly following *de novo* synthesis. Sympathetic and (some) sensory neurons require NGF for survival and growth, and to regulate neurotransmitter synthesis during development and in adulthood [21].

NGF secretion by vascular smooth muscle and NGF expression in neurons is regulated by activity and neurotransmitter receptors. Excitatory agents, including platelet-derived growth factor (PDGF), prostaglandin (PG)$E_{2\alpha}$ and PGF_2 increase the expression or secretion of NGF. Inhibitory agents, including β-adrenergic agonists and CGRP, cause a decrease in NGF secretion [71]. Muscle activity *per se* may regulate NGF production. Increased bladder activity associated with experimentally-induced diuresis increases tissue NGF [72]. In the obstructed bladder, distension of the bladder wall may be the signal for smooth muscle cells to induce cell growth and synthesise NGF. Mechanical stretch of bladder smooth muscle cells *in vitro* results in enhanced accumulation of NGF in the culture medium [73]. In cell culture, the bladder body secretes less NGF than does the bladder base, and the base secretes less than the urethra. A similar gradient in growth rate occurs *in vitro*. The urethral cells being most active. However, no regional difference is found in bladder tissue NGF content, despite significant variations in norepinephrine levels [74]. Innervation of the bladder and lower urinary tract varies in different regions. In the rat, the bladder body is innervated by excitatory cholinergic and rare inhibitory adrenergic nerves, whereas, in the bladder base and urethra, adrenergic nerves are more prevalent [75, 76]. Tissue levels of NGF do not vary in these different regions, suggesting that NGF tissue levels are not correlated with specific phenotypes, functions or innervation patterns. Basal NGF secretion rates vary in a regional fashion, but inversely to growth, with the bladder body highest and urethra lowest in this respect.

> **Key Points**
> - NGF tissue levels do not correlate with phenotype/function or innervation pattern.
> - Basal rate of NGF secretion varies by region and inversely to growth.
> - NGF may be an endogenous mediator in persistent pain.
> - NGF may have a role in neurotrophic effects associated with bladder outlet obstruction.

Change of NGF in pathological conditions

In a study of chemical cystitis using a rat model, it was found that pretreatment with a systemic NGF antagonist can largely prevent reflex excitability of the bladder [77]. Furthermore, treatment with the NGF antagonist partially and significantly reversed established inflammatory changes in the bladder. The NGF antagonist has no significant effect on bladder reflex excitability in the uninflamed state [77].

NGF may be an endogenous mediator in some states of persistent pain. The stimulus-response function of afferent A_δ and C fibres is evaluated with a series of isotonic distensions of the bladder. After intravesical instillation of NGF, more afferent fibres are sensitised, as shown by the development of ongoing activity and a leftward shift of stimulus-response functions compared with the rat treated with vehicle solution only. Intravesical NGF instillation can also elicit a dose-dependent extravasation of Evans' Blue into the bladder [78]. Acute pharmacological effects of NGF include reduced activation threshold for small-diameter myelinated afferents [72].

Partial urethral ligation in rats produces changes in the neural control of the lower urinary tract, including bladder hyperactivity and facilitation of a spinal micturition reflex pathway. Urethral obstruction produces increased voiding frequency and hypertrophy of the urinary bladder with profound increments in the dimensions of afferent and efferent neurons supplying the bladder in the rat. A significant increase in the size of bladder postganglionic neurons in the major pelvic ganglia is found in rats with partial urethral ligation. Neuronal hypertrophy is not associated with a change in the number of major pelvic ganglia neurons in the ligated rats [79]. Hypertrophied bladder samples from rat and humans contain significantly more NGF per milligram wet weight, protein and DNA than do normal bladder samples. The temporal correlation between NGF content, neuronal hypertrophy, and bladder weight is consistent with a role for NGF in the neurotrophic effects associated with obstruction. Blockage of NGF by autoimmunisation abolished the hypertrophy of NGF-sensitive bladder neurons in the pelvic ganglia after obstruction. These findings indicate that parenchymal cells in the hypertrophied bladder can synthesise NGF and act to alter the size and function of neurons in animals and humans [73].

Alterations in the reflex pathway controlling micturition are observed after bladder outlet obstruction [80]. This neural and reflex plasticity is mediated by NGF, since obstructed rats immunised against NGF and with high titres of circulating anti-NGF activity do not show enlargement of dorsal root ganglia neurons, increased voiding, or an enhanced micturition reflex [73,81].

NGF levels in the urinary bladder have been measured following unilateral ganglionectomy (bladder denervation) or separation of the postganglionic bladder neurons from the central nervous system of the rat (bladder and ganglion decentralisation). These interruptions of the neural input to half of the bladder gave rise to histological evidence of smooth muscle growth, increased bladder weight, transient increases in tissue NGF up to ten-fold and hypertrophy of the neurons in the pelvic ganglia supplying the bladder. This indicates that neural input has a significant role in regulating growth of the bladder and that innervation influences tissue levels of NGF in the bladder [82].

Epidemiological studies have shown that hypertensive men are more likely to undergo surgical intervention for irritative voiding symptoms from benign prostatic hyperplasia than age-matched controls. The spontaneously hypertensive rat has been used to investigate the roles of the sympathetic pathway of micturition. Elevated NGF derived from vascular and bladder smooth muscle cells appears to direct morphological, biochemical and functional change. The spontaneously hypertensive rat has a lower bladder capacity and micturition volume, with increased urinary frequency together with the presence of unstable contractions. It is likely that upregulation of NGF production causes sensory (and possibly noradrenergic) pathways to elicit hyperactive voiding [83].

References

1. Morrison JFB. Sensations arising from the lower urinary tract. In: M Torrens, JFB Morrison (eds). *The Physiology of the Lower Urinary Tract*. Heidelberg: Springer Verlag, 1987, 89–132.
2. de Groat WC. Spinal cord projections and neuropeptides in visceral afferent neurons. *Prog Brain Res* 1986; 67: 165–87.
3. de Groat WC. Neuropeptides in pelvic afferent pathways. *Experimentia* 1987; 43: 801–13.
4. Maggi CA. The role of peptides in the regulation of micturition reflex, an update. *Gen Pharmacol* 1991; 22: 1–24.
5. Hulsebosch CE, Coggeshall RE. An analysis of the axon populations in the nerves to the pelvic viscera in the rat. *J Comp Neurol* 1982; 211: 1–10.
6. de Groat WC. Nervous control of the urinary bladder of the cat. *Brain Res* 1975; 87: 201–11.
7. Mallory B, Steers WD, de Groat WC. Electrophysiological study of micturition reflexes in rats. *Am J Physiol* 1989; 257: R410–21.
8. Steers WD, Ciambotti J, Etzel B et al. Alterations in afferent pathways from the urinary bladder of the rat in response to partial urethral obstruction. *J Comp Neurol* 1991; 310: 401–10.
9. Maggi CA, Lecci A, Santicioli P et al. Cyclophosphamide cystitis in rats: involvement of capsaicin-sensitive primary afferents. *J Auton Nerv Syst* 1992; 38: 201–8.
10. Tramontana M, Del Bianco E, Cecconi R et al. Veratridine evokes release of calcitonin gene-related peptide from capsaicin-sensitive nerves of rat urinary bladder. *Eur J Pharmacol* 1992; 212: 137–42.

11. Maggi CA, Santicioli P, Geppetti P *et al*. Simultaneous release of substance P and calcitonin gene-related peptide (CGRP)-like immunoreactivity from isolated muscle of the guinea pig urinary bladder. *Neurosci Lett* 1988; 87: 163–7.

12. Hua XY, Theoddorson-Norheim E, Brodin E *et al*. Multiple tachykinins (neurokinin A, neuropeptide K and substance P) in capsaicin-sensitive sensory neurons in the guinea-pig. *Regul Pept* 1985; 13: 1–19.

13. Fowler CJ, Beck R, Gerrard S *et al*. Intravesical capsaicin for treatment of detrusor hyperreflexia. *J Neurol Neurosurg Psychiatry* 1994; 57: 169–73.

14. Geirsson G, Fall G, Sullivan L. Clinical and urodynamic effects of intravesical capsaicin treatment in patients with chronic traumatic spinal detrusor hyperreflexia. *J Urol* 1995; 154: 1825–9.

15. De Ridder D, Chandiramani V, Dasgupta P *et al*. Intravesical capsaicin as a treatment for refractory detrusor hyperreflexia: a dual center study with long-term follow-up. *J Urol* 1997; 158: 2087–92.

16. Birder LA, de Groat WC. Increased *c-fos* expression in spinal neurons after irritation of the lower urinary tract in the rat. *J Neurosci* 1992; 12: 4878–89.

17. Creedon DJ, Tuttle JB. Nerve growth factor synthesis in vascular smooth muscle. *Hypertension* 1991; 18: 730–33.

18. Furukawa S, Furukawa Y, Satoyoshi E, Hayashi K. Nerve growth factor secreted by mouse heart cells in culture. *J Biol Chem* 1984; 259: 1259–64.

19. Furukawa S, Furukawa Y, Satoyoshi E, Hayashi K. Synthesis and secretion of nerve growth factor by mouse astroglial cells in culture. *Biophys Res Commun* 1986; 136: 57–63.

20. Gorin PD, Johnson EM, Jr. Effects of long term nerve growth factor deprivation on the nervous system of the adult rat. An experimental autoimmune approach. *Brain Res* 1980; 198: 27–30.

21. Sann H, Walb G, Pierau FK. Postnatal development of the autonomic and sensory innervation of the musculature in the rat urinary bladder. *Neurosci Lett* 1997; 236: 29–30.

22. Ekstrom J, Ekman R, Hakanson R. Ontogeny of neuropeptides in the rat urinary bladder. *Regul Pept* 1994; 50: 23–8.

23. Yokokawa K, Sakanaka M, Shiosaka S *et al*. Three dimensional distribution of substance P-like immunoreactivity in the urinary bladder. *J Neurol Transm* 1985; 63: 209–22.

24. Su HC, Wharton J, Polak JM *et al*. CGRP immunoreactivity in afferent neurons supplying the urinary tract, combined retrograde tracing and immunohistochemistry. *Neuroscience* 1986; 18: 727–47.

25. Yokokawa K, Tohyama M, Shiosaka S *et al*. Distribution of CGRP-containing fibers in the urinary bladder of the rat and their origin. *Cell Tissue Res* 1986; 244: 271–8.

26. Maggi CA, Giuliani S, Santicioli P *et al*. Species-related variations in the effects of capsaicin on urinary bladder functions, relation to bladder content of substance P-like immunoreactivity. *Naunyn Schmiedebergs Arch Pharmacol* 1987; 336: 546–55.

27. Crowe R, Haven AJ, Burnstock G. Intramural neurons of the guinea-pig urinary bladder, histochemical localization of neurotransmitters in cultures and newborn animals. *J Auton Nerv Syst* 1986; 15: 319–39.

28. Lincoln J, Burnstock G. Autonomic innervation of the urinary bladder and urethra. In: Maggi CA (ed). *Nervous Control of the Urogenital System*. Philidelphia: Harwood Academic Publishers 1993; 33–68.

29. Dixon JS, Jen PY, Gosling JA. Immunohistochemical characteristics of human paraganglion cells and sensory corpuscles associated with the urinary bladder. A developmental study in the male fetus, neonate and infant. *J Anat* 1998; 192(3): 407–15.

30. Smet PJ, Moore KH, Jonavicius J. Distribution and colocalization of calcitonin gene-related peptide, tachykinins, and vasoactive intestinal peptide in normal and idiopathic unstable human urinary bladder. *Lab Invest* 1997; 77: 37–39.

31. Jen PY, Dixon JS, Gosling JA. Co-localisation of tyrosine hydroxylase, nitric oxide synthase and neuropeptides in neurons of the human postnatal male pelvic ganglia. *J Auton Nerv Syst* 1996; 59: 41–50.

32. Dixon JS, Jen PY, Gosling JA. A double-label immunohistochemical study of intramural ganglia from the human male urinary bladder neck. *J Anat* 1997; 190: 125–34.

33. Crowe R, Chapple CR, Burnstock G: The human prostate gland: a histochemical and immunohistochemical study of neuropeptides, serotonin, dopamine beta-hydroxylase and acetylcholinesterase in autonomic nerves and ganglia. *Br J Urol* 1991; 68: 53–61.

34. Chapple CR, Crowe R, Gilpin SA *et al*. The innervation of the human prostate gland-the changes associated with benign enlargement. *J Urol* 1991; 146: 1637–44.

35. Dixon JS, Canning DA, Gearhart JP, Gosling JA. An immunohistochemical study of the innervation of the ureterovesical junction in infancy and childhood. *Br J Urol* 1994; 73: 292–7.

36. Burcher E, Zeng XP, Strigas J et al. Autoradiographic localization of tachykinin and calcitonin gene-related peptide receptors in adult urinary bladder. *J Urol* 2000; 163: 331–7.

37. Maggi CA, Santicioli P, Patacchini R et al. Regional differences in the motor response to capsaicin in the guinea-pig urinary bladder: relative role of pre- and post-junctional factors related to neuropeptide-containing sensory nerves. *Neuroscience* 1988; 27: 675–88.

38. Maggi CA. The dual, sensory and efferent function of the capsaicin-sensitive primary sensory neurons in the urinary bladder and urethra. In: Maggi CA (ed) *Nervous Control of the Urogenital System*. Philidelphia: Harwood Academic Publishers, 1993; 383–422.

39. Maggi CA, Meli A. The sensory-efferent function of capsaicin-sensitive sensory neurons. *Gen Pharmacol* 1988; 19: 1–43.

40. Burcher E, Buck SH. Multiple tachykinin binding sites in hamster, rat and guinea-pig urinary bladder. *Eur J Pharmacol* 1986; 128: 165–77.

41. Nimmo AJ, Morrison JFB, Whitaker EM. A comparison of the distribution of substance P and CGRP receptors in the rat bladder. *Q J Exp Physiol* 1988; 73: 789–92.

42. Maggi CA, Santicioli P, Abelli L et al. Regional differences in the effects of capsaicin and tachykinins on motor activity and vascular permeability of the rat lower urinary tract. *Naunyn Schmiedebergs Arch Pharmacol* 1987; 335: 636–45.

43. Maggi CA, Giuliani S, Santicioli P et al. Visceromotor responses to CGRP in the rat lower urinary tract, evidence for a transmitter role in the capsaicin-sensitive nerves of the ureter. *Eur J Pharmacol* 1987; 143: 73–82.

44. Andersson PB, Malmgren A, Uvelius B. Functional responses of different muscle types of the female rat urethra *in vivo*. *Acta Physiol Scand* 1989; 140: 365–67.

45. Watts SW, Cohen ML. Effect of bombesin, bradykinin, substance P and CGRP in prostate, bladder body and neck. *Peptides* 1991; 12: 1057–62.

46. Abelli L, Conte B, Somma V et al. The contribution of capsaicin-sensitive sensory nerves toluene-induced visceral pain in conscious, freely moving rats. *Naunyn Schmiedebergs Arch Pharmacol* 1988; 337: 545–51.

47. Callsen-Cencic P, Mense S. Expression of neuropeptides and nitric oxide synthase in neurones innervating the inflamed rat urinary bladder. *J Auton Nerv Syst* 1997; 65: 33–44.

48. Saban MR, Saban R, Bjorling DE. Kinetics of peptide-induced release of inflammatory mediators by the urinary bladder. *Br J Urol* 1997; 80: 742–7.

49. Shaker HS, Tu LM, Kalfopoulos M et al. Hyperreflexia of the urinary bladder: possible role of the efferent function of the capsaicin sensitive primary afferents. *J Urol* 1998; 160: 2232–9.

50. Shaker HS, Wang Y, Loung D et al. Role of C-afferent fibres in the mechanism of action of sacral nerve root neuromodulation in chronic spinal cord injury. *BJU Int* 2000; 85: 905-10.

51. Crowe R, Vale J, Trott KR et al. Radiation-induced changes in neuropeptides in the rat urinary bladder. *J Urol* 1996; 156: 2062–66.

52. Banasiak D, Burcher E. Effect of capsaicin on distribution of binding sites for tachykinins and calcitonin gene-related peptide in rat urinary bladder: a quantitative autoradiographic study. *Peptides* 1994; 15: 333–9.

53. Mathison R, Davison JS. Attenuated plasma extravasation to sensory neuropeptides in diabetic rats. *Agents Actions* 1993; 38: 55–9.

54. Chapple CR, Milner P, Moss HE, Burnstock G. Loss of sensory neuropeptides in the obstructed human bladder. *Br J Urol* 1992; 70: 373–81.

55. Birder LA, Roppolo JR, Iadarola MJ, de Groat WC. c-fos as a marker for subsets of visceral second order neurons in the rat lumbosacral spinal cord. *Soc Neurosci Abstr* 1990; 16: 703.

56. Herdegen T, Kovary K, Leah J, Bravo R. Specific temporal and spatial distribution of Jun, Fos and Krox-24 proteins in spinal neurons following noxious transsynaptic stimulation. *J Comp Neurol* 1992; 313:178–91.

57. Wang Y, Zhou Y, Mourad MS, Hassouna MM. Neuromodulation reduces urinary frequency in rats with hydrochloric acid-induced cystitis. *BJU Int* 2000; 86: 726–30.

58. Hunt SP, Pini A and Evan G. Induction of c-fos-like protein in spinal cord neurons following sensory stimulation. *Nature* 1987; 328: 632–4.

59. Cruz F, Avelino A, Coimbra A. Desensitization follows excitation of bladder afferents by intravesical, as shown by c-fos activation in the rat spinal cord. *Pain* 1996; 64: 553–56.

60. Wu YP, Ling EA. Induction of Fos-like immunoreactivity in the hypothalamic, medullary and thoracic spinal cord neurons following middle cerebral artery occlusion in rats. *Neurosci Res* 1988; 30: 145–53.

61. Birder LA, Roppolo JR, Iadarola MJ, de Groat WC. Electrical stimulation of visceral afferent pathways in the pelvic nerve increases *c-fos* in the rat lumbosacral spinal cord. *Neurosci Lett* 1991; 129:193–6.

62. Wang Y, Hassouna MM. Neuromodulation reduces *c-fos* gene expression in spinalized rats: a double-blind randomized study. *J Urol* 2000; 163–65.

63. Chang CJ, Huang ST, Hsu K *et al*. Electroacupuncture decreases *c-fos* expression in the spinal cord induced by noxious stimulation of the rat bladder. *J Urol* 1998; 160: 2274–9.

64. Callsen-Cencic P, Mense S. Increased spinal expression of *c-fos* following stimulation of the lower urinary tract in chronic spinal cord-injured rats. *Histochem Cell Biol* 1999; 112: 63–72.

65. Vizzard MA. Increased expression of spinal cord Fos protein induced by bladder stimulation after spinal cord injury. *Am J Physiol Regul Integr Comp Physiol* 2000; 279: R295–305.

66. Avelino A, Cruz F, Coimbra A. Lidocaine prevents noxious excitation of bladder afferents induced by intravesical capsaicin without interfering with the ensuing sensory desensitization: an experimental study in the rat. *J Urol* 1998; 159: 567–70.

67. Cruz F, Avelino A, Lima D, Coimbra A. Activation of the *c-fos* proto-oncogene in the spinal cord following noxious stimulation of the urinary bladder. *Somatosens Mot Res* 1994; 11: 319–20.

68. Al-Chaer, ED, Lawand NB, Westlund KN, Willis WD. Visceral nociceptive input into the ventral posterolateral nucleus of the thalamus: a new function for the dorsal column pathway. *J Neurophysiol* 1996; 76: 2661–74.

69. Al-Chaer, ED, Lawand NB, Westlund KN, Willis WD. Pelvic visceral input into the nucleus gracilis is largely mediated by the postsynaptic dorsal column pathway. *J Neurophysiol* 1996; 76: 2675–90.

70. Nahin RL, Madsen AM, Giesler GL, Jr. Anatomical and physiological studies of the gray matter surrounding the spinal cord central canal. *J Comp Neurol* 1983; 220: 321–35.

71. Lewin GR, Mendell LM. Nerve growth factor and nociception. *Trends Neurosci* 1993; 16: 353–9.

72. Steers WD, Kolbeck S, Creedon DJ, Tuttle JB. Nerve growth factor in the urinary bladder of the adult regulates neuronal form and function. *J Clin Invest* 1991; 88: 1709–15.

73. Persson K, Sando JJ, Tuttle JB, Steers WD. Protein kinase C involvement in stretch-induced nerve growth factor production by urinary tract smooth muscle cells. *Am J Physiol* 1995; 269: C1018–24.

74. Persson K, Steers WD, Tuttle JB. Regulation of nerve growth factor secretion in smooth muscle cells cultured from rat bladder body, base and urethra. *J Urol* 1997; 157: 2000–6.

75. Kluck P. The autonomic innervation of the human urinary bladder neck and urethra: a histochemical study. *Anat Rec* 1980; 198: 439–47.

76. Johnson JM, Skau KA, Gerald MC, Wallace LJ. Regional noradrenergic and cholinergic neurochemistry in the rat urinary bladder: effect of age. *J Urol* 1988; 139: 611–15.

77. Dmitrieva N, Shelton D, Rice AS, McMahon SB. The role of nerve growth factor in a model of visceral inflammation. *Neuroscience* 1997; 78: 449–51.

78. Dmitrieva N, McMahon SB. Sensitization of visceral afferents by nerve growth factor in the adult rat. *Pain* 1996; 66: 87–90.

79. Steers WD, Ciambotti J, Erdman S, de Groat WC. Morphological plasticity in efferent pathways to the urinary bladder of the rat following urethral obstruction. *J Neurosci* 1990; 10: 1943–51.

80. Steers WD, de Groat WC. Effect of bladder outlet obstruction on micturition reflex pathways in the rat. *J Urol* 1988; 140: 864–71.

81. Steers WD, Creedon DJ, Tuttle JB. Immunity to NGF prevents afferent plasticity following urinary bladder hypertrophy. *J Urol* 1996; 155: 379–85.

82. Tuttle JB, Steers WD, Albo M, Nataluk E. Neural input regulates tissue NGF and growth of the adult rat urinary bladder. *J Auton Nerv Syst* 1994; 49: 147–58.

83. Steers WD, Clemow DB, Persson K *et al*. The spontaneously hypertensive rat: insight into the pathogenesis of irritative symptoms in benign prostatic hyperplasia and young anxious males. *Exp Physiol* 1999; 84: 137–47.

7 Pretreatment diagnostic evaluation

V. Grünewald and K. Höfner

Basic principles of pretreatment diagnostic evaluation

The purpose of the diagnostic evaluation prior to treatment of an individual patient by sacral neuromodulation has several different aspects. Pretreatment diagnostic evaluation should:

- establish a sound and reliable diagnosis underlying the patient's clinical symptoms;
- establish the presence of an appropriate indication for treatment of the diagnosed condition by sacral neuromodulation;
- rule out contraindications for treatment by sacral neuromodulation and conditions requiring other forms of treatment;
- objectively identify and quantify the patient's symptoms in order to enable comparison to be made during development as treatment progresses (peripheral nerve evaluation [PNE] and following permanent implantation);
- try to identify potential risk factors and prognostic factors to allow the individual patient sound informed consent to treatment by sacral neuromodulation.

Although sacral neuromodulation has become an established treatment modality for lower urinary tract dysfunction, it is still (and should be) a continuously changing and developing field of significant scientific and clinical interest. However, since few prospective experimental and clinical studies are available [1–3], many issues in this field have not yet been elucidated and many questions remain unanswered. For this reason it is currently difficult to present a generally accepted concept of the diagnostic evaluation prior to treatment by sacral neuromodulation. Problems start with terminology, increase when it comes to indications and contraindications, and sometimes become numerous when the experiences of individual users of the technique and its modifications become involved.

In this chapter we therefore try to present information acceptable to most users of sacral neuromodulation and we are careful to indicate our own, subjective, views in the text where necessary.

Terminology, definition and classification of SNS treatment indications

Sacral neuromodulation has been shown to have a positive effect on both impaired storage and voiding function of the lower urinary tract [1–5]. For diagnostic evaluation before sacral nerve stimulation

> **Key Points**
> - Pretreatment evaluation of SNS patients is multipurpose.
> - As SNS is a dynamic field, recommendation of a universally accepted diagnostic evaluation is difficult.

(SNS) it is, therefore, useful to discriminate between disturbances of these two basic functions, and to classify the treatment indications and their clinical workup accordingly.

Impaired storage function

Whereas inadequate function of the urethral sphincter mechanism alone, as one cause of impaired storage function (urinary stress incontinence), has not become a generally accepted indication for sacral neuromodulation, combined (mixed incontinence or stress/urge incontinence with a prominent urge component) and particularly isolated bladder-related causes of storage problems (bladder hyperactivity and bladder hypersensitivity) are currently the main indications for SNS therapy [5]. Terms used synonymously for bladder (or detrusor) hyperactivity, characterised by involuntary detrusor contractions during filling cystometry, are detrusor instability (when used as a generic term), motor urge/motor urge incontinence (in cases with a suspected non-neurogenic aetiology of involuntary detrusor contractions), or detrusor hyperreflexia (in cases of known neurogenic aetiology) [6]. Both in bladder hyperactivity and in bladder hypersensitivity (sensory urge/sensory urge incontinence sometimes being used as a synonym for this condition, lacking the presence of involuntary detrusor contractions during filling cystometry) patients complain about similar symptoms (lower urinary tract symptoms [LUTS], storage symptoms) which are also termed 'irritative' and include urgency, frequency, nocturia, and urge incontinence [7]. Particularly in patients with bladder hypersensitivity, pain is a frequently associated symptom, which also might respond well to neuromodulation therapy. Symptoms associated with bladder hyperactivity or hypersensitivity, are as follows:

- urgency
- frequency
- nocturia
- urge incontinence
- pain

As sacral neuromodulation is predominantly indicated for symptomatic treatment of refractory neurogenic or non-neurogenic primary (idiopathic) urge/urge incontinence, one of the main functions of the diagnostic evaluation is to rule out secondary (symptomatic) urge/urge incontinence, which will usually allow causal treatment of the underlying problem. Potential causes of secondary (symptomatic) urge/urge incontinence are as follows:

- non-specific urinary tract infection (UTI)
- specific cystitis (tuberculosis, bilharziasis), irradiation cystitis
- cyclophosphamide cystitis
- oestrogen deficit
- infravesical obstruction
- congenital malformations
- urethral diverticulum

- urethral prolapse
- foreign bodies
- bladder stones
- tumours (bladder, urethra, prostate)
- pelvic floor insufficiency (mixed stress urge/incontinence).

Impaired voiding function

Voiding dysfunction can be caused by infravesical obstruction (mechanical or functional due to unphysiological sphincter activity during micturition), by disturbances of the bladder function (detrusor hypoactivity or inactivity, detrusor hyposensitivity or insensitivity) or a combination of these. Terms used synonymously for functional infravesical obstruction are detrusor–sphincter dyscoordination (generic term), detrusor–sphincter dysfunction (non-neurogenic aetiology) and detrusor–sphincter dyssynergia (neurogenic aetiology). Detrusor hypoactivity or inactivity (generic term) can be called detrusor hypocontractility or acontractility in the case of non-neurogenic aetiology or detrusor hyporeflexia or areflexia in the case of known neurogenic aetiology [7].

Symptoms of voiding dysfunction (lower urinary tract voiding symptoms, 'obstructive' symptoms) include weak flow, straining, prolonged voiding time, hesitancy, intermittency, post-void dribbling, incomplete evacuation, overflow incontinence and complete urinary retention in extreme cases [7].

Whereas the cause of a voiding disorder can be appropriately differentiated by specific urodynamic tests (pressure–flow measurement and analysis) as long as an individual is still able to void during the test [8, 9], there is currently no way by which to differentiate the underlying mechanisms of the voiding disorders in the state of complete urinary retention, which will urodynamically always present as detrusor acontractility or areflexia (terminology depending on the presence or absence of a known neurogenic aetiology).

One important function of the diagnostic evaluation is to rule out mechanical infravesical obstruction as a cause of voiding dysfunction, because that is not an indication for sacral neuromodulation therapy. Another important function is to differentiate detrusor 'acontractility' from detrusor areflexia, because complete destruction of the peripheral innervation will not allow neuromodulation therapy to be effective.

One of the most frequent reasons for voiding dysfunction in patients treated by SNS is non-neurogenic detrusor–sphincter dysfunction. In our opinion, non-physiological afferent impulses from the intermittently or continuously contracted pelvic floor/urethral sphincter indirectly cause detrusor hypocontractility or acontractility, because they inhibit an adequate detrusor contraction, so that either it cannot be initiated at all or it can no longer be maintained at a sufficient level and/or for an appropriate time interval. Thus, in our opinion, both detrusor hypocontractility or acontractility and detrusor–sphincter dysfunction reflect a common pathophysiological mechanism, which should also account for complete urinary retention.

Key Points
- Urodynamic tests reveal causes of voiding disorders.
- Complete urinary retention precludes such tests.
- Mechanical infravesical obstruction must be ruled out.
- Detrusor acontractility and areflexia must be differentiated.
- Detrusor hypo-/acontractility, detrusor–sphincter dysfunction, and urinary retention may have a common pathophysiological mechanism.

Diagnostic tests

Medical history

Meticulous evaluation of the individual medical history is the basis for any further diagnostic test and an essential part of the evaluation before considering SNS for treatment of lower urinary tract dysfunction.

First the patient must be questioned about his or her symptoms; their quality, duration, and time of onset; and the consequences for quality of life. Micturition habits, quality of voiding, and incontinence episodes should be evaluated in detail. This part should also include sexual life anamnesis, history and type of UTIs and their treatment, and evaluation of defecation habits. A more precise evaluation can be achieved by standardised and validated questionnaires (see next sections).

Also important is the assessment of previous and current diseases or surgical procedures potentially affecting lower urinary tract function. The patient should be asked particularly about known urological, neurological and gynaecological diseases or surgical procedures performed in these areas. In female patients evaluation of number and type of deliveries and potential complications is mandatory.

Detailed documentation of all previous diagnostic tests, and particularly of treatments including date, duration, and their effect on the patient's condition, is necessary in order to establish an appropriate indication for sacral neuromodulation, which is at present essentially based on the fact that the patient's condition had been refractory to all prior treatments.

Several drugs may affect lower urinary tract function (Table 7.1); evaluation of all drugs currently used, the duration of their use, and their dosage, as well as any known drug allergies, is absolutely necessary. The patient should also be sytstematically asked about use of anticholinergic and cholinergic drugs, α blockers, finasteride, and antispasmodics in the past, because these products are frequently used in urological practice for treatment of lower urinary tract dysfunction and many patients may have forgotten about their use, especially if such drugs were ineffective.

Voiding diary

Systematic documentation by the patient of each micturition — including time, voided volume, and (if possible) residual urine, together with number, time and severity of incontinence episodes over a period of 3–7 days — is simple, cheap, and one of the most effective tests for objective assessment of lower urinary tract function. If always performed in the same way, it is a perfect tool for evaluation of the efficacy of any type of treatment. In SNS, comparison of the pretreatment diary parameters with those obtained during PNE will provide the key information for deciding whether and how to perform a permanent implant.

Questionnaires

Questionnaires allow an objective qualitative and quantitative assessment of symptoms and/or their effects on quality of life and are useful for monitoring therapy [10–12]. Even though a

Table 7.1   *Drugs affecting lower urinary tract function*

Drug group	Drugs	Mechanism of action	Effect
Direct parasympathomimetics	Carbachol, bethanechol	Increase of detrusor contractility	Urge incontinence
Indirect Parasympathomimetics	Physostigmine, neostigmine, pydridostigmine, distigmine		
β blockers	Atenolol, sotalol, metoprolol, propanolol (etc.)		
Prostaglandins	Prostaglandin E2, prostaglandin 2α		
α blockers	Phentolamine, doxazosin, terazosin, phenoxybezamine	Reduction of sphincter tonus and of bladder outlet resistance	Stress incontinence
Muscle relaxants	Baclofen, dantrolene, flavoxate		
Anticholinergics (parasympatholytics)	Atropine, trospiumchloride, oxybutynin, tolterodine, etc.	Inhibition of detrusor by direct or indirect anticholinergic effect or relaxation of detrusor smooth muscle	Residual urine, urinary retention, overflow incontinence
Tricyclic antidepressants	i.e. Imipramine, amitriptyline, nortryptiline, desipramine		
Neuroleptics: phenothiazines	Chlorpromazine, fluphenazine, promethazine, thioridazine, etc.		
Neuroleptics: butyrophenone derivatives	Haloperidol, droperidol		
Neuroleptics: thioxanthenes	Chlorprothixene		
Hypnotics: barbiturates	Hexobarbitone, phenobarbitone, pentabarbitone, etc.		
Hypnotics: benzodiazepines	Nitrazepam, diazepam, flurazepam, etc.		
Hypnotics: alcohols and aldehydes	Chloral hydrate, paraldehyde		
Hypnotics: chinazolines	Methaqualone		
Hypnotics: piperidine derivatives	Gluthehimide, methyprylon		
α sypathomimetics:	Adrenaline, noradrenaline, etilefrine, norfenefrine, etc.		
α sympathomimietics (direct/indirect)	Phenylephrine, synephrine, etc.		
β sympathomimetics	Isoprenaline, orciprenaline, etc.		
Calcium antagonists	Verapamil, nifedipine, diltiazem, etc.		
Alcohol		Sedation, relaxation of smooth muscle, diuresis	Residual urine, urinary retention
Diuretics	Furosemide, ethacrynic acid, triamterene, amiloride	Increased diuresis	Deterioration of pre-existing incontinence

generally accepted questionnaire for global assesment of voiding and incontinence is currently not available, many questionnaires fulfil the requirements of a well-investigated test — offering sufficient validity, reliability, stability, consistency and reproducibility — and are therefore recommended by the First International Consultation on BPH and the First International Consultation on Incontinence [11,12].

Clinical examination

The clinical examination in patients with lower urinary tract dysfunction will focus on the urogenital tract and include rectal and vaginal inspection and palpation. In men, clinical evaluation of the prostate and detection of enlargement of the gland or clinical signs of prostate cancer are the most important findings, while in women clinical signs of genital descensus (prolapse) are frequent and may influence the decision about further treatment, particularly in women with mixed stress and urge incontinence.

Several clinical tests for assessment and quantification of urinary incontinence have been described. Useful tests in our opinion are the stress test and the bladder-neck elevation test for clinical demonstration of incontinence, the Q-tip test [13] for discrimination between urethral hypermobility and sphincter insufficiency as a cause of urinary stress incontinence, and (particularly) the pad test [14], which objectively quantifies involuntary urine loss under standardised conditions and allows objective grading of urinary incontinence. In our opinion the modification of the test described by Hahn and Fall in 1991 [15] is a good compromise between accuracy and clinical practicability.

Another important part of the clinical examination is a basic neurological examination with a focus on the lumbosacral peripheral innervation. Pathological findings and corresponding clues from the medical history should be a reason for referring the patient to a neurologist for further detailed evaluation and specific neurophysiological testing.

Laboratory tests

If a urinary tract infection (UTI) is present, urinalysis, urine culture and antibiogram are mandatory tests in any patient with lower urinary tract dysfunction. Particularly in the elderly, such UTIs are the most frequent cause of urgency/urge incontinence and also a frequent complication in patients with significant voiding dysfunction. Association with fever should always indicate the need for further evaluation of the upper urinary tract, particularly searching for evidence of reflux or obstruction. UTIs must be ruled out or appropriately treated for a sufficient period of time before invasive transurethral instrumentation, endoscopy or urodynamic investigations are performed.

Laboratory blood tests should (at least) include serum sodium and potassium levels, as well as urea and creatinine levels for orientation about upper urinary tract function. Pathological findings should prompt additional tests such as creatinine clearance, renal scintigraphy, and ultrasonographic (US) or radiological imaging.

The serum prostate-specific antigen (PSA) level should be determined in all men of more than 40 years old for early detection of prostate cancer.

Ultrasonographic and radiological imaging

Ultrasonographic imaging for determination of post-void residual urine and evaluation of the upper urinary tract should be performed in all patients presenting with symptoms of lower urinary tract dysfunction. Pathological findings should lead to further radiological investigation by intravenous pyelography (IVP), retrograde urethrograpy (only male patients) or voiding cystourethrography (VCUG).

Whereas in the presence of a normal US test, IVP and retrograde urethrography are not necessary as routine tests in the pretreatment diagnostic workup of patients prior to sacral neuromodulation, VCUG or at least cystography (if the patient is in complete urinary retention) should, in our opinion, be carried out in all patients not undergoing videourodynamic studies. The VCUG provides much essential morphological and functional information (such as detection of congenital malformations of the spine and the sacrum, reflux, prolapse, dyssynergic voiding, bladder-neck sclerosis, stones, foreign bodies, diverticula, fistulae and more) that cannot be detected with any other test at the same time in such an easy, rapid and safe manner.

Endoscopy

The main indication for urethrocystoscopy in the pretreatment diagnostic evaluation of patients prior to SNS is to rule out bladder cancer as a potential cause of urgency/urge incontinence and to exclude other secondary aetiologies of urgency/urge incontinence, including fistulae and congenital malformations. For definite exclusion of carcinoma *in situ* of the bladder, this should be combined with random biopsies from the bladder mucosa, requiring anaesthesia in most cases. Each individual physician must decide whether this is necessary in every patient with lower urinary tract symptoms, or if it should be restricted to elderly patients with risk factors such as smoking or additional pathological findings on VCUG, urine cytology and US. We routinely perform urethrocystoscopy in all patients, if this is possible, without anaesthesia; we would do this with an anaesthetised patient only if associated pathological findings would require endoscopic verification or treatment, or if bladder biopsies are considered necessary in individual patients.

Urodynamic investigation

Urodynamic studies are the most important tool in the diagnostic evaluation of lower urinary tract dysfunction [16–18]. The urodynamic investigation, together with other clinical aspects, will determine the final diagnosis of the disorder and will therefore be one of the most important sources of information for deciding whether to treat a patient by sacral neuromodulation. We do not, here, intend to discuss special urodynamic techniques and how to interpret them; instead we prefer to focus on basic principles of urodynamic studies

Key Points
- Ultrasonographic imaging and voiding cystourethrography are most helpful.
- Endoscopy helps to exclude bladder Ca and other secondary causes of urgency/urge incontinence.
- Urodynamics are crucial in diagnosis.

Key Points

- Urodynamics must include uroflowmetry/residual filling cystometry, and pressure–flow measurement.

and their relevance for baseline or follow-up investigations of patients before or after SNS.

All urodynamic studies should be conducted according to the standards (and using the terminology) of the International Continence Society (ICS) in order to make them comparable [19, 20]. Urodynamic studies in potential SNS patients should always investigate both storage and voiding function of the lower urinary tract, regardless of whether only one of the functions is clinically affected. Exclusion of UTI prior to the investigation is mandatory.

The urodynamic investigation should begin with *free uroflow-metry and determination of residual urine* by US or catheterisation immediately after the flow. Flowmetry will serve as a screening test for voiding dysfunction and enable the patient's voiding behaviour to be assessed without catheters irritating the urethra. For comparison, at least one other flowmetry reading should be obtained on a separate occasion.

After the catheters have been inserted, *filling cystometry* investigating storage function should be the next step. Because of individual variations and the fact that the patient will adapt to the artificial setting of the test situation, filling cystometry should be repeated at least once. Provocative tests for eliciting detrusor instability (instillation of iced water) should be performed if urgency/urge incontinence is the patient's main complaint. Simultaneous registration of a pelvic floor electromyogram (EMG) during cystometry is useful; however, it is more important to perform this when the patient is voiding. For practical reasons the equipment is usually installed before the filling cystometry is started.

If the patient is able to void, *pressure–flow measurement*, precisely investigating voiding function, should be the next step. If the patient is in complete urinary retention, provocative tests, such as the subcutaneous injection of carbachol (carbachol test, Lapides test) can be performed, in order to differentiate between neurogenic detrusor areflexia and non-neurogenic detrusor acontractility [21]. However, in our view, a PNE test (which should be performed in such patients anyway) will provide more precise and valid information about the integrity of the innervation of the lower urinary tract and should, therefore, be preferred. For the same reasons as were discussed for cystometry, pressure–flow studies should be repeated at least once. Owing to increased adaptation to the test and the transurethral catheter, there is a tendency for every patient to void with less detrusor sphincter dysfunction (and therefore less infravesical obstruction) when the study is repeated. If the patient is able to void at least 20–30ml, this will be of significant relevance for discrimination between mechanical infravesical obstruction, functional infravesical obstruction and detrusor hypocontractility, which can now be easily identified by pressure–flow analysis. For additional morphological information from the lower urinary tract during filling and voiding, particularly in neurogenic lower urinary tract dysfunction, it can be useful to perform a videourodynamic study or separate VCUG (the latter not being the same as the former because the urodynamic data cannot be assigned exactly to a defined phase of the VCUG). As with videourodynamic studies, simultaneous EMG recording will supply additional information about the behaviour of the striated musculature in the bladder outlet during voiding; however, most information will already have been obtained from the pressure–flow study and its analysis. Because different concepts of pressure–flow analysis are currently under discussion [20], each investigator should decide on one concept only in order to facilitate comparison between individual studies, including follow-up studies of the same patient. However, most of the new computerised urodynamic units offer many different types of pressure–flow analysis in their built-in software packages, which take this into account [17].

Whereas filling cystometry and pressure–flow studies are mandatory, and a minimal programme for sound urodynamic investigation, flowmetry is a useful additional screening test. Other urodynamic tests are optional, mainly because of a lack of general acceptance or standardisation. Some tests have been especially developed to give better urodynamic proof of urinary stress incontinence, as it is often very difficult to provide evidence of low-grade stress incontinence during cystometry. Urethral pressure profilometry, leak-point pressure measurements [22, 23] and other techniques have been developed to achieve this. Although, in our opinion, these tests provide useful confirmation of the presence of stress incontinence (and therefore enable investigators to exclude these patients from neuromodulation therapy), others are content to diagnose stress incontinence by merely excluding urge incontinence. Detection of urethral instability as a cause of urge incontinence, by simultaneous urethral pressure measurement during cystometry and/or a pressure–flow study, is also a technique used by many investigators; however, others deny the existence of urethral instability as an independent pathophysiological mechanism of incontinence, regarding it as a subtype of detrusor instability.

PNE test

Next to, or even combined with an urodynamic test, percutaneous nerve evaluation is the other important diagnostic tool, which should be used in each individual scheduled to be treated by sacral neuromodulation.

Percutaneous test stimulation of the sacral spinal nerves is carried out for three reasons:

- assessment of functional integrity of the sacral spinal nerves;
- assessment of individual variations in lower urinary tract innervation;
- assessment of clinical efficacy of sacral nerve neuromodulation in an individual patient.

Assessment of functional integrity of the sacral spinal nerves and the peripheral innervation of the lower urinary tract, arising from the sacral spinal segments S2–S4, can be performed both for the somatic and the autonomic innervation. Whereas the somatic nerves (afferent and efferent) can be easily tested under local anaesthesia as part of the standard procedure [24] described in other chapters

> **Key Points**
> - PNE should always precede implantation.
> - PNE assesses function of somatic/autonomic innervation.
> - Local anaesthesia is needed for somatic nerve tests.
> - Visceromotor nerve tests call for general anaesthesia plus urodynamics.

of this book, visceromotor nerves can usually be studied only under general anaesthesia with simultaneous urodynamic recording of stimulation-induced detrusor contractions (stimulation is painful for patients without neurological disease, because high stimulation intensities are necessary for recruiting non-myelinated visceromotor autonomic fibres).

In patients with confirmed detrusor instability, it is often also possible to test whether SNS will reduce (or suppress) detrusor instability. This can be done without anaesthesia under urodynamic test conditions. However, even though a positive response during this test might indicate a favourable outcome, it does not prove that individuals without detectable changes during this test will not respond clinically to neuromodulation therapy as well.

Apart from a positive clinical response during PNE (for which there is also no ideal correlation), no clinical or urodynamic factors have been identified that can predict a positive outcome for any individual patient with a permanent implant.

Percutaneous test stimulation should, in our opinion, always be carried out at least on the S3 sacral spinal nerves and, if possible also, at the S4 level, as the latter sometimes has a very good clinical effect and far fewer side effects (for instance, co-stimulation of the leg and foot muscles).

The PNE test should always be performed both uni- and bilaterally, in both the acute and the subchronic phase of the test. Despite many current problems with test-electrode dislocation, this is the only way to find out whether an individual patient will be adequately treated by a unilateral implant, or if it would be more appropriate to choose a primary, bilateral, two-channel implant (at double the expense). Our current procedure is to perform a unilateral implant in all those patients with a 100% clinical response during PNE (what more could be achieved by a bilateral implant as long as no greater long-term efficacy can be confirmed in prospective studies?). We would place a bilateral two-channel implant in those patients gaining additional benefit from bilateral test stimulation compared with unilateral stimulation, as well as in those where even a partial response (less than 50%) can be achieved only by bilateral but not by unilateral test stimulation.

References

1. Schmidt RA, Jonas U, Oleson KA et al. Sacral nerve stimulation for treatment of refractory urinary urge incontinence. Sacral Nerve Stimulation Study Group. *J Urol* 1999 Aug; 162: 352–7.

2. Bosch JL, Groen J. Sacral nerve neuromodulation in the treatment of patients with refractory motor urge incontinence: long-term results of a prospective longitudinal study. *J Urol* 2000; 163: 1219–22.

3. Jonas U, Fowler CJ, Cantazarro F et al. Efficacy of sacral nerve stimulation (SNS) in urinary retention: results up to 18 months following implantation. *J Urol* 2001; 165: 15–19.

4. Thon WF, Baskin LS, Jonas U et al. Neuromodulation of voiding dysfunction and pelvic pain. *World J Urol* 1991; 9: 138–41.

5. Grünewald V, Höfner K, Thon WF et al. Sacral electrical neuromodulation as an alternative treatment option for lower urinary tract dysfunction. *Rest Neurol Neurosc* 1999; 14: 189–93.

6. Grünewald V, Jonas U. Neurogenic abnormalities. In: JM Fitzpatrick, JR Krane (eds.) *The Bladder*. London: Churchill Livingstone, 1995, 195–211.

7. Grünewald V, Jonas U. Blasenentleerungsstörung. In: K Höfner, CG Stief, U Jonas (eds) *Benigne Prostatahyperplasie — Ein Leitfaden für die Praxis* Heidelberg: Springer Verlag, 2000, 110–36.

8. Schäfer W. Basic principles and clinical application of advanced analysis of bladder voiding function. *Urol Clin North Am* 1990; 17: 553–66.

9. Höfner K, Kramer AEJL, Tan HK *et al*. CHESS classification of bladder outflow obstruction: a consequence in the discussion of current concepts. *World J Urol* 13; 1995; 59–64.

10. Barry MJ, Fowler FJ, O'Leary M *et al*. The American Urological Association symptom index for benign prostatic hyperplasia. *J Urol* 1992; 148: 1549–55.

11. Mebust W, Roizo R, Shroeder F, Villers A. Correlations between pathology, clinical symptoms and the course of the disease. In: ATK Cockett, Y Aso, C Chatelain, L Denis, K Griffiths, S Khoury, G Murphy (eds) *Proceedings of the 1st International Consultation on BPH*. Jersey: Scientific Communication International Ltd, 1992, 53–62.

12. Donovan J, Naughton M, Gotoh M *et al*. Symptom and quality of life assessment. In: P Abrams, S Khoury, A Wein (eds) *Proceedings of the 1st International Consultation on Incontinence*. Jersey: Health Publication Ltd, 1999; 295–331.

13. Crystle CD, Charme LS, Copeland WE. Q-tip-test in stress urinary incontinence. *Obstet Gynecol* 1971; 38: 313–15.

14. Sutherst J, Brown M, Shawer M. Assessing the severity of urinary incontinence in women by weighing perineal pads. *Lancet* 1981; 1: 1128–30.

15. Hahn I, Fall M. Objective quantification of stress urinary incontinence: a short, reproducible, provocative pad-test. *Neurourol Urodyn* 1991; 10: 475–81.

16. Höfner K. Urodynamic evaluation of lower urinary tract dysfunction. *Curr Opin Urol* 1992; 2: 257–62.

17. Höfner K, Kramer G, Tan HK *et al*. Advances in urodynamics. *Eur Urol Update Series 1993; 2, No. 5*: 34–9.

18. Jonas U, Heidler H, Höfner K, Thüroff, JW (eds) *Urodynamik*. Volume 2. Stuttgart: Ferdinand Enke Verlag, 1998.

19. Abrams P, Blaivas JG, Stanton SL, Andersen JT. The standardisation of terminology of lower urinary tract function. *Scand J Urol Nephrol Suppl* 1988; 114: 5–19.

20. Griffiths D, Höfner K, van Mastrigt R *et al*. Standardization of terminology of lower urinary tract function: pressure–flow studies of voiding, urethral resistance and urethral obstruction. International Continence Society Subcommittee on Standardization of Terminology of Pressure–Flow Studies. *Neurourol Urodyn* 1997; 16: 1–8.

21. Lapides J, Friend CR, Ajemian EP, Reus WF. A new test for neurogenic bladder. *J Urol* 1962; 88: 245–7.

22. McGuire EJ, Cespedes RD. Leak-point pressures. *Urol Clin North Am* 1996; 23: 253–62.

23. Höfner K, Oelke M, Wagner T, Efer J, Jonas U. Computerunterstützte Messung und Standardisierung des leak-point-pressure beim Husten (cough leak point pressure — CLPP) zur Diagnostik der Streßinkontinenz. *Aktuel Urol* 1999; 30: 321–8.

24. Schmidt RA, Senn E, Tanagho EA. Functional evaluation of sacral spinal nerve root integrity. *Urology* 1990; 35: 388–92.

8 Hardware: development and function

M. Gerber, J. Swoyer and C. Tronnes

Key Points
- The implantable pulse generator stimulates sacral nerves by regular, programmed, electrical pulses.
- A long-life battery is encased in biocompatible material.
- The implanted battery/wires/electrodes stimulate a specific body site.
- Pacemaker technology has led to neurostimulator development.
- SNS requires test stimulation hardware and a chronic, implantable system.

History

The basic concept behind the implantable pulse generator (IPG) that provides stimulation to the sacral nerve is not far removed from the concepts behind cardiac pacing. A long-lived battery encased in biocompatible material is programmed to deliver pulses of electricity to a specific region of the body through an electrode at the end of an encapsulated wire.

Medtronic, the manufacturer of the InterStim neurostimulator, has over 40 years' experience in developing and manufacturing IPGs. Earl Bakken, the founder of the company, first created a wearable, battery-operated pacemaker at the request of Dr. C. Walton Lillehei, a pioneer in open-heart surgery at the University of Minnesota Medical School Hospital, who was treating young patients for heart block.

Since the early 1970s, Medtronic has applied and adapted the technology behind pacemakers to the development of neurostimulators. Neurostimulation technology was first used for spinal cord stimulation with bipolar leads, shortly followed by its use for deep brain stimulation for the relief of pain. In the late 1970s, peripheral nerve stimulation was applied to the treatment of phantom limb and sciatic nerve pain, followed in the 1980s by its application to the problem of foot drop. The Itrel I, the first-generation neurostimulator, was introduced in 1983. Current versions are used for the treatment of incontinence, pain and movement disorders (Fig. 8.1).

Vast resources are critical to any company seeking new applications for this technology. The development of neurostimulators requires physiology laboratories for research, materials, science specialists, battery-development and manufacturing facilities, and semiconductor development and production facilities.

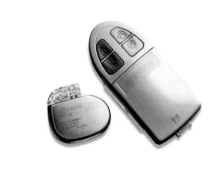

Figure 8.1 The original Itrel was commercially introduced in 1983; current versions are used for the treatment of incontinence and movement disorders.

System overview

The use of sacral nerve stimulation (SNS) requires test stimulation hardware and a chronic, fully implantable system. Generally, a test stimulation is done and, if this is successful, a chronic system is implanted. An alternative method uses a staged testing/implant procedure, where a chronic lead is implanted and connected to a percutaneous extension and test stimulator. All three systems are discussed in this section.

Acute testing hardware

The testing hardware consists of a needle, test lead, test stimulator, interconnect cabling and a ground pad (Fig. 8.2).

Needle

A 20-gauge foramen needle with a bevelled tip is used to gain access to the sacral nerve for placing the test stimulation lead. The stainless steel needle is depth-marked along its length and electrically insulated along its centre length. The portion near the hub is exposed to allow connection to the test stimulator. By stimulating through the uninsulated tip of the needle, the physician can determine the correct SNS site for the test stimulation lead.

Test lead

The initial test lead was a peripheral nerve evaluation (PNE) fluoro-polymer-coated, 11-stranded straight wire. An exposed metal tip at the distal end served as an electrode. The Medtronic 3057 test stimulation lead was developed to reduce the effects of lead migration.

The model 3057 test lead is a coiled, seven-stranded stainless-steel wire coated with fluoropolymer. Its electrode was extended to 10mm (0.4ins) to increase the length of coverage and reduce the effects of minor migration. Depth indicators help to align the lead electrode with the needle tip. The lead contains its own stylet, which is removed once the correct position has been found, leaving the lead flexible and stretchable, to mitigate migration.

Test stimulator

The model 3625 test stimulator is used both for patient screening, where the patient is sent home with the device, and for intraoperative usage in determining lead placement thresholds. It provides output characteristics that are similar to those of the implantable neurostimulator and can be operated in either monopolar or bipolar modes. An off-the-shelf, 9V battery provides power. Amplitude control is accessible to the patient when it is being used as a screening device. The physician can set amplitude limits to ensure patient safety and the validity of the test.

The test stimulator has several safety features. An automatic output shut-off occurs when the amplitude is turned up too rapidly, as when the control is inadvertently bumped. A loose device battery will also cause output shut-off to prevent intermittent stimulation and shock to the patient. Sensors, which detect when electrocautery is being used, shut the

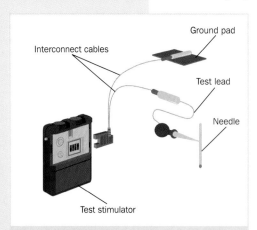

Figure 8.2 *The test stimulation hardware consists of the test stimulator, test lead, needle, interconnect cables and ground pad.*

Interconnect cables

Ground pad

Test lead

Needle

Test stimulator

output off. Protection circuitry can be reset by turning the test stimulator off for a minimum of 3 seconds.

Interconnect cables

Single-use electrical cables are used to hook the test stimulation lead to the model 3625 test stimulator during the test stimulation procedure in the physician's office and when the patient goes home for the evaluation period.

The patient cable is used to deliver acute stimulation during the test procedure. The insulated tin-plated copper cable has a 2mm socket at one end and a spring-activated mini-hook at the other end. The mini-hook makes a sterile connection to the foramen needle, test stimulation lead, or implant lead. The socket end is connected to the test stimulator by a long screener cable, the latter being a two-wire cable with a single connector to the model 3625 test stimulator at one end; one of the wires is connected to the patient cable and the other to the ground pad. After the test stimulation, the patient cable is removed and a short screener cable is substituted for at-home use. This cable is connected to the ground pad and directly to the test lead. It is designed to withstand the rigours of home use and can be disconnected, to facilitate changing clothes.

Ground pad

The ground pad provides the positive polarity in the electrical circuit during the test stimulation and the at-home trial. It is made of silicone rubber and is adhered to the patient's skin. As described above, for the at-home trial a short screener cable is substituted for the long screener cable and connected directly to the lead.

Test stimulation kit

Although it is not a required part of the testing hardware, a test stimulation kit is available containing most of the materials needed for one test stimulation. Drapes, iodine, anaesthetic needle, syringe, wound dressing and other supplies are combined in a sterile wrap for ease of use.

Percutaneous extension hardware

Percutaneous extension hardware is available for those who wish to use an alternative method of patient screening (Fig. 8.3). This method, which is also known as a staged implant, may be used when there is need for positive fixation of the test lead, or if acute testing has given inconclusive results.

The chronic lead is implanted in the normal manner and is connected to a percutaneous extension (model 3550-05). The extension is designed to provide a connection between the chronic lead and the external test stimulator. Positive contact is made using four set screws; the connection is sealed with a silicone boot that covers the set screws. The percutaneous extension, which is intended for temporary use, features four insulated wires, wound together and sized for a small incision, so that they can be brought through the skin. The percutaneous extension is then connected to the screener cable, as described above.

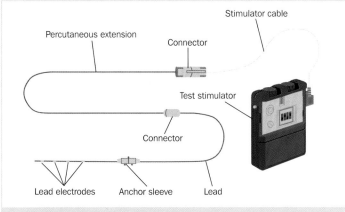

Figure 8.3 *The percutaneous extension and connector cable are useful for staged testing and implantation.*

Chronic system

The chronic system consists of an implantable neurostimulator, a lead, an extension, a physician programmer and a patient programmer.

Neurostimulator

The implantable neurostimulator (Medtronic model 3023) weighs about 42g and has a volume of 22cm^3 (about the size of a stopwatch) (Fig. 8.4) It comprises about 70% battery and 30% electronics. The physician has unlimited access to programmable parameters such as amplitude, frequency and pulse width. Each parameter can be changed by means of an external, physician programmer that establishes a radio-frequency (RF) link with the implanted device. A patient programmer provides limited access to allow the patient to turn the neurostimulator on and off, or to change amplitude within a range established by the physician (via the physician programmer). The neurostimulator can also be programmed to turn on/off using a strong magnet; however, magnetic sources such as purse magnets, theft-detection systems and airport screening systems are strong enough to switch the device on and off, and this feature can be disabled by means of the physician programmer. Electromagnetic interference (EMI) can be a problem, but that generated by common sources, such as microwave ovens, televisions, and cellular telephones should not affect the implanted neurostimulator. However, if the patient will be working around strong electromagnetic sources, such as a radio tower, the manufacturer should be contacted beforehand for advice.

The neurostimulator 'can' (the external titanium container of the neurostimulator) may be used in either a monopolar configuration (lead negative, can positive) or a bipolar configuration, which will result in marginally better longevity. Typically, neurostimulators will last 7–10 years, depending on the mode as well as on

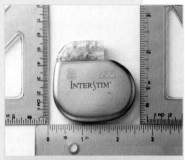

Figure 8.4 *The model 3023 neurostimulator is similar in size to a stopwatch.*

programming of the amplitude, frequency, and pulse width. Additionally, the use of more than one active electrode will reduce longevity. During follow-up visits, the physician's programmer will detect an end-of-life indicator before the battery depletes. Those patients who are not participating in follow-up visits will become aware when the battery needs replacement, through the patient programmer or on the return of symptoms. When the device is replaced, it should be returned to the supplier for analysis and proper disposal; Medtronic tests all returned products.

Implantable lead system

The lead is a quadripolar design, with four separate electrodes that can be individually programmed to plus, minus or off. This allows the physician to optimise the electrode configuration for each patient and to change programming, without additional surgery, at a later date, to adapt to minor lead migration or changing disease states. The electrode sizes, spacing, and configurations have been designed specifically for SNS.

The lead is supplied with multiple stylets and anchors, to accommodate physician preferences. A stylet (straight or bent) is inserted into the lumen of the lead to provide extra stiffness during implant. Two different degrees of stiffness provide the physician with options to tailor the handling and steering properties of the lead, as preferred. The stylet must be removed before connection with the mating component.

The physician also has a choice of anchors, which allow fixation of the lead to stable tissue to prevent dislodging of the lead after implantation. Three anchor configurations are available: a silicone rubber anchor fixed in place on the lead has wings, holes and grooves to facilitate suturing; a second type, also made of silicone, slides into place anywhere along the lead body, and must be sutured to the lead to hold it in place; a new plastic anchor is also available, which can be locked in place anywhere along the lead body without a suture to the lead.

Quadripolar extension

After the lead has been implanted and anchored, it is attached to an extension, which provides the interface to the neurostimulator. This extension, which is available in varying lengths to facilitate flexibility in IPG placement, is designed to provide a sealed connection to the lead. Positive contact is made with four set screws, and the connection is sealed with a silicone boot that covers the set screws, as described in the section on percutaneous extension hardware.

Physician programmer

The console programmer (Medtronic model 7432) is a microprocessor-based system that the physician uses to programme the implanted neurostimulator non-invasively. The programmer uses an application-specific memory module, installed by means of a plug-in software module.

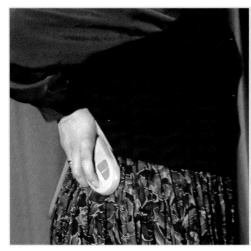

Figure 8.5 *The patient places the programmer over the site of the neurostimulator in order to adjust the frequency of the device or to turn it on or off.*

Patient programmer

The patient programmer also communicates with the implanted neurostimulator by an RF link (Fig. 8.5). The patient can adjust stimulation parameters within the range set by the physician. This is intended to allow the patient to turn the device on or off, and to change amplitude for comfort (as during postural changes), without returning to the physician's office.

Control magnet

The control magnet allows the patient to turn the neurostimulator on and off; however, since the introduction of the patient programmer (which has the same function), the control magnet is not often used.

Materials

All the materials used in the implanted system have a long history of use in cardiac stimulation and spinal cord stimulation. Materials are chosen for three reasons:

1. *Biocompatibility* — the materials must not cause an adverse reaction in the human body.
2. *Biostability* — the materials should not degrade while in the hostile environment of the body.
3. *Performance* — the materials and component designs must meet rigorous performance standards.

Implantable neurostimulator

The 'can' of the implantable neurostimulator is constructed of titanium, which is highly resistant to corrosion and is compatible with the human body. Titanium has been used in cardiac pacemakers since the 1980s. Everything but the front of the neurostimulator (which faces away from muscle) is coated with a parylene insulating coating, to avoid muscle stimulation when the stimulator is operated in a monopolar mode.

Lead system

The implanted lead body is made from polyurethane plastic. Polyurethane is a tough polymer, allowing for a small-diameter lead that is both strong and resistant to cuts. The implantable lead stylets are polymer-coated metal wires with plastic handles. The electrodes on the lead system are made from a platinum alloy. As well as being very resistant to corrosion, platinum has other qualities that make it a good choice for electrodes: it can deliver electrical current to the tissue while being directly exposed to body fluids, with little degradation over long periods, whereas materials such as stainless steel would eventually dissolve under similar conditions. Platinum also shows up well in fluoroscopy and radiography, thus facilitating imaging.

The conductors are individually coiled wires, one wire running from each electrode to a connector contact. The wire material is a specialized nickel alloy, which is more corrosion-resistant than stainless steel and can withstand the high stress associated with an implant. The coiled design enhances the lead's ability to withstand the bending and flexing stresses incurred during the patient's normal life. Each wire is insulated with an inert fluoropolymer, which is an excellent insulator. The extension (interconnect cable) has coiled nickel alloy wires, and is insulated with silicone rubber; silicone is very compliant and has a long history of successful use as an implantable material.

Future direction of the therapy hardware

The ongoing development of tools and hardware is driven by the desire to reduce the invasiveness of the implant and the likelihood of adverse events. Development efforts are concentrated on system components and tools that will allow implantation of the lead system through small incisions or percutaneous approaches. It is inevitable that the size of the neurostimulator will be reduced as future generations of the device are developed; more efficient power batteries and packaging will drive this aspect of development.

A rechargeable power battery may allow a smaller device. Although a smaller device would be welcomed, attaining this goal with a rechargeable battery is not seen as the best approach. A rechargeable neurostimulator would require the patient frequently to recharge the unit; this would inconvenience the patient and could reduce patient compliance. Additionally, a rechargeable battery would be more expensive than a non-rechargeable one owing to the technology required and the additional equipment necessary for recharging. Furthermore, this would not eliminate the need for periodic replacement of the neurostimulator every 5–10 years.

System components will be optimised for the therapy, to reduce the time needed for management of both implant and patient. The

Key Points

- Increased effectiveness and physician control are probable near-future developments.
- Long-term software loading is a future possibility.
- Improved test leads may allow longer test periods.
- SNS-application research may involve pelvic disorders and spinal cord injury.

incorporation of microprocessors and implementation of features such as a battery gauge will provide additional operational information while decreasing the time needed to manage the patient. Physicians will be able to analyse system use, lead status and other parameters. The addition of sensing technology may provide an opportunity to create a closed-loop system that captures data to optimise both diagnosis and functioning.

Bilateral stimulation may provide more efficacious therapy. There is considerable interest in this approach, and it seems to be a probable avenue of research in the near future. However, any use of bilateral stimulation would have to justify the larger neurostimulator, the extra lead system, and the additional costs associated with this approach; at present, there is no scientific experience to support this approach.

Apart from a reduction in the size of the implanted device, enhanced physician control is the most likely development to occur in the foreseeable future. Graphics-based programming and control will simplify device programming; it will allow more complex features to be incorporated in the neurostimulator without adding undue complexity to the physician programmer. Management of patient data files will become easier as additional data-management features are added to the programmer; the physician will be able to obtain a patient-programming history and other patient-management data. It is conceivable that, in the not-so-distant future, the physician may be able to access patient-device data over the Internet, thus making unnecessary some clinic visits and allowing for remote follow-up of patients who are on holiday or have moved house.

Future devices may allow software loading in a non-invasive manner, to upgrade the device long after implantation. Such capability could be used to provide new therapy algorithms as well as new therapy waveforms.

The future will also bring enhanced test stimulation devices, which will provide improved fixation during the test stimulation period. The development of new leads is one such focus with the aim of allowing a longer test stimulation period without lead migration.

Future applications of the hardware

The future application of SNS is dependent on new clinical research. Pelvic disorders, such as pelvic pain and sexual dysfunction, appear likely to be the first areas of investigation; sacral anterior root stimulation for spinal cord injury may also provide a worthwhile avenue of enquiry. The development of these applications — or of any other, for that matter — will potentially require new waveforms and the development of new therapy algorithms. The future is as open as the availability of resources and the application of science allow.

9 Indications and predictive factors

W.A. Scheepens and

P.E.V. van Kerrebroeck

Introduction

Sacral neuromodulation is an established treatment modality for patients with chronic voiding dysfunction. Since the late 1980s and early 1990s this therapy has evolved in an effective but mainly empirically-based way, as the precise mechanisms of its action are still unknown. Another factor that impairs understanding of the treatment is that no predictive factors have, as yet, been identified and that patient indications are expanding [1]. Urologists that have been sceptical are, therefore, becoming more so, despite the fact that sacral neuromodulation is a US FDA-approved therapy. It must not be forgotten that, for patients treated with sacral neuromodulation, all conservative treatment possibilities have been exhausted and such patients face lifelong self-catheterisation or invasive abdominal surgery. Any patient at that stage must be offered a trial stimulation period to evaluate whether sacral neuromodulation is a possible treatment option, before resorting to an invasive procedure.

This chapter discusses patient indications and predictive factors in selecting the right patient for sacral neuromodulation.

Indications

The US FDA have approved three indications for patients with chronic voiding dysfunction, refractory to appropriate conventional treatments, which generally fit into one of the following categories:

1. urinary urge incontinence;
2. urgency–frequency syndrome;
3. voiding difficulty:
   - incomplete voiding or incomplete retention (>50ml residual);
   - complete retention; unable to initiate normal micturition.

Refractory – Unresponsive applied to a condition that fails to respond satisfactorily to a given treatment.

Lower urinary tract dysfunctions

Urinary urge incontinence, from a urodynamic point of view, can be caused by detrusor instability or detrusor hyperreflexia. There are some similarities between detrusor hyperreflexia and detrusor instability, which suggest that both can have a neurological cause. Detailed neurophysiological testing and imaging has, as yet, failed to show any such deficit in idiopathic instability; the term 'non-neurogenic' therefore refers to the fact that a neurogenic abnormality is not evident. Owing to the complexity of neuromuscular control of vesico-urethral function, a subtle neurogenic cause (central or peripheral) cannot be excluded.

The origin of detrusor instability remains obscure, because idiopathic detrusor instability represents a complex web of many contributory causes.

Congenital (immature bladder)

The development of normal urinary control involves a complex physiological relationship dependent on maturation and also on behavioural influences. The persistence of spontaneous instable detrusor contraction, and the child's response to this, plays a key role in the origin of many paediatric urological conditions. Enuresis, recurrent cystitis, vesico-ureteral reflux and Hinman's syndrome may all be manifestations of dysfunctional voiding patterns that are associated with persistent detrusor instability. The degree of structural damage to the urinary tract depends on the frequency, magnitude and duration of elevated intravesical pressures and on the degree of obstruction that is produced by uncoordinated sphincter contraction. The main expression of the immature bladder, however, is persistence of detrusor instability.

Various theories have been proposed to explain the cause of this dysfunctional voiding. McGuire and Savastano state that the primary abnormality is detrusor instability [2]. The detrusor–sphincter dyssynergia that occurs simultaneously originates as a result of sudden unanticipated detrusor contractility. Contraction of the pelvic floor musculature is a normal response to control urgent urination and results in reflex inhibition of the detrusor. After a period of time, these pelvic floor contractions become customary and carry over to voluntary voiding, resulting in an intermittent urinary stream and residual urine.

Ageing

In the elderly, detrusor instability is more common and the prevalence of urge incontinence increases with age, independent of outflow obstruction or neurological disorder. Older men have the same symptoms as women, suggesting that lower urinary tract symptoms are a manifestation of ageing in both sexes. However, the boundaries between detrusor instability and detrusor hyperreflexia are uncertain in this group of patients, since age-associated neurological diseases such as subclinical cerebrovascular disorders, autonomic neuropathy and chronic brain failure (dementia) commonly occur. Functional brain scanning using single-photon emission computed tomography has shown that there is underperfusion of the cortex as a whole, and of the frontal lobes in particular, in geriatric patients with detrusor instability. The subperfusion is particularly noticeable in the right superior lobe [3]. Thus, detrusor instability has been linked with both cognitive impairment and decreased perfusion of the frontal lobes.

On the other hand, abnormal cell-to-cell communications have been reported in elderly people with detrusor instability. Electron microscopy of detrusor biopsies carried out by Elbadawi *et al.* [4] revealed a characteristic structural pattern. The main features of this dysfunctional pattern are abundant protrusion junctions and abutments, which mediate in electrical coupling between muscle cells, generating myogenic contractions.

Psychosomatic factors

There is little current support for a psychological cause for detrusor instability in women. Previous support has been based on the response to behavioural treatment and on the fact that certain psychological factors may trigger urge incontinence, such as the sound of running water, a stressful event, or an event such as turning the key in the front door. Although these events certainly do act as triggers, there is no evidence that the mechanism is primarily psychogenic. By triggering the emotional motor system in the brain, it is possible to influence micturition. This emotional motoric system is located in the limbic systems and gives rise to a descending system that is completely separate from the somatic motor system. All emotionally-related activities together are crucial for the survival of the individual or its species. Parts of this emotional centre represent specific functions such as vocalisation, blood pressure, sexual behaviour and micturition [5].

Hypersensitivity disorders

There is evidence that neuropeptide-containing sensory nerves innervate the human bladder. These sensory afferents are capsaicin-sensitive unmyelinated C fibres and usually transmit sensations of bladder fullness, urgency and pain. Local release of tachykinin and other peptides from sensory nerves in the bladder wall has been shown to produce diverse biological effects, such as bladder smooth muscle contractions, facilitation of neural transmission and increased vascular permeability. These properties of bladder sensory nerves may suggest that increased afferent activity can induce bladder overactivity in patients with hypersensitivity disorders. Since capsaicin can suppress C-fibre sensory neuron activity, Maggi *et al.* instilled capsaicin intravesically in patients with hypersensitive disorders of the lower urinary tract, resulting in the abolition or marked attenuation of their symptoms [6,7]. This result may support the above hypothesis, but knowledge of the sensory function of the bladder is still limited.

Current theories of bladder overactivity

Current thinking explains all forms of bladder overactivity in the light of two principal hypotheses — the myogenic and neurogenic theories. Separation into these two groups is useful when attempting to explain the aetiology of the disorder; however, the division is artificial, as muscle and nerve function are so intimately linked that a disorder in one system will produce secondary changes in the other. Mechanisms of bladder overactivity vary with different aetiologies (neurogenic bladder, outflow obstruction, ageing, hypersensitivity, etc.); it is not easy, therefore, to find a common feature that underlies detrusor overactivity. In this respect, Brading and Turner have emphasised the myogenic changes (regardless of aetiology) [8,9]. On the basis of observations that denervation is consistently found in detrusor biopsy specimens from patients

Key Points
- Bladder overactivity has been explained as myogenic or neurogenic.

Key Points

- It may stem from changes in smooth muscle, leading to detrusor contraction.
- Bladder overactivity may arise from several neural alterations.
- Antimuscarinic drugs can improve symptoms of detrusor overactivity.
- Activation of postganglionic neurons, from any cause, may produce unstable detrusor contraction.
- SNS is effective therapy for urge incontinence.

with various forms of detrusor instability, they proposed that partial denervation of the detrusor may alter the properties of smooth muscle, leading to increased excitability and increased coupling of cells. Thus, local contraction that occurs at some point in the detrusor will spread throughout the bladder wall, resulting in coordinated myogenic contraction of the whole detrusor. However, what actually triggers this local contraction is not resolved. As Brading [9] has stated, the changes in smooth muscle properties seem to be a necessary prerequisite for the production of instable detrusor contraction.

Bladder overactivity may be caused by (a) decreased inhibitory control in the central nervous system (CNS), (b) reorganisation of spinal reflex pathways, (c) increased afferent activity, (d) increased sensitivity to efferent stimulation in the detrusor or (e) a combination of these factors. Whichever factors are involved, it is important to note that unstable detrusor contraction is actually induced by postganglionic neurons in the detrusor. From a clinical point of view it is clear that, in any form of detrusor overactivity, antimuscarinic drugs can improve symptoms, reduce urgency, and increase bladder capacity; this may suggest that postganglionic cholinergic neurons are activated, leading to detrusor instability. Even in the myogenic theory of detrusor instability, the neurogenic factors are required to trigger such instability. Thus, in the case of detrusor instability, some activation of postganglionic neurons (cholinergic or purinergic) may occur during bladder filling, whereas this activation can be directly caused by an uninhibited micturition reflex (supraspinal or spinal) in the case of detrusor hyperreflexia.

Both neurogenic and myogenic mechanisms may be involved in the pathogenesis of bladder overactivity. Although the cause of overactive bladder differs in neurogenic bladder dysfunction, aetiology-related detrusor instability, idiopathic detrusor instability, and activation of postganglionic neurons may finally produce the same effect on bladder behaviour — instable detrusor contraction.

Urinary urge incontinence

The urinary bladder has two functions — the storage of urine and the evacuation of urine at socially convenient times. The most common problem with urine storage arises when the bladder fails to remain relaxed until an appropriate time for micturition is present. As previously stated this bladder overactivity can be caused by detrusor hyperreflexia or detrusor instability on the basis of the presence or absence of a clinically-detectable neurological disorder; however, abnormal bladder behaviour in both situations is characterised by the same urodynamic entity — involuntary detrusor contraction. Urge incontinence is defined as an involuntary loss of urine with urge sensations, which causes social and hygienic problems [10]. Patients with detrusor instability can have urge incontinence.

Several prospective studies have shown the efficacy of sacral neuromodulation in refractory urge-incontinent patients. Sacral nerve stimulation therapy appeared to provide sustained clinical benefit, defined as a greater than 50% reduction in symptoms, for 18–72 months after implantation [11–13]. Single-centre and multicentre studies have demonstrated a significant therapeutical effect in urge incontinence, varying from 41% to 100% [11–23].

In August 1997 the US FDA approved the implantation of a sacral neuromodulation system for patients with refractory urge incontinence.

Urgency–frequency syndrome

The urgency–frequency syndrome is another manifestation of the overactive bladder. It is characterised by an uncontrollable urge to void, resulting in frequent, small amounts of urine voided as often as every 15 minutes. Patients report that they do not feel empty after voiding. Often, but not always, pain or discomfort accompanies this condition. Incontinent episodes may occur but are not the primary complaint. Other urological conditions associated with this syndrome are urethral syndrome, pelvic pain such as prostatodynia, orchalgia and interstitial cystitis; related non-urological conditions include irritable bowel, proctalgia and anal sphincter instability.

From a urodynamic point of view, these patients do not demonstrate an unstable detrusor contraction on provocative cystometry; they have thus been diagnosed as having sensory as opposed to motor urgency — the urgency–frequency syndrome.

Because the aetiology of irritative voiding symptoms such as urgency–frequency remains unknown, knowledge of the relevant pathophysiology is still fairly limited. Current theories have recognised this syndrome as a significant indication of increased fragility or excitability in the sacral reflex neural regulation of voiding. It is considered to be the result of an imbalance between the facilitatory and excitatory control systems, causing a hyperexcitable micturition reflex. Pelvic floor spasticity seems to be the main consequence of augmentation of sensory input into the CNS (for example, peripheral inflammation) or a loss of intrinsic CNS inhibitory circuits due to neural pathology.

There are few effective treatments for refractory urinary urgency–frequency. Urgency–frequency symptoms can have a marked impact on the quality of life of patients [24]. Therefore, in patients in whom the urgency–frequency syndrome is refractory a trial stimulation must be considered. A multicentre study by Hassouna *et al.* on the efficacy and safety of this proceedure has shown a significant increase in voided volume per void and a decrease in number of voids per 24 hours and degree of urgency prior to voiding: in 56% of the patients a significant reduction was achieved; 32% of the patients obtained a slight reduction; sustained clinical benefit was achieved for 2 years after the implantation [24]. Other studies have also shown clinical benefits of sacral neuromodulation in the urgency–frequency syndrome, in 43–83% of patients [25–31].

Urinary retention

Patients with bladder-emptying problems can experience voiding symptoms (for example, hesitancy, loss of force of the urinary stream, decrease of the calibre of the stream), incomplete voiding (more than 50ml residual urine in the bladder after voiding) or

Key Points

- Urgency–frequency is of unknown aetiology.
- It probably results from a hyperexcitable micturition reflex.
- As urgency–frequency affects QoL, SNS must be tried.
- SNS has given good results in patients with urgency–frequency.

Key Points

- Bladder-emptying problems can have one of two causes.
- These are impaired detrusor contraction and bladder outlet obstruction.
- Both can have functional or organic causes.
- Organic causes respond to surgery; functional causes are difficult to treat.
- Toilet-training problems may lead to non-neurogenic bladder hypo/acontractility.
- Detrusor contractility decreases with age in both sexes.

complete retention (inability to initiate a void). Functionally, micturition is a result of two factors — detrusor contraction and urethral resistance; bladder-emptying problems can be caused, therefore, by impaired detrusor contraction (weak or no bladder contraction) or bladder outlet obstruction (high urethral resistance). Both can have organic or functional causes. Impaired detrusor contractions secondary to benign prostatic hyperplasia or high urethral resistance due to strictures are examples of organic causes and can be surgically treated. In functional causes, however, no organic defects can be demonstrated, so that the treatment of these disorders very often does not address the cause. Detrusor hypocontractility or acontractility and/or spastic pelvic floor syndrome may be responsible for failure to empty the bladder. The underlying pathophysiology of these functional causes has not been clearly elucidated and is probably multifactorial.

Bladder hypocontractility or acontractility

The acontractile detrusor is one that does not demonstrably contract during urodynamic studies. In cases where no neurogenic disease is evident, the hypocontractility is considered to be idiopathic.

Non-neurogenic bladder hypocontractility/acontractility

Idiopathic non-obstructive bladder hypocontractility/acontractility is a perplexing entity in modern urological practice. Some functional disorders during the maturation phase, such as poor voiding habits or the results of forced toilet training, can become manifest over time. The desire to void is a sensation which, in the developed child, is incorporated into daily life so that voiding takes place at an appropriate time and place. Problems with training or psychological difficulties can have a great impact on the results. Misuse of the pelvic floor may cause a change in dynamics of the lower urinary tract function. If the neural reflexes are not conditioned appropriately as a result of constant misuse (e.g. voiding by using abdominal muscle instead of relaxing pelvic floor muscles), these neural reflexes may undergo a permanent change. Since inhibitory reflexes are learned during maturation of the nervous system, proper use of the pelvic floor is critical to correct development of these behavioural reflexes. Some parents send their child to the toilet many times, although the bladder may be empty. Voiding in these circumstances can only be achieved by abdominal straining. As the child will be rewarded on production of even the smallest amount of urine, the result may be an abnormal voiding pattern. The same is true when children receive negative feedback related to voiding. Children with a lazy bladder void infrequently, the result usually being urinary tract infection and overflow incontinence. Long-standing overactivity of the pelvic floor is thought to be responsible for decompensation of the detrusor, leading to a non-contractile bladder. However, no data are available to support this theory.

A mild degree of bladder weakness occurs quite commonly in older individuals. There is a clear and significant reduction in detrusor contractility with age, both in women and in men. In the absence of previous obstruction, the detrusor is characterised at the cellular level by widespread degenerative changes of both muscle cells and axons, without accompanying regenerative changes. These degenerative changes can easily explain the limited capacity of muscle cells to generate contraction, as well as being an impediment of the neural mechanism that triggers it at the muscle cell level.

Pelvic floor muscle-urethral external sphincter overactivity

The sacral micturition reflex is a positive feedback system that is poised to empty the bladder unless acted on by inhibitory reflexes. Any deficiency in the inhibitory reflexes acting on the detrusor are likely to result in bladder overactivity, including urge incontinence and urgency–frequency. One of the best-known inhibitory reflexes of the detrusor results from external sphincter contraction. Weaknesses in the pelvic floor that prevent sufficient contraction of the sphincter may, therefore, result in an uninhibited detrusor. The converse is also true in patients with voiding dysfunction: if the pelvic floor muscles and sphincter are tetanically contracted, the detrusor is inhibited to the point of overfilling and distending the bladder.

Some cases of voiding dysfunction are associated with some degree of hyperactivity of the pelvic floor and external urethral sphincter muscles. These patients have a lack of pelvic control, as shown by their inability to localise the pelvic floor. A theory is that, in these patients, there is overinhibition of the voiding reflex through a pathological reflex [30]. Schmidt has suggested that neuromodulation may function through directing the patient to relocalise the pelvic floor and, hence, to regain the capability of relaxing it and initiating voiding [32].

Fowler's syndrome

In 1988, Fowler and colleagues described a syndrome in young women in whom urinary retention was the predominant clinical feature and electromyography (EMG) of the striated muscle of the urethral sphincter revealed abnormal activity [33]. The EMG activity is localised exclusively to the urethral sphincter and consists of a type of activity that would be expected to cause inappropriate contraction of the muscle in which it is found. The EMG activity has many features of myotonia, a condition in which a striated muscle remains in a state of sustained activity following contraction. However, detailed EMG analysis shows that there are significant differences and that sphincter activity consists of two components — complex repetitive discharges and a decelerating burst. Why this type of EMG activity should develop in the urethral sphincter is unknown. The observation by Fowler that women with urinary retention also often have polycystic ovaries raises the possibility that the activity is linked in some way to hormonal imbalance, perhaps impairing muscle membrane stability and allowing a direct spread of electrical impulses throughout the muscle. Whatever the cause or nature of the abnormal EMG, urinary retention seems to be produced by impaired sphincter relaxation. Although the hypothesis that urinary retention in these young women is the result of a primary failure of relaxation of the

Key Points

- Sacral micturition reflex imbalance may cause bladder overactivity or detrusor inhibition.
- Voiding dysfunction may arise from lack of pelvic control.
- SNS may help patients to localise and relax the pelvic floor.
- In Fowler's syndrome, impaired sphincter relaxation causes urinary retention.

Key Points

- SNS may benefit patients with Fowler's syndrome.
- PNE is the only way to assess potential success of SNS.
- Patients with positive (>50%) PNE results are candidates for implantation.
- However, a positive PNE test does not guarantee success after implantation.

sphincter remains to be proved, some indirect findings support this idea. Thus evidence has been provided showing the existence of a group of women with an abnormally high urethral pressure profile and obstructed voiding, in whom ultrasound studies focusing on sphincter volume showed local muscle hypertrophy.

Patients diagnosed as having the Fowler syndrome are good candidates for sacral neuromodulation [34].

Predictive factors

Clinical parameters for selecting the right patient for sacral neuromodulation have not yet been well defined; therefore, before a permanent implant is placed, a temporary lead is implanted to evaluate any advantageous effects of the sacral neuromodulation system. Koldewijn and colleagues showed that bladder overactivity and urethral instability gave the best response to test stimulation but were not predictors of success; neither could gender, patient age, history or diagnosis qualify as a predictive factor [1]. The only way to assess the potential success of sacral neuromodulation after a permanent implant is by peripheral nerve evaluation (PNE). If a PNE test reveals a positive (more than 50%) improvement in a patient's key voiding parameters according to baseline and PNE-test voiding diaries, that patient is a candidate for implantation.

Success rates after implantation have been mentioned previously in different indications. It is not possible, however, to conclude that a positive PNE test is a predictive factor, as those patients who did not have a positive PNE test did not receive an implant; these patient categories, therefore, cannot be compared. Further research in exploring predictive factors is essential to improve the therapy and patient indications.

References

1. Koldewijn EL, Rosier PF, Meuleman EJ et al. Predictors of success with neuromodulation in lower urinary tract dysfunction: results of trial stimulation in 100 patients. *J Urol* 1994; 152: 2071–5.
2. McGuire EJ, Savastano JA. Urodynamic studies in enuresis and the nonneurogenic/neurogenic bladder. *J Urol* 1984; 132(2): 299–302
3. Blok BF, Willemsen AT, Holstege G. A PET study on brain control of micturition in humans. *Brain* 1997; 120: 111–21.
4. Elbadawi A, Yalla S, Resnick N. Structural basis of geriatric voiding dysfunction. Aging detrusor: normal vs impaired contractility. *J Urol* 1993; 150: 1657.
5. Blok BFM, Holstege G. Neuronal control of micturition and its relation to the emotional motor system. *Prog Brain Res* 1998; 107:113–26
6. Maggi CA. Tachykinins and calcitonin gene-related peptide (CGRP) as co-transmitters released from peripheral endings of sensory nerves. *Prog Neurobiol* 1995; 45(1): 1–98.
7. Maggi CA, Barbanti G, Santicioli P et al. Cystometric evidence that capsaicin-sensitive nerves modulate the afferent branch of micturition reflex in humans. *J Urol* 1989; 142(1): 150–4
8. Brading AF, Turner W. The unstable bladder: towards a common mechanism. *Bri J Urol* 1994; 73: 3.
9. Brading AF. A myogenic basis for the overactive bladder. *Urology* 1997; 50 (Suppl 6A): 57–67.

10. Abrams P, Blaivas JG, Stanton SL, Andersen JT. The standardisation of terminology of lower urinary tract function. The International Continence Society Committee on Standardisation of Terminology. *Scan J Urol Nephrol* 1988; 114: 5–19.

11. Schmidt RA, Jonas U, Oleson KA *et al*. Sacral nerve stimulation for treatment of refractory urinary urge incontinence. Sacral Nerve Stimulation Study Group. *J Urol* 1999; 162: 352–7.

12. Bosch JL, Groen J. Sacral nerve neuromodulation in the treatment of patients with refractory motor urge incontinence: long-term results of a prospective longitudinal study. *J Urol* 2000; 163: 1219–22.

13. Weil EH, Ruiz Cerdá JL, Eerdmans PH *et al*. Sacral root neuromodulation in the treatment of refractory urinary urge incontinence: a prospective randomized clinical trial. *Eur Urol* 2000; 37: 161–71.

14. Bemelmans BL, Mundy AR, Craggs MD. Neuromodulation by implant for treating lower urinary tract symptoms and dysfunction. *Eur Urol* 1999; 36: 81–91.

15. Bosch JL, Groen J. Sacral (S3) segmental nerve stimulation as a treatment for urge incontinence in patients with detrusor instability: results of chronic electrical stimulation using an implantable neural prosthesis. *J Urol* 1995; 154: 504–7.

16. Bosch JL, Groen J. Neuromodulation: urodynamic effects of sacral (S3) spinal nerve stimulation in patients with detrusor instability or detrusor hyperflexia. *Behav Brain Res* 1998; 92: 141–50.

17. Braun PM, Boschert J, Bross S *et al*. Tailored laminectomy: a new technique for neuromodulator implantation. *J Urol* 1999; 162 :1607–9.

18. Ishigooka M, Zermann DH, Doggweiler R, Schmidt RA. Sacral nerve stimulation and diurnal urine volume. *Eur Urol* 1999; 36: 421–6.

19. Malouf AJ, Vaizey CJ, Nicholls RJ, Kamm MA. Permanent sacral nerve stimulation for fecal incontinence. *Ann Surg* 2000; 232: 143–8.

20. Bosch JL, Groen J. Treatment of refractory urge urinary incontinence with sacral spinal nerve stimulation in multiple sclerosis patients. *Lancet* 1996; 348: 717–9.

21. Shaker H, Hassouna MM. Sacral root neuromodulation in the treatment of various voiding and storage problems. *Int Urogynecol J Pelvic Floor Dysfunct* 1999; 10: 336–43.

22. Tanagho EA. Prinzipien und indikationen der elektrostimulation der harnblase. *Urologe [A]* 1990; 29: 185–90.

23. Weil EH, Ruiz Cerdá JL, Eerdmans PH *et al*. Clinical results of sacral neuromodulation for chronic voiding dysfunction using unilateral sacral foramen electrodes. *World J Urol* 1998; 16: 313–21.

24. Hassouna MM, Siegel SW, Lycklama á Nijeholt AAB *et al*. Sacral neuromodulation in the treatment of urgency–frequency symptoms: a multicenter study on efficacy and safety. *J Urol* 2000; 163: 1849–54.

25. Hassouna MM, Group NSS. Effect of sacral neuromodulation on urinary urgency–frequency. *J Urol* 1999; 162: 254.

26. Weil EHJ, Ruiz Cerdá JL, Eerdmans PH *et al*. Clinical results of sacral neuromodulation for chronic voiding dysfunction using unilateral sacral foramen electrodes. *World J Urol* 1998; 16: 313–21.

27. Hasan ST, Neal DE. Neuromodulation in bladder dysfunction. *Curr Opin Obstet Gynecol* 1998: 10(5) 395–9.

28. Bower WF, Moore KH, Adams RD, Shepherd R. A urodynamic study of surface neuromodulation versus sham in detrusor instability and sensory urgency. *J Urol* 1998; 160: 2133–6.

29. Walsh IK, Johnston RS, Keane PF. Transcutaneous sacral neurostimulation for irritative voiding dysfunction. *Eur Urol* 1999; 35(3): 192–6.

30. Elabbady AA, Hassouna MM, Elhilali MM. Neural stimulation for chronic voiding dysfunctions. *J Urol* 1994; 152: 2076–80.

31. Chai TC, Zhang C, Warren JW, Keay S. Percutaneous sacral third nerve root neurostimulation improves symptoms and normalizes urinary HB-EGF levels and antiproliferative activity in patients with interstitial cystitis. *Urology* 2000; 55: 643–6.

32. Schmidt R. Advances in genitourinary neurostimulation. *Neurosurgery* 1986; 19: 1041–44.

33. Fowler CJ, Christmas TJ, Chapple CR *et al*. Abnormal electromyographic activity of the urethral sphincter, voiding dysfunction, and polycystic ovaries: a new syndrome? *Br Med J* 1988; 297: 1436–8.

34. Swinn M, Kitchen N, Goodwin R, Fowler CJ. Sacral neuromodulation for women with Fowler's syndrome. *Eur Urol* 2000; 38: 439–443.

10 Sacral nerve stimulation: PNE

S.W. Siegel

Temporary sacral nerve stimulation: PNE

Peripheral nerve evaluation (PNE) is the first step needed to determine whether sacral nerve stimulation (SNS) for the control of lower urinary tract dysfunction is appropriate for a given patient. It is a temporary application of neuromodulation, both as a therapy and a diagnostic test — yielding accurate information about the location, integrity and function of the sacral nerves, the nature of a patient's symptoms, and the likelihood that SNS will ultimately improve the symptoms and quality of life. If symptoms improve significantly, this is an indication that they are neuromuscular in nature and that there is a high degree of probability that a permanent implant will be effective. Thus, PNE uniquely provides an objective demonstration of the potential benefit of SNS to the patient and clinician, allowing them both to make an informed choice about the therapy.

Patient preparation

Once the appropriate pretreatment diagnostic studies have been completed, the patient with intractable voiding dysfunction is offered the option to undergo PNE. It is important to explain fully the rationale of PNE — the procedure specifics, potential risks and benefits — and to prepare the patient to limit activities and make objective observations during the length of the trial. Patients must complete accurate voiding diaries prior to the test; these will then be used as a comparative baseline. Specific, relevant instruction and review of the diaries prior to the PNE is essential. Patients should maintain their usual fluid intake and medications as the trial is conducted. It is also important that they limit physical activities that may reduce the length of time needed to judge the efficacy of the trial: we advise the patients to avoid exercise, to move with care so as not to displace the temporary electrodes, and to limit bathing for the first 3 days of a trial. If patients are curious to see the impact of the trial stimulation on symptoms of dyspareunia, we encourage them to wait to have intercourse until at least 3 days of diary data have been collected.

For very anxious or sensitised patients, it may be helpful to give them premedication with a benzodiazepine, or to apply a topical anaesthetic such as EMLA cream (lignocaine plus prilocaine) to the presacral skin 30 minutes before testing. It is also important to make patients aware of how and where they may feel the temporary stimulation during the conduct of the trial: they may be told that the stimulation should feel like a 'pulling' or a 'vibration' in the rectal or genital areas. Appropriately positioned foramen needles and test electrodes

Key Points
- PNE objectively shows patients and clinician the potential benefit of SNS.
- Patient information, explanation and preparation is important.
- Patients must complete accurate voiding diaries before PNE.
- Voiding diaries give baseline information; they must be reviewed before PNE.
- During the trial, patients should limit exercise, movement and bathing.
- Patients must be told how and when they may feel the temporary stimulation.

Key Points

- Stimulation should be comfortable/soothing, not painful/shock-like.
- Patients should be helped to relax during the trial.
- An assistant must be present to operate the hand-held screener and attend to the patient.
- Patients are positioned prone on a flat, padded table, with hips supported.
- Necessary materials are included in the Medtronic PNE kit.
- The S3 foramen is located in several ways by bony landmarks.

should be comfortable or soothing when stimulated: painful or shock-like sensations indicate that an ideal position relative to the nerve has not been achieved. Patients should be given examples and encouragement to use specific anatomical terms in describing the location of paraesthesiae. Above all, it is important to help patients to remain as relaxed as possible during the trial, keeping them well informed about what to expect as the trial progresses.

Location

The PNE can reasonably be performed in an office or hospital setting; this will depend on individual concerns such as space, equipment, cost and personal preference (for example, whether fluoroscopy or intravenous sedation is to be used during the procedure). It is essential to have an assistant to operate the hand-held screener and to tend to the patient's comfort. Ideally, there should be room to allow a friend or family member to be present near the patient during the procedure, if requested.

Positioning and preparation

A flat, padded table is essential. The patient should be positioned prone, using pillows for the face, hips, and shins (Fig. 10.1). The hips should be supported in order to flatten the back and minimise lumbar lordosis. The assistant must have ready access to the feet and calves in order to report the physical responses during stimulation. Some practitioners prefer to tape the buttock cheeks open in order to allow direct visualisation of the anus during acute stimulation, but this is not necessary in order to see a 'bellows' response (inward rolling of the intergluteal fold), and is uncomfortable and extremely embarrassing for the patient; it is therefore the author's strong preference not to do this. The test stimulation product supplied by Medtronic (Table 10.1) contains the materials needed to prepare and drape the presacral area and to perform the entire procedure; a few additional supplies such as a local anaesthetic and basic instruments (scissors, forceps) are needed. The area below the posterior superior iliac crests, between the lateral edges of the greater sciatic notches and above the crease between the buttocks and upper thighs, is draped off after preparation with a warmed antiseptic solution. The grounding pad is affixed to the patient's heel, where it can be easily checked. The patient screener is connected by the cables supplied to the ground pad and to the patient screener cable.

Performing the procedure

Bony landmarks are used to identify the S3 foramen; several different methods can be employed simultaneously in order to assess its location (Table 10.2). First, the midline is determined by palpating the central spinous processes and drawing a line through the middle of the sacrum. Next, the level of the

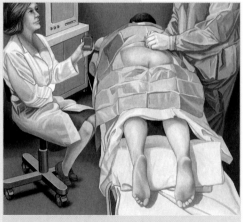

Figure 10.1 Patient position and preparation.

Table 10.1 *Materials required*

Test stimulation lead kit	Test stimulator kit	Test stimulation cables
Preparation supplies	*Non-sterile*	*Non-sterile*
Surgical drapes	1 test stimulator	Long cable is used in the
PVP solution	1 9V battery	office short cable is used
Swab stick	1 attachment clip	duringthe test period
Sterile marker	1 operator manual	when the patient is at
Control syringe		home
Gauze		
Bandages		
Needle for local anaesthetic		
Sterile procedural supplies		
2 foramen needles (3.5"/9cm)		
1 test stimulation lead		
1 patient cable		
Non-sterile procedural supplies		
Ground pads		
Product literature		

greater sciatic notches is located by direct palpation. This can be simplified by tracing along the lateral edge of the sacrum until the traced outline becomes perpendicular to the midline, which is the sciatic notch (Fig. 10.2); the S3 foramen is one finger-breadth lateral to the midline at the level of the greater sciatic notch. A method of cross-checking is to sight across the patient, and to estimate the point at which the sacrum is parallel to the floor; this high point, or crest of the sacrum, is typically at S4, or one fingerbreadth caudal to the S3 foramen. A third method of identification is to measure a point in the midline 9cm (about one hand's breadth) cephalad from the tip of the coccyx; this correlates with S4. By combining these methods, the skin over the S3 foramen can usually be identified quickly and accurately. In cases where there is difficulty, fluoroscopy (if it is readily available) may be used to locate the foramen. Typically, the medial edge of the foramen can be identified with a PA view and, if a C-arm is used, the radiographic plane can be sighted down the shaft of the needle in order to direct

Table 10.2 *Methods of locating the S3 foramen*

• Greater sciatic notches and central spinous process
• Crest or high point of sacrum
• Measure up 9cm from tip of coccyx
• Fluoroscopy

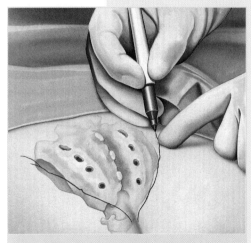

Figure 10.2 *Identification of bony landmarks.*

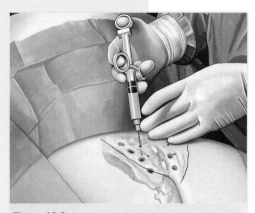

Figure 10.3 *Local anaesthesia of skin and periosteum.*

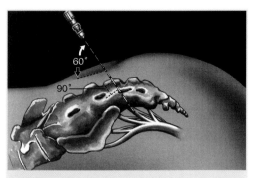

Figure 10.4 *Appropriate needle orientation within S3.*

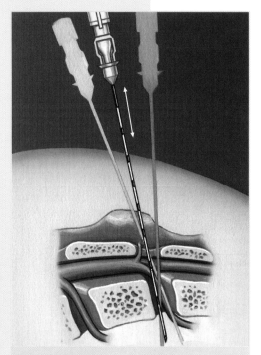

Figure 10.5 *Adjustment of needle orientation within foramen to improve acute responses.*

its position further. A lateral view with fluoroscopy is also useful in estimating the depth of needle or electrode placement relative to the anterior sacral surface.

The skin over S3 is infiltrated with 1–2ml 1% lignocaine, using a fine-gauge needle. It is important to create a skin weal or 'peau d'orange' appearance in order to achieve adequate skin analgesia. Deeper layers may be infiltrated; however, other than skin, the most important area to anaesthetise is the posterior sacral periosteum, which typically is very sensitive. The foramen needle is passed through the skin and, when the periosteum is touched, 5–10ml lignocaine is placed at that level. During infiltration, it is helpful to probe the sacral surface gently with the tip of the foramen needle, making sure that a broad area is covered (Fig. 10.3). This is also an initial opportunity to locate the foramen; if it is identified at this point, further infiltration should cease.

Once the posterior sacral surface has been anaesthetised, it can be safely probed with the needle tip without fear of patient discomfort. The needle depth is checked upon first touching the sacral surface, and a note should be made of the level. When the foramen has been entered, the further depth of insertion should be about 1.5–2cm from this point. A line parallel and one finger-breadth lateral to the sacral midline is probed by 'walking' the tip of the foramen needle (with stylet inserted to minimise the potential for tissue shearing) along the sacrum, until a 'drop-off' into the foramen is detected. If no foramen is identified, the landmarks should be rechecked and a line slightly lateral or medial to the first should be probed. It is important to pay attention to the orientation of the foramen needle relative to the skin surface: correct orientation within the S3 foramen should be parallel to the midline, at approximately a 60-degree angle to the skin (Fig. 10.4). Orientation within S2 is usually more acute; within S4, it is almost perpendicular to the skin surface. By maintaining such an orientation within the appropriate foramen, the ideal contact between the needle/lead and the nerve ramus can be achieved. If the tip of the needle is orientated medially there is a risk of mechanical stimulation of the nerve, which is perceived as a painful shock to the patient and must be resolved by immediate repositioning within the foramen (Fig. 10.5). For example, if the needle is orientated too perpendicularly it is possible to stimulate S2 within the S3 foramen.

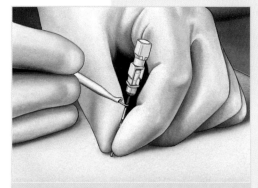

Figure 10.6 *The uninsulated portion of the needle is stimulated with the patient screener cable.*

Acute simulation

Once the needle has been positioned within the foramen, the patient screener cable should be attached to the uninsulated portion of the foramen needle, which is located immediately beneath the hub (Fig 10.6). This area must be separated from the skin by an insulated segment of the needle. To do this may require pushing the skin near the needle hub down during stimulation; alternatively, in very obese patients, a 12cm foramen needle must be used. The amplitude of stimulation is gradually increased from zero, checking for the first sensation registered by the patient. It can then be increased slowly, observing for physical responses, but only to the point where the patient perceives the stimulation as strong but not painful. Care must be taken to avoid 'zapping' the patient by ramping up too quickly; this procedure must be individualised to each patient because of the variable positioning between the needle and nerve, and the sensitivity of the subject. If stimulation is painful at low levels, the needle should almost always be repositioned more lateral to the nerve. Ideally, the patient should perceive stimulation as comfortable and soothing. If pelvic pain is a part of the clinical presentation, it is encouraging if the patient feels the stimulation as paraesthesia in the area of the pain.

Responses

Typical responses (Table 10.3) at S3 are a 'bellows' movement of the pelvic floor, which is a rolling-inward motion of the intergluteal fold; plantar flexion of the great toe (or toes) should also be seen. Patients will feel paraesthesiae in the rectum, perineum, scrotum or vagina. Responses at S2 include a 'clamp' movement, or a twisting and pinching of the anal sphincter, which may also be noticed as a pulling-down of the coccyx. The lower-extremity motions associated with S2 include plantar flexion of the entire foot, lateral rotation of the heel and calf cramping; usually there is also obvious gluteal contraction and/or hip movement. Patients feel stimulation in the genital area and in the leg. The S4 responses include a 'bellows' motion of the pelvic floor and no lower-extremity activity, with patients typically sensing pulling in the rectum only.

Key Points

- Correct needle/skin angle is 60° in S3; less in S2; almost 90° in S4.
- Medial orientation of the needle tip may stimulate the nerve mechanically.
- This gives the patient a painful shock and mandates needle repositioning.
- Acute stimulation must be increased slowly until perceived as strong, *not* painful.
- Responses to stimulation differ according to the foramen penetrated.

Table 10.3 *Responses of patient to stimulation*

Nerve innervation	Response		Sensation
	Pelvic floor	Foot/calf/leg	
S2 Primary somatic contributor of pudendal nerve for external sphincter, leg, foot	'Clamp'* of anal sphincter	Leg/hip rotation, plantar flexion of entire foot, contraction of calf	Contraction of base of penis, vagina
S3 Virtually all pelvic autonomic functions and striated muscle (levator ani)	'Bellows'** of perineum	Plantar flexion of great toe, occasionally other toes	Pulling in rectum, extending forward to scrotum or labia
S4 Pelvic, autonomic, and somatic. No leg or foot	'Bellows'**	No lower-extremity motor stimulation	Pulling in rectum only

*Clamp: contraction of anal sphincter and, in males, retraction of base of penis. Move buttocks aside and look for anterior/posterior shortening of the perineal structures.

**Bellows: lifting and dropping of pelvic floor. Look for deepening and flattening of buttock groove.

The site yielding an S3 response is usually the most appropriate for subchronic stimulation. If S2 or S4 responses are determined upon initial needle positioning, a site below or above the initial site should be selected, the skin and periosteum should be infiltrated with anaesthetic, and the procedure should be repeated.

Placement of the temporary electrode

The temporary electrode is placed once S3 has been identified by acute stimulation. The depth of the electrode is marked on the surface for both 7 and 12cm foramen needles. The foramen needle stylet is removed and the temporary electrode is gently threaded into the lumen until the point marked on the electrode just disappears into the hub, or when resistance from the tissue beyond the needle tip is met. Stimulation of the temporary electrode is helpful in confirming its accurate positioning. At this point, the electrode is stabilised with fingers or a forceps as the needle is withdrawn around it. It may be helpful to continue to stimulate the temporary electrode and constantly to monitor the patient response during this process; this can help to ensure that the electrode is not inserted too deeply or has accidentally been pulled back during needle withdrawal. Once the temporary electrode has been advanced beyond the tip of the foramen needle, the needle should never be pushed back down along the temporary electrode, as this may result in the tip shearing off. If the electrode has been inserted too deeply after needle withdrawal, it is possible to stimulate and withdraw the temporary electrode simultaneously while its stylet is still in place, until the appropriate responses are seen again. Once responses are confirmed, the electrode is grasped and stabilised while the foramen needle and electrode stylet are completely removed. If the acute stimulation responses cannot be duplicated, it is usually necessary to remove the temporary electrode, replace the foramen needle, and reposition the temporary electrode. Once the stylet from the temporary electrode has been withdrawn, it is necessary to use a new electrode if repositioning is required.

The temporary electrode is secured to the skin using the benzoin solution and breathable membrane dressings supplied in the kit. The ground pad is positioned on the patient's back, near the site of the lead placement, and the connections are made to the appropriate patient screener cable. All redundant portions of the electrode and the connection to the ground pad are covered with a dressing (Fig 10.7).

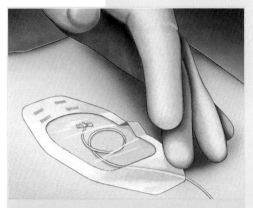

Figure 10.7 *Breathable membrane dressing over test lead insertion site.*

Documentation of responses and radiographic confirmation

It is essential to record the acute responses accurately and to obtain AP and lateral sacral films (or hard copy from fluoroscopy) to confirm the electrode position after placement. These will be helpful for intraoperative comparison during the implantation phase.

Patient screener

The patient is given instructions regarding the use of the screener (Fig. 10.8). The rate dial is usually set at 10–15pps and taped over so that it cannot be adjusted. The patient is instructed to turn the amplitude up or down, as needed, to maintain a strong but comfortable level of stimulation at all times; adjustment may be needed depending on position (for instance, sitting versus standing) or as the trial progresses. Basic troubleshooting information should also be reviewed carefully with the patient in order to optimise the trial phase. It is important that the patient should be reminded to keep diaries throughout the trial phase and to report any difficulties in using the device as soon as possible.

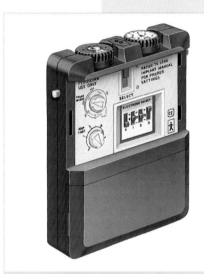

Figure 10.8 *Patient screener.*

Patient selection

The response to the subchronic phase of PNE is used to determine whether a patient's symptoms are sufficiently altered by neuromodulation, and whether the patient should go on to the implantation phase. Baseline and subchronic phase diaries are therefore essential; at least 2 or 3 days of each are needed to make the comparison. If key patient variables (such as the number of incontinent

Key Points

- Electrode stimulation during adjustment may facilitate correct positioning.
- When the stylet has been removed, a new electrode must be used if replacement is needed.
- Records of responses and X-ray confirmation of electrode position are essential.
- Remind patients that accurate diaries and reports of screener-use problems are important.

Key Points

- Comparison of baseline and subchronic diaries is crucial.
- Changes (≥ 50%) in patient variables indicate a good candidate for implantation.
- Changes <50% call for an individual decision or repeat test stimulation.
- Marked bowel-symptom improvement is highly predictive of benefit of implantation.
- Electrodiagnostic monitoring and routine 'staged' implants may be future options.

episodes, pads used, degree of incontinence, number of voids, voided or catheterised volumes) change by at least 50%, such patients are excellent candidates for implantation; if the degree of change is less than 50%, the decision can be individualised, or the test stimulation can be repeated. A dramatic impact on bowel symptoms is also a highly predictive sign that the device will be of benefit. Whether to implant on the basis of a decrease of pain symptoms is less certain, and care should be taken to ensure that an objectively measurable parameter (such as those mentioned) is also improved.

Future directions

Future directions include the addition of electrodiagnostic monitoring during the procedure, which will give an electronic signature of the nerves stimulated. If the trial phase is successful, that signature can then be duplicated during the implantation phase, further ensuring a similar level of success. Other measures to be explored include the more routine performance of a 'staged' implant, which involves permanent implantation of the lead electrode, externalised via a tunnelled lead extension, as the first step. If patients respond favourably, the next phase involves removal of the lead extension, and connection and implantation of the implantable pulse generator. However, the relative ease and low cost make the PNE, as described, an invaluable diagnostic tool.

11 Electrophysiological monitoring of sacral nerve stimulation

J.T. Benson

Introduction

Sacral nerve stimulation (SNS) is a surgical therapy involving neural pathways and may be monitored by electrophysiological techniques.

Electrophysiological monitoring of neural function during surgery began with electrocorticographical monitoring of therapeutic surgery for epilepsy at the Mayo Clinic over 30 years ago. The first consortium of people working independently on intraoperative monitoring of neural function met at a workshop in Cleveland, Ohio, at the Case Western Reserve University School of Medicine in September 1977, and the field of electrophysiological monitoring began a rapid growth which is still evolving. Monitoring is now used for patients undergoing a variety of surgical procedures involving the cerebral cortex, brain stem, spinal cord and the cranial and peripheral nerves.

Monitoring of surgical procedures involving peripheral nerves is not new, as surgeons have for many years used the presence or absence of a visible muscle twitch following electrical stimulation of the supplying nerve as an indicator of the nerve's integrity. Such biological monitoring is currently used with SNS, but electrophysiological techniques have made monitoring of many peripheral nerve procedures, including SNS, more sophisticated.

Surgical monitoring is now widely available. In most institutions, the monitoring is provided by clinical neurophysiological staff and specially trained technicians. Although most of these monitors are not currently familiar with the techniques of monitoring SNS, the principles are the same as those for other peripheral nerve monitoring, and the techniques are easily learned. Surgeons practising SNS, unless specifically trained in the electrodiagnostic medicinal techniques specific to peripheral nerve monitoring, would do well to gain the assistance of such monitoring staff.

What is electrophysiological monitoring?

Electrophysiological monitoring can be applied to many procedures, so what does it comprise, especially where it applies to SNS?

The central and peripheral nervous system function can be monitored by various electrophysiological techniques. The techniques particularly valuable for monitoring peripheral nerve function, including the sacral nerves, are the recording of compound muscle action potentials (CMAPs) and electromyography (EMG).

Key Points
- SNS surgeons should call on staff trained in electrophysiological monitoring (EPM).
- Techniques for monitoring peripheral nerve function are compound muscle action potentials (CMAP) and electromyography (EMG) recording.

Key Points

- CMAPs indicate the number of intact axons and functioning muscle fibres.
- CMAPs also indicate function of the neuromuscular junction.

Compound muscle action potentials are the responses evoked by direct stimulation of a nerve while recording from a muscle it innervates. The muscle is composed of many parallel muscle fibres, each capable of conducting an action potential along its length. If the fibres are activated synchronously by an external stimulus, the small action potentials of individual fibres summate to generate a CMAP, which is recordable with standard electrodiagnostic equipment.

The nerve stimulus requires current flow between two electrodes, which goes through the nerve fibres to depolarise the nerve's axons. The two electrodes are the cathode (negative electrode), at which the depolarisation occurs, and the anode (positive electrode). If both stimulating electrodes are located on the nerve, the stimulation is 'bipolar'. Stimulation may also be performed with the cathode on the nerve and the anode situated some distance away — a 'monopolar' stimulus. The latter is the case with sacral test stimulation, with a 'ground pad' acting as the anode and the mini-hook (applied to the foramen needle or the lead) being the cathode. After surgical implantation, the stimulation may be bipolar (using any two of the quadripolar electrodes) or monopolar (using a lead electrode as the cathode and the implanted pulse generator as the anode). Stimulation thresholds may be measured using the stimulus at which a response is first recognised or the stimulus at which all axons in the nerve are activated. The latter parameter is defined as the stimulus at which the response no longer increases, assuming that the stimulus does not spread to another nerve ('supramaximal' response). The stimulator may be a 'constant voltage' stimulator, with a relative scale of 1–10, or a 'constant current' stimulator, which computes resistance and corrects voltage to supply a known level of current which is measured in amperes. The amount of current required to obtain a supramaximal response is a function of how near the stimulating electrode is to the nerve.

The CMAP recording is performed with pairs of electrodes. The electrodes for recording SNS are surface electrodes of varying types. These include patches, applied to the perineum or para-anally and composed of disposable chlorided silver discs mounted on self-adhesive stickers, useful for recording at the anal sphincter. Catheter-mounted ring electrodes are used for urethral recording (Fig.11.1). Sponge-mounted electrodes may be placed transvaginally or transrectally to record the activity of the levator ani.

If properly recorded, CMAPs are reproducible, measurable, biphasic waveforms (Figs.11.2 and 11.3) produced as a nerve conduction study, hence requiring the stimulation to be via the stimulator which is part of the electrodiagnostic equipment. CMAP surface amplitudes are a gauge of the number of intact axons, number of functioning muscle fibres and function of the neuromuscular junction.

Electromyography is a method of monitoring SNS after the stimulating electrodes have been

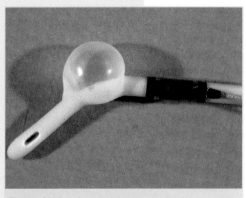

Figure 11.1 *Foley catheter ring electrode: two lengths of platinum wire protected by a plastic coating and positioned 1cm distal to the Foley balloon.*

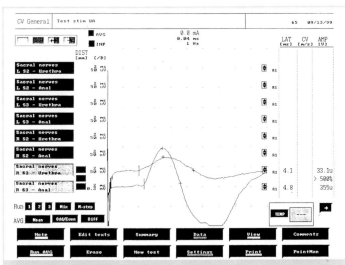

Figure 11.2 *Compound muscle action potentials: stimulation of the right third sacral nerve via a foramen needle. The top waveform (urethra) is the supramaximal, biphasic waveform recorded with the catheter ring electrode. The lower waveform (anal) is recorded with the para-anal surface electrodes. The latency (LAT) of the response is its start, as measured in milliseconds from the time of the stimulus at the beginning of the line. The amplitude is the 'height' of the initial phase, measured in microvolts.*

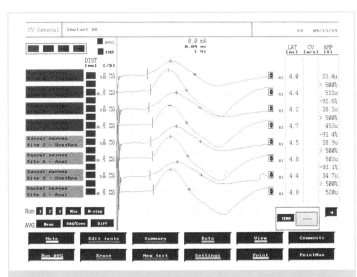

Figure 11.3 *Compound muscle action potentials: study performed during sacral stimulation implant surgery. Stimulation via the four electrodes located on the quadripolar lead: electrode 0, stimulation at top two lines; electrode 1, lines three and four; electrode 2, lines five and six; electrode 3, lines seven and eight. At each stimulation site, recording is performed with a ring electrode in the urethra for urethral CMAP and a sponge located transanally at the levator for anal CMAP. Note moderately large amplitude responses obtained with all four stimulating electrodes, indicating optimal placement of the quadripolar lead.*

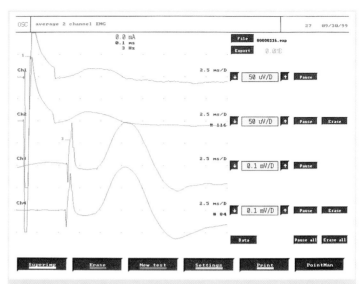

Figure 11.4 *EMG recording of patient with implanted electrode: the top line is the individual CMAP recorded from a urethral lead, held in place on the screen by a 'trigger' marked 1. The trigger is located on the stimulus artefact, which is produced by volume conduction of the current produced by the implanted pulse generator. The second line is the averaged waveform of 116 individual CMAPs from line one. The third line is an individual CMAP obtained from a recording of levator electrodes, held in place on the screen by a 'trigger' marked 3. The fourth line is the averaged waveform from 84 individual CMAPs from line three.*

placed (either with test stimulation or with surgical implantation). This, again, is a process of recording composite muscle fibre activity with surface electrodes but differs from the above-described CMAP in that it is not a nerve conduction study because the stimulation is via the external or implanted generator and not by the stimulator of the electrodiagnostic equipment. The described surface electrodes are applied to the muscle of interest (urethra, levator, anal sphincter) and activity occurring in those muscles is recorded. The recording is displayed on an oscilloscope and requires a 'trigger' that holds the image of interest in a fixed position on the screen. A computer 'averager' can display a mean of several waveforms if variability is present (Fig.11.4).

Why is electrophysiological monitoring necessary?

As SNS can be monitored by biological signs (motor effects of 'bellows', toe movement, etc. and sensory effects of patient description of where sensations are felt), then why should electrophysiological monitoring be performed?

Electrophysiological monitoring provides direct and immediate feedback about the function of neural structures. Such feedback is helpful in (a) identifying which nerve is being stimulated, (b) determining proximity of the stimulating electrodes to the nerve, (c) isolating nerve tissue to help to protect neural struc-

Table 11.1 Results of SNS in various areas.

Area	Nerve root stimulated (mean percentage amplitude) and latency (in ms)		
	Primary root	Secondary root	Tertiary root
Urethra	S3 (65%) 3.5	S4 (23%) 3.1	S2 (12%) 3.8
Levator ani	S3 (73%) 4.0	S4 (23%) 2.9	S2 (4%) 3.4
EAS*	S3 (47%) 3.4	S2 (29%) 4.0	S4 (24%) 3.0
Abductor hallucis	S2 (90%) 23.9	S3 (8%) 24.8	S4 (0%) 26

*EAS, external anal sphincter.

Key Points

- EPM enables stimulation of the sacral nerve that gives the best clinical response.
- EPM ensures selection of the sacral nerve most affecting areas of interest.
- EPM enables precise placement of stimulating electrodes.

tures from operative injury and (d) quantifying the number of axons within the nerve that are being stimulated.

Stimulating the sacral nerve that will give the best clinical response for the patient is a valuable function of electrophysiological monitoring. Although exact mechanisms of sacral stimulation therapy are poorly understood, it is clear that nerves to the levator ani, the urethra and the anal sphincters need to be stimulated selectively. Therefore, in a given patient, monitoring helps to select which sacral nerve in that patient is the principal one supplying these areas. Electrical stimulation of a nerve creates volleys of action potentials, which flow in both directions in the nerve (orthodromic and antidromic). The orthodromic efferent activity is measurable at the target muscle and it is this effect that is measured by monitoring CMAPs. The antidromic afferent activity is instrumental in affecting reflex activation of pelvic nerves and is possibly the more important factor in the mechanisms of action with SNS therapy. This afferent activity is known to be produced when the measurable efferent activity is created.

The most common sacral nerve supplying the sacral areas of interest for SNS therapy is the third sacral nerve, as indicated by Clark *et al* [1], (Table 11.1). However, sacral neuroanatomy is very variable, more so than many other areas of the peripheral nervous system [2, 3]. The use of electrophysiological monitoring ensures selection of the sacral nerve with the greatest effect on the areas of interest, thus increasing the efficacy of SNS therapy. Although the third sacral nerve is the selection of choice in most patients, in some patients the fourth may be a better choice; this decision can be made when using electrophysiological monitoring.

Another reason for using electrophysiological monitoring is for precise placement of the stimulating electrodes. Movement of the stimulating electrode by as little as a millimetre can make an observable and measurable difference to the amount of stimulation received by the nerve. Optimal placement of the stimulating electrode in the sacral foramen can be determined using electrophysiological monitoring.

During surgical implantation for SNS, tissues may be identified as neural by electrical stimulation with electrophysiological monitoring. Such identification assists in protecting the nerve tissue from operative trauma, especially when dissecting near or within the sacral foramina, where nerve visualisation is poor.

Most nerves are a collection of motor and sensory axons of variable size and function. The responses observed with electrophysiological monitoring provide data directly related to the number of axons within the nerve that are being stimulated in response to a known intensity of electrical stimulus. This quantifiable stimulus and response makes the process of SNS therapy objectively measurable. This objectivity is useful in management of an individual patient and extremely valuable in research into SNS therapy.

When should electrophysiological monitoring be used?

As there are many steps or phases to SNS therapy, when is electrophysiological monitoring useful?

Electrophysiological monitoring of SNS may be used in the test stimulation phase, the operative implant stage and for programming after implantation.

During test stimulation, the monitoring ensures that the sacral nerve most involved with innervation of the desired target structures (urethra, levator muscle, anal sphincter) is the one chosen for stimulation. It further assists in localisation of the stimulating lead to the optimal site for stimulating the selected nerve. It makes it possible to verify that the lead wire has remained in position for correct nerve stimulation after the wire has been placed and connected to the external stimulator. This verification may be made immediately after placement of the lead and also at any time during the testing phase if lead wire migration is a possibility. After completion of the test phase, monitoring may be repeated to ascertain that the stimulus was correctly located throughout the testing period.

During surgical implantation, monitoring can assure the surgeon that the nerve selected for stimulation by the implanted quadripolar lead is identical to that selected and stimulated during the test procedure. This can be done by comparing the electrophysiological responses obtained at surgery with those obtained during test stimulation. Comparison of these reproducible physiological results obviates comparison of radiographic studies, which are anatomical only and not necessarily functionally related. Monitoring during surgery also usefully identifies neural tissue, so that dissection or cauterisation injury to the nerve is prevented. However, the chief value of monitoring during implantation is in assisting precise localisation of the quadripolar lead; a minor alteration in the direction or depth of insertion of the lead into the foramen can cause major fluctuations in the observed responses with electrophysiological recording. Analysing the responses enables the lead to be positioned to gain the maximal effect from stimulation with each of the four electrodes located on the lead. The distance of each of the electrodes from the nerve can be ascertained. Optimal positioning of each of the four electrodes in relation to the nerve increases the options for programming the therapy for the patient after implantation.

With programming, objective parameters may be used when applying electrophysiologic monitoring, markedly increasing the efficacy of programming. EMG monitoring of patients with implanted sacral stimulators conveys information regarding the number of axons within the nerve that are being stimulated (what portion of the supramaximal CMAP amplitude is present), the frequency of stimulation, the on–off cycle, and the location of the stimulating electrode in relation to the nerve (a factor of the amount of stimulation required to produce a supramaximal response). Data collected by Mutone *et al.* [4] suggest that measurable monitoring parameters (chiefly amplitude of the CMAP) are correlated with clinical improvement. Therefore, instead of varying a parameter with the programming and waiting to see if the patient improves, the response can be monitored and the parameters varied to alter the response in a manner that correlates with clinical improvement.

Technique of electrophysiological monitoring of SNS

Although precise technical details are beyond the scope of this chapter, how is electrophysiological monitoring of SNS performed in general?

For electrophysiological monitoring of SNS, a standard electrodiagnostic instrument with two channels for recording, trigger and delay line, and averaging capabilities is optimal.

Test stimulation

Stimulation is via the electrodiagnostic instrument nerve conduction programme. The stimulator of the electrodiagnostic instrument is connected to the 'ground patch' surface electrode (anode) and the mini-hook (cathode), which will be attached to the foramen needle and subsequently to the lead wire. The stimulation is single, of duration 0.5ms, negative polarity, at a frequency of 1Hz, and the stimulus triggers the recorded waveform with no delay. Recording is by two channels, one recording from the urethral electrodes and one from the levator muscle by either transanal or transvaginal electrodes. Leads from these electrodes are connected to the two pre-amplifier channels. Parameters for both channels are a sweep speed of 2ms per division, sensitivity (gain) of 50μV per division, low-frequency filter setting of 2Hz and high-frequency filter setting of 10 kHz, with the speaker on for both channels. The sensitivity settings usually have to be changed during the test stimulation, depending on the magnitude of the responses of the individual patient.

The test stimulation is directed at various sacral foramina (via the foraminal needle). The choice of nerve for the test stimulus is made by comparison of results of the data, choosing the one with the largest-amplitude CMAPs relative to the intensity of stimulating current. After the optimum nerve has been chosen, the lead wire is placed using electrophysiological monitoring *during* the lead placement (by stimulating through the lead wire) to ensure that the lead electrode remains in contact with the nerve. After placement of the

Key Points

- EPM allows response to parameter variation to be altered to maximum clinical effect.
- SNS EPM requires a 2-channel standard electrodiagnostic instrument.
- An instrument with trigger and delay line and averaging capabilities is optimal.

lead wire, the wire is connected to the external pulse generator that the patient will use during the test stimulation and EMG recording is performed with the same recording parameters as described for the lead placement. The patient adjusts the external pulse generator to a level of stimulus tolerable for the test stimulation period and the CMAPs generated are observed objectively by attaching the urethral and levator electrode leads to the two pre-amplifier channels and selecting an oscilloscope or EMG screen. Throughout the test period, the EMG recording may be repeated to confirm correct nerve stimulation. At the end of the test period, EMG recording can verify that the lead has remained in the correct location for nerve stimulation.

Surgical implantation

Once the foramen needle has been passed, a stimulus is given through the needle in the same manner as the test stimulus to verify that the resulting waveforms are similar to those obtained with the successful test stimulus. Once the nerve has been selected and the quadripolar lead placed surgically, each of the four electrodes is tested, the lead being manipulated to obtain optimal responses at each electrode. A permanent record of the data is made to assist with later programming; data of particular interest include latency and amplitude of the CMAP and the required stimulus (in mA) to obtain supramaximal CMAP at each of the four electrodes.

Programming

Compound muscle action potentials are obtained by the same technique as that described for the use of EMG recording after lead placement for the test stimulation. If the patient is not doing well clinically, the stimulus parameters are adjusted in order to increase the amplitude of the CMAP obtained. Initial results suggest that such a change in an individual patient is associated with clinical improvement, although these initial impressions require further verification. Stimulus parameters that can be altered to effect an increase in CMAP amplitude include (1) stimulus intensity (limited by patient's perception of pain), (2) stimulus frequency, (3) length of on–off cycles, (4) pulse width, (5) replacement of the electrode used as the cathode, and (6) changing the mode of stimulation from bipolar to unipolar or vice versa.

Conclusions

SNS is an exciting and effective therapy. At present the procedure is in its infancy, and many modifications are to be expected. The use of electrophysiological monitoring is a modality that can enhance this efficacious therapy.

References

1. Clark MH, Fuller E, Benson JT. Human sacral neuroanatomy: electrophysiologic determination. *American Urogynecological Society Annual Meeting*, October 2000, poster 35.
2. Jünemann KP, Lue TF, Schmidt RA *et al*. Clinical significance of sacral and pudendal nerve anatomy. *J Urol* 1988; 139: 74.
3. Borirakchanyauat S, Aboseif SR, Carroll PR *et al*. Continence mechanism of the isolated female urethra: an anatomic study of the intrapelvic somatic nerves. *J Urol* 1997; 158: 822–6.
4. Mutone N, Fuller E, Benson JT. Relationship of levator and urethral compound muscle action potentials and clinical response to sacral nerve neuromodulation. *American Urogynecological Society Annual Meeting*, October 2000, poster 39.

12 Atlas of peripheral nerve evaluation (PNE)

V. Grünewald and U. Jonas

Percutaneous nerve evaluation (PNE test)

The aims of percutaneous neurostimulation testing (peripheral nerve evaluation; PNE) are to check the neural and functional integrity of the sacral nerves, to determine whether neurostimulation is beneficial for each particular patient, and to clarify which sacral spinal nerves must be stimulated to achieve the optimum therapeutic effect in each individual case.

After administration of local or general anaesthesia (avoiding long-acting muscle relaxants), the patient is placed in the prone position with 45-degree flexion of the hip and knee joints (Fig. 12.1a). The operative area is covered with a sterile sheet, leaving the surgeon a clear view of the anal region and the lower extremities for detection of typical reflex contractions (Fig. 12.1b).

A local anaesthetic is injected into the subcutaneous fatty tissue and the muscles, (but not into the sacral foramen itself), and the sacral foramen S3, found approximately one finger-breadth lateral to the median line (Fig. 12.2), is then localised on one side with a 20-gauge foramen needle (Fig. 12.3). The Medtronic stainless steel foramen needle has a bevelled tip, is depth-marked along its length and electrically insulated along the centre portion of its needle length in order to avoid inadvertent stimulation of the back and gluteal muscles. The needles are available in 9 and 12cm lengths. The portion near the hub is exposed to allow connection to the test stimulator. By stimulating through the uninsulated tip of the needle, the physician can find the correct sacral nerve stimulation site for placement of the test stimulation lead. Generally, the surgeon starts with foramen S3, which is located at the level of the sciatic notch; when the first foramen has been successfully located, tracing the other foramina (each at a distance of approximately one finger-breadth in the vertical line) becomes easier.

Keeping the needle at a 60-degree angle to the skin surface with a rostrocaudal and slightly lateral pointing tip of the needle (Figs. 12.3 and 12.4), will ensure that the needle is inserted into the targeted foramen. Once the resistance caused by the sacroiliac ligament just above the foramen has been overcome, the puncture should progress parallel to the course of the sacral nerve, which normally enters at the upper medial margin of the foramen. With this method one achieves optimal positioning of the needle for stimulation and avoids injuring the spinal nerve. The insulated needle (cathode) is then connected to an external, portable pulse generator (Medtronic model 3625 test stimulator) via a connection cable. The pulse generator itself is connected to a neutral electrode (anode) attached to the shoulder.

As the sensitivity of each individual patient varies, the voltage used for stimulation usually ranges between 1 and 6V. By intermittent touching of the uninsulated part of the foramen needle near the hub, with slowly increasing voltage at 20Hz frequency, the sensory and motor responses evoked by the stimulation can be observed (Fig. 12.4). Stimulation of S3 evokes contraction of the levator ani muscle and the sphincter urethrea (the 'bellows' effect). Plantar flexion of the hallux, of all the toes or of the entire foot of the ipsilateral extremity, can be observed. Patients have reported a dragging sensation in the rectal and vaginal region, at times extending to the scrotum or the labia. If plantar flexion of the entire foot is observed, the gastrocnemius muscle should be palpated, because a strong contraction usually indicates stimulation of S2 fibres and should be avoided.

Stimulation of S2 generally causes the whole leg to rotate. Sensorimotor activity in the perineal region is limited to superficial contraction of the superficial transversus perinei muscle (the 'clamp' effect).

Stimulation of S3, with its connections to the bladder, the pelvic floor, and the urethral sphincter, generally produces the most beneficial effect. Furthermore, most patients will not tolerate the permanent external rotation of the leg caused by stimulation of S2. Occasionally, stimulating S4 also causes clinical improvement. Stimulation of S4 provokes a strong contraction of the levator ani muscle, accompanied by a dragging sensation in the rectal region. Reflex responses in the area of the ventral pelvic floor (including the urethral spincter mechanism) or of the lower extremities are exceptional. If stimulating one side produces an inadequate response, the contralateral side should be tested; the aim is to obtain a typical painless stimulatory response. In our department, both sides are routinely tested and we try to place temporary leads in all S3 and S4 foramina.

Once the optimal stimulation site has been identified, the obturator is removed from the foramen needle, and a temporary wire test lead (Medtronic model 3057 test lead) is inserted through the lumen of the needle (Fig. 12.5). The model 3057 test lead is a coiled, seven-stranded, stainless-steel wire coated with fluoropolymer. Its electrode has been extended to 10mm (0.4 inches) to increase the length of coverage and reduce the effects of minor migration. Depth indicators help to align the lead electrode with the needle tip. Before the test lead is inserted into the needle lumen, the needle should be advanced as far as possible in order to maintain a stimulation effect, even with minor displacement of the test electrode. Once the test lead has been inserted into the needle, the latter must not be advanced any further in order to avoid severing the lead, which may have already passed beyond the sharp tip of the needle. The needle is then carefully removed from the sacral foramen, leaving the test lead in place (Fig. 12.6). The stimulation is then repeated to check the correct position of the test electrode. To mitigate migration the lead contains its own stylet which is removed once the correct position has been found, leaving the lead flexible and stretchable. The needle can be completely detached from the test lead only after the stylet has been removed; once this has occurred, the stylet cannot be repositioned. A repetition of the test stimulation, confirming the correct position of the test lead, is therefore mandatory at this stage, otherwise the test lead cannot be re-inserted.

After correct positioning, the test lead is coiled on the skin (Fig. 12.7) and fixed with adhesive transparent film (Tegaderm®) (Fig. 12.8). Finally, the correct position of the wire is radiologically confirmed and the portable external impulse generator is connected.

During the following 3–6 days the patient is able to control the setting of the stimulatory current within a preprogrammed range, so that it produces a pleasant, painless, sensation in the region of the pelvis and genitalia. During this period the patient controls the test stimulation under ordinary day-to-day conditions. The impulse generator will be turned off only for micturition.

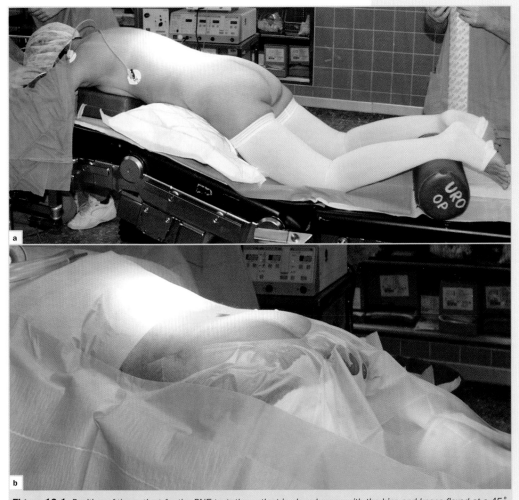

Figure 12.1 *Position of the patient for the PNE test: the patient is placed prone with the hips and knees flexed at a 45° angle, with the surface of the sacrum exactly horizontal. The buttocks are spread with a wide tape to enable inspection of the anus, legs and feet during stimulation of the sacral spinal nerves (optional, depending on the surgeon's preference).*

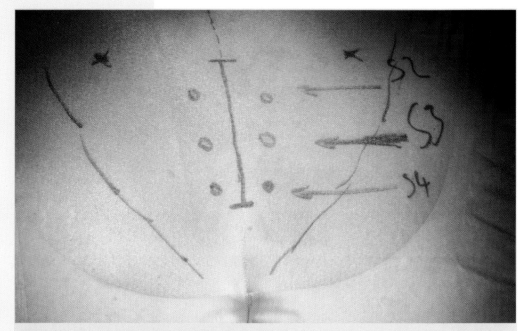

Figure 12.2 *After skin sterilisation and draping, using transparent film to cover the anal region and the legs, the positions of the S2, S3 and S4 foramina are marked on the skin on both sides. As shown here, the lateral margins of the sacrum, the midline and the position of the posterior iliac spina are also outlined. The S3 foramen is located about one finger-breadth lateral to the midline at the level of the sciatic notch, or three finger-breadths caudal to the posterior iliac spina. The S2 and S4 foramina are located one finger-breadth cranial or caudal to the S3 foramen.*

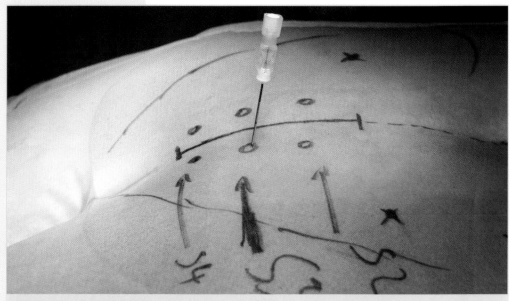

Figure 12.3 *A 20-gauge Medtronic foramen needle, 9 or 12cm long, is inserted into the right S3 foramen. The skin is punctured at the medial border of the mark and the needle is advanced at a 60° angle to the skin surface in the sagittal plane, with the needle tip pointing caudally. In the vertical plane the needle should be at a 5–10° angle to the skin surface, with the needle tip pointing slightly laterally.*

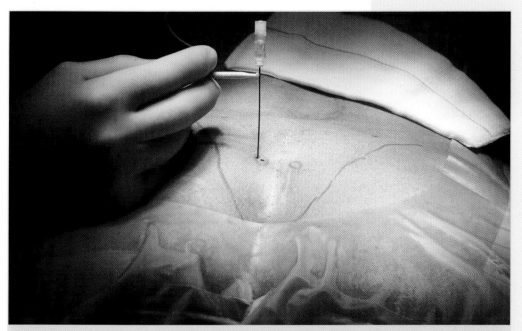

Figure 12.4 *After insertion of the needle into the foramen, test stimulation is performed by touching the most proximal non-insulated part of the needle with the stimulator clamp, which is the negative pole (cathode) of the external stimulator.*

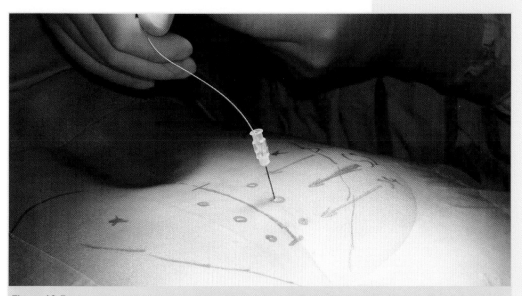

Figure 12.5 *After removal of the obturator of the foramen needle, a Medtronic test stimulation electrode is inserted into the lumen of the needle and advanced until it reaches the tip where it cannot be advanced any further. At this stage, the needle itself must not be inserted any further, as this movement might sever the electrode tip, preventing its subsequent removal. Test stimulation is repeated by touching the proximal end of the electrode; this should have the same result as direct stimulation of the needle.*

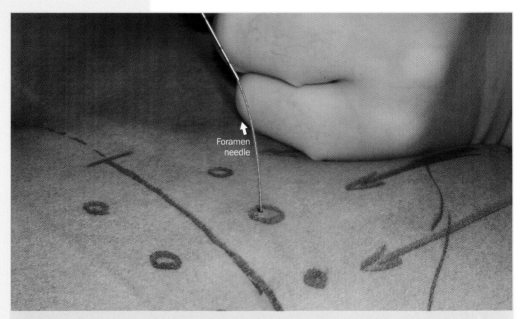

Figure 12.6 *While the test stimulation electrode is held in place, the foramen needle is gently pulled back. Test stimulation is repeated and should give the same results as before. If this is not the case, the test electrode can be removed and re-used at this stage, because the stylet is still in place, giving the electrode sufficient rigidity for its reinsertion through the foramen needle after the latter has again been inserted into the foramen. If the stimulation response is adequate, the stylet of the test electrode can then be removed. Only at this stage can the foramen needle be pulled over the proximal end of the test electrode and removed, leaving the distal end of the test electrode in place. The test electrode is now very flexible and can no longer be reinserted, because the stylet cannot be precisely repositioned.*

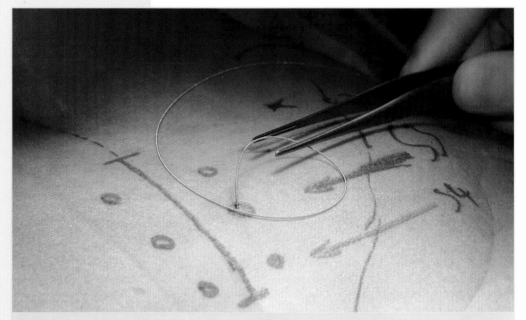

Figure 12.7 *The test electrode is coiled and attached to the skin in order to prevent dislocation of the electrode by inadvertent traction. Subsequently, it should be fixed to the skin with an adhesive sterile spray dressing.*

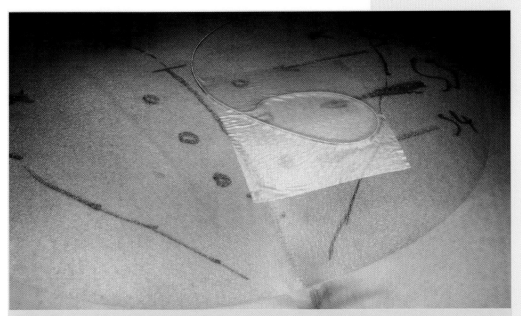

Figure 12.8 *The electrode is finally fixed to the skin with sterile adhesive transparent film, secured by a wide tape. Several test electrodes can be placed and fixed in the same way during a single procedure; electrodes should be placed in at least both S3 foramina.*

13 Atlas of implantation
U. Jonas and V. Grünewald

Permanent unilateral sacral foramen implant

The sacral foramen electrode and impulse generator are implanted under general anaesthesia (intubation anaesthesia). Long-acting muscle relaxants must not be used, as these would impair the intra-operative electrostimulation. As a prophylactic measure, antibiotics (usually third-generation cephalosporins) are administered intra-venously as a single bolus 30 minutes before starting the surgical procedure, without continuation postoperatively. On each of the 2 preoperative days, and on the day of surgery itself, the patient is fully immersed in a bath to which an iodine disinfectant solution has been added to ensure sterile conditions.

The patient is placed in the prone position with a 45-degree flexion of the hip and knee joints. The sacral, flank, and perineal regions are carefully disinfected and the operative field is draped in the same manner as for percutaneous stimulatory testing, to give the surgeon a clear view of the perineum and lower extremities (Fig. 13.1). A 8cm-long midline incision is made above the sacrum, reaching one-third caudal and two-thirds cranial from the S3 fora-men (Fig. 13.2). The S3 foramen, which is the site used mainly for implantation, is traced using the bony orientation points described in the previous chapter.

After transection of the subcutaneous fat, the muscle fascia (thoracolumbar fascia) is incised approximately 1cm lateral of the midline in a longitudinal direction. As an additional point of orientation, one can use the gluteus maximus muscle which originates at the lower margin of the S3 foramen. Usually, the gluteus maximus has to be incised over a length of 1–2 cm for good exposure of the S3 foramen and a little further caudal if implantation of the S4 foramen is intended. The paraspinal muscles are then divided longitudinally and the dorsal aspect of the sacrum is exposed. At this stage it is important to preserve the tight ligaments overlying the sacral periosteum in order to have sufficient material to which the permanent lead can be sutured at a subsequent stage of the procedure. Self-retaining retractors (for example, a ring retractor [Lone-Star Inc.]) will keep the incision open and enable the procedure to be performed with only one assistant, or with the assisting nurse. Intraoperative test stimulation, using the same equipment as described in the previous chapter, will confirm the precise location of the foramen selected (Fig. 13.3). With few excep-tions, selection of the implantation site depends substantially on the result of the percutaneous test stimulation.

Once the chosen sacral foramen has been located, the perma-nent electrode (Medtronic quadripolar lead, model 3080) is rinsed in an antibiotic solution of bacitracin and gentamycin, and the wound itself is irrigated using the same solution. Meanwhile the foramen needle is left in place to avoid re-localisation of the foramen while preparing the permanent electrode for implantation. Proximal to the four contact points of the permanent electrode, a silicon rubber cuff is glued to the electrode body. The cuff is fitted with three eyelets to accommodate non-absorbable atraumatic needle-armed sutures (for example, Ethibond®), which are now positioned, tied and armed with mosquito clamps (Fig. 13.4). After removal of the foramen needle, the electrode is gently inserted into the foramen (Fig. 13.5). No major resistance should be experienced; if necessary, the opening should be carefully enlarged by spreading it with cardiovascular forceps or a mosquito clamp. Renewed test stimulation will determine the most effective contact point between the electrode and spinal nerve; the most distal contact point is termed '0', with the subsequent three being numbered 1–3 sequentially. An identical motor response at all four contact points is ideal. If only one contact gives a satisfactory response, the electrode should be repositioned at a different angle to the foramen and the test stimulation repeated. The pre-attached sutures are then used to secure the electrode to the ligaments overlying the periosteum of the sacral bone (Fig. 13.6). Test stimulation should be repeated at this stage to confirm an appropriate postion of the electrode after fixation.

A small skin incision is now made in the flank between the iliac crest and the twelfth rib on the side where the electrode has been placed. With the aid of a 12Fr thorax drain (part of the implant kit supplied by the manufacturer), a subcutaneous tunnel is formed between the two wounds, starting from the flank incision and running towards the sacral incision (Fig. 13.7). The obturator of the tunnelling device is removed and the silicone sheath (which is open at both ends) left in place. The free end of the electrode is guided through the sheath to the flank incision, after the stylet has been removed from the electrode (Fig. 13.8). This stylet gives the electrode rigidity for placement in the foramen. The silicone sheath is now removed from the flank incision, the proximal end of the electrode is marked with a suture, and the electrode is buried in a subcutaneous pocket which has been created at the site of the flank incision (Fig. 13.9). The flank incision is temporarily closed, leaving the marking suture exposed between the skin sutures. The flank incision with the protruding marker suture is then covered with a sterile, transparent dressing.

The sacral incision is then irrigated with a solution of bacitracin and gentamycin, closed in layers and covered with a sterile dressing (Figs. 13.10 and 13.11).

The patient is now positioned on the contralateral flank (Fig. 13.12). The flank and abdomen on the side chosen previously for placement of the Medtronic InterStim model 3023 implantable pulse generator (Fig. 13.13) are disinfected and the surgical field is draped with a sterile cover. A subcutaneous pocket is subsequently created in the lower abdomen to host the pulse generator (Fig. 13.14). The site chosen should be easily accessible to the patient and should not be covered by an excessive amount of fatty tissue as this could impede both the on/off switching mechanism of the generator and the telemetric programming. The flank incision is now reopened, the proximal end of the electrode is exposed and the marking suture is removed. Using a 12Fr thoracic drain, a subcutaneous tunnel is again created between the flank incision and the subcutaneous pocket in the lower abdomen (Fig. 13.15), through which a connecting extension cable (Medtronic quadripolar extension, model 3095) between electrode and impulse generator is guided (Fig. 13.16). Extensions are available in different lengths (25, 40, and 51cm). Once the electrode has been connected to the extension cable in the area of the flank incision by tightening of the screws on the extension cable (Fig. 13.17), the contact point is sealed with a silicone cover, fixed with two sutures and placed subcutaneously. After irrigation, the flank incision is closed in layers and covered with a sterile dressing.

Finally, the other end of the connecting cable is attached to the impulse generator, also by tightening the small screws on the pulse generator (Fig. 13.18). The generator is attached to the rectus fascia using two non-absorbable sutures (Fig. 13.19). The uninsulated surface of the generator bearing the label should face outwards in order to avoid contraction of the rectus abdominis musculature on unipolar stimulation.

After the abdominal incision has been irrigated with an antibiotic solution, the wound is closed in two layers and covered with sterile dressings (Fig. 13.20).

On the first postoperative day, anterior–posterior (Fig. 13.21) and lateral (Fig. 13.22) radiographs of the implant are obtained to verify that all components are correctly positioned and will act as a control for comparison in case of subsequent problems (for instance, dislocation of the electrode).

Modifications of the surgical procedure include placement of the pulse generator in the gluteal area thus avoiding repositioning of the patient during the procedure (Fig. 13.23. See also Chapter 16, page 193) and implantation of bilateral electrodes, which should be powered by a two-channel pulse generator (Medtronic Synergy, model 7427, Fig. 13.24) for adequate synchronous independent stimulation of each side.

The implant remains deactivated at least until the day following surgery and will be activated by a telemetric programming unit (Medtronic Console Programmer, model 7432, Fig. 13.25), allowing programming of all features of the implant by the physician during the initial activation and follow-up stages. This might be necessary in cases where unilateral stimulation alone is not sufficient.

Whereas, previously, patients could only turn first-generation pulse generators on or off by using a control magnet (Fig. 13.25), the pulse generators currently available also allow the patient to re-adjust stimulation intensity, frequency, and pulse width within limits preset by the physician. This is done by means of a special patient programmer device (Medtronic patient programmer, model 3031A, Fig. 13.25), which is comparable to a remote control unit.

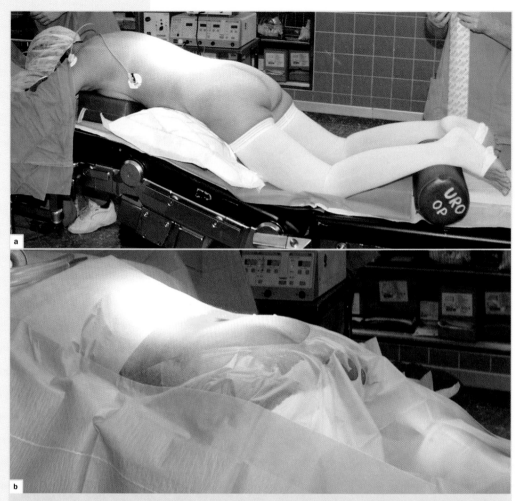

Figure 13.1 *(a) The patient is placed prone with the hips and knees flexed at a 45° angle and with the surface of the sacrum exactly horizontal. The buttocks are spread with a wide tape to enable inspection of anus, legs and feet during stimulation of the sacral spinal nerves (optional, depending on the surgeon's preference). (b) After skin disinfection the operative field is draped, using transparent film to cover the anal region and the legs.*

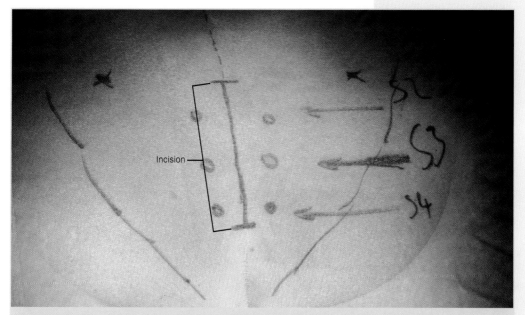

Figure 13.2 *The positions of the sacral S2, S3, and S4 foramina are marked on the skin on both sides. As shown, the lateral margins of the sacrum, the midline, the location of the incision and the position of the posterior iliac spina are also outlined. The S3 foramen is located about one finger-breadth lateral to the midline at the level of the sciatic notch, or 3 finger-breadths caudal to the posterior iliac spina. The incision is about 8cm long in the midline, extending one-third caudal and two-thirds cranial from the S3 foramen.*

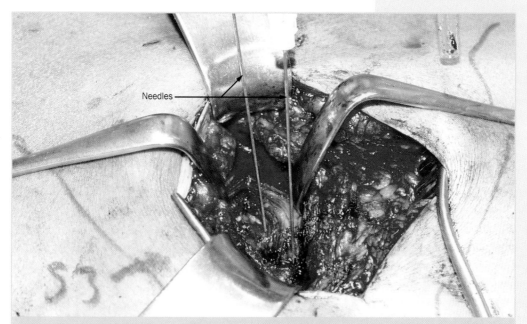

Figure 13.3 *After incision of the skin and transsection of the subcutaneous fat, the thoracolumbar fascia is exposed and incised in a craniocaudal direction 1cm lateral to the midline. The deep spinal muscles are divided and the sacral surface is exposed, leaving the overlying ligaments intact. As shown, the sacral surface is exposed and two 9mm Medtronic foramen needles are placed in the S2 (cranial) and the S3 (caudal) foramina for intraoperative test stimulation.*

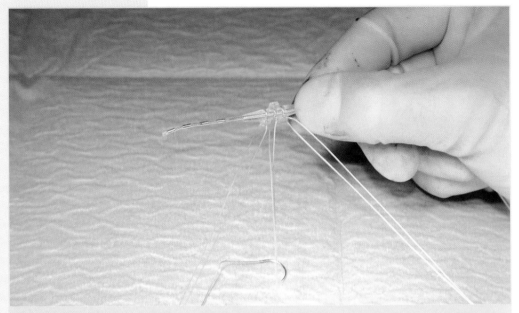

Figure 13.4 *The permanent sacral foramen electrode (Medtronic quadripolar electrode) is prepared for implantation. Proximal to the four contact points of the electrode (called '0-1-2-3' from distal to proximal), the silicone rubber cuff is seen glued to the electrode body. The cuff has three buttonholes to accommodate non-absorbable 2/0 sutures, which are then tied to the cuff and armed with small mosquito clamps. The previously fixed sutures are subsequently used for fixation of the electrode to the ligaments overlying the sacral periosteum (see Fig. 13.6). The tip of the electrode is slightly bent.*

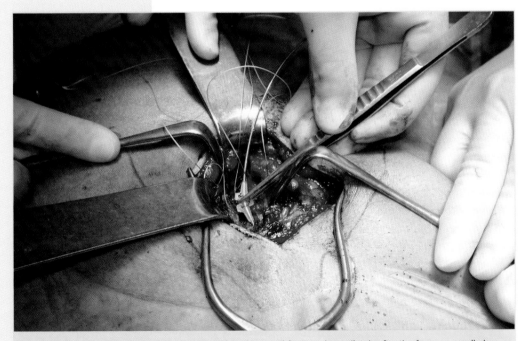

Figure 13.5 *The electrode is now gently inserted into the sacral foramen immediately after the foramen needle has been removed. The bent tip of the electrode should point laterally and insertion should be accomplished without any force being applied.*

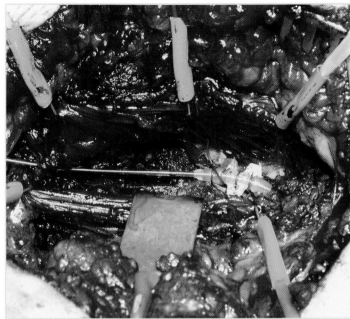

Figure 13.6 *After the correct position of the electrode has been confirmed by repeated, separate stimulation of all four contact points (which, ideally, should all give the same response), the electrode is attached to the ligaments overlying the sacral periosteum, using the non-absorbable sutures previously attached to the electrode (Fig. 13.4). The electrode is usually inserted into the foramen as far as possible, with the distal edge of the fixation cuff being located exactly at the entrance to the posterior opening of the sacral foramen.*

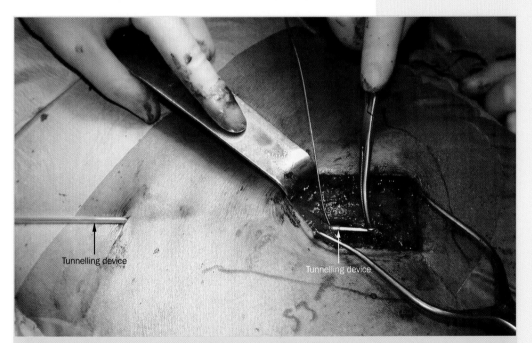

Figure 13.7 *After electrode fixation, a small incision is made at the ipsilateral flank halfway between the 12th rib and the rim of the iliac bone (in order to avoid contact of the electrode with these bony structures). A small subcutaneous pocket is created, allowing sufficient space for the later connection between the electrode and the extension cable. The incision should be positioned as far laterally as possible, but close enough to allow the electrode to reach the flank incision and with sufficient length to perform the connection (at least 2cm). This can be estimated by holding the electrode over the skin in the direction of the planned incision. The tunnelling device is shown in place; it has been advanced subcutaneously from the flank incision towards the sacral incision; at this stage its sharp tip is removed.*

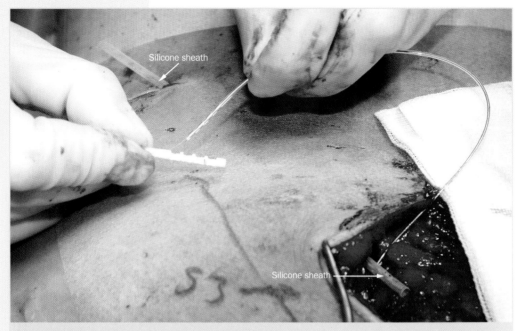

Figure 13.8 *The tunnelling tool of the tunnelling device is removed and the silicone sheath is seen. After removal of the electrode stylet, the proximal end of the electrode is guided through the sheath. The sheath itself is subsequently removed.*

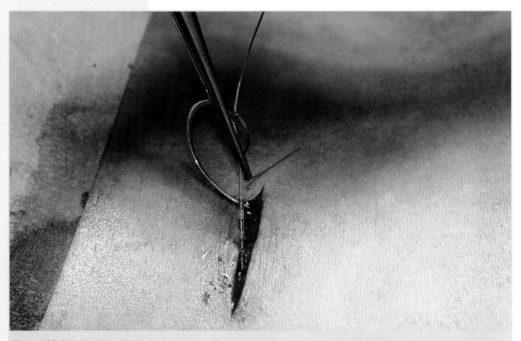

Figure 13.9 *The proximal end of the electrode is marked with a non-absorbable suture and the electrode is temporarily inserted subcutaneously. The flank incision is temporarily closed, with the marking suture exposed. The incision is covered with a sterile transparent film.*

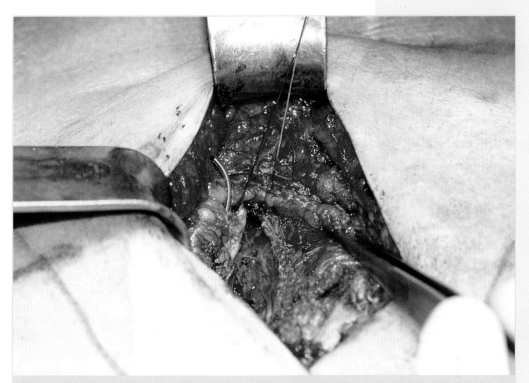

Figure 13.10 *The sacral incision is closed in layers, carefully avoiding any harm to the electrode as this could cause an insulation defect and inadvertent painful stimulation of the deep spinal muscles.*

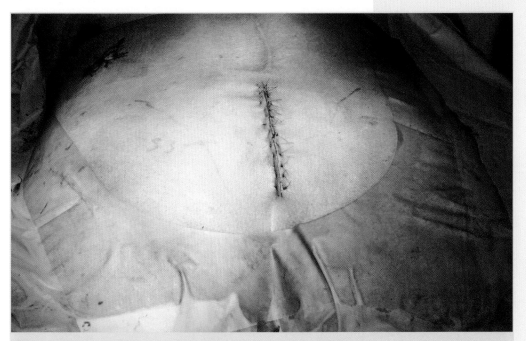

Figure 13.11 *The skin is closed with interrupted, non-absorbable, monofilament sutures to allow drainage of fluid into the sterile dressing. No drain is placed.*

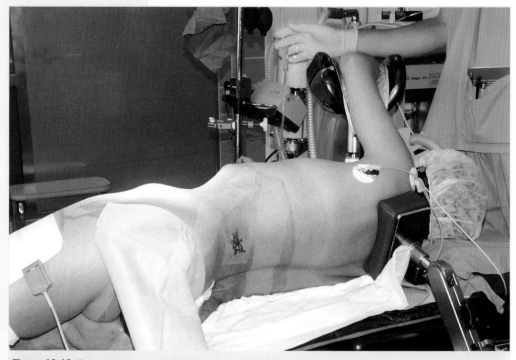

Figure 13.12 *The patient is repositioned on the contralateral flank. The transparent film covering the small flank incision is removed and the flank and lower abdomen are scrubbed.*

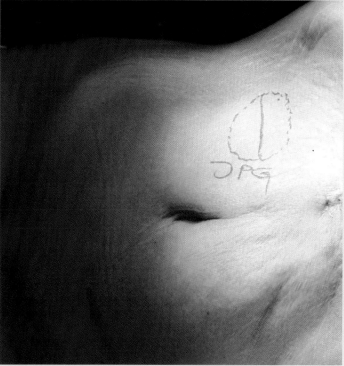

Figure 13.13 *The site for subcutaneous placement of the pulse generator in the area of the lower abdomen should be preoperatively marked. It should be easily accessible by the patient, should not interfere with clothing, and positioned away from bony structures to avoid pressure and pain. There should be sufficient subcutaneous fat to avoid bulging of the skin.*

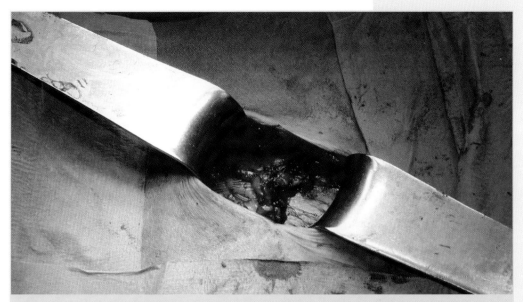

Figure 13.14 *After thorough scrubbing and draping of the flank and lower abdomen, a subcutaneous pocket is created in the area marked preoperatively (see Fig. 13.13). The fascia is exposed and the pocket enlarged sufficiently to host the pulse generator without tension.*

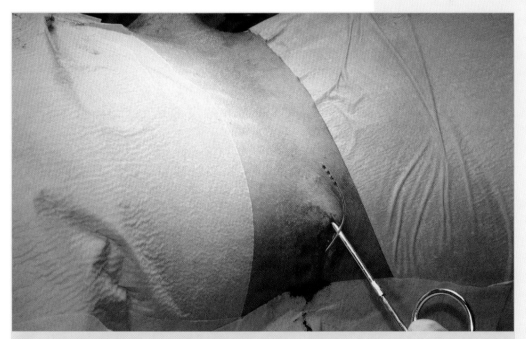

Figure 13.15 *The flank incision is reopened and the electrode exposed. The marking suture is removed, care being taken to avoid damage to the insulation. Another tunnelling device is used to create a subcutaneous tunnel between the flank incision and the abdominal pocket incision starting from the flank incision. For obese patients, the device can be extended to gain sufficient length to reach the abdominal incision; for slim patients, the device can be bent to follow the curvature of the flank.*

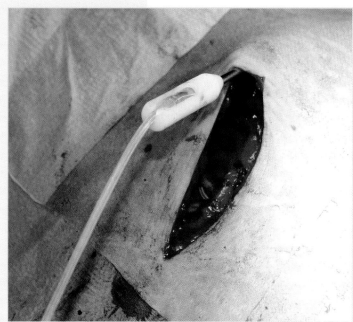

Figure 13.16 *The plastic tip of the tunnelling device is removed and replaced by a special cover, into which the flank-connector end of the extension cable is inserted and pulled towards the flank incision. The extension cable must be long enough to allow tension-free connection.*

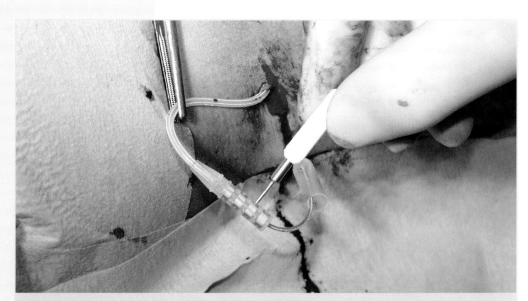

Figure 13.17 *After removal of the tunnelling device, the electrode is inserted into the connector slot of the extension cable, after an insulating silicone sheath has been pushed over the free end of the electrode. The four screws of the extension cable connector are tightened after confirmation that the proximal electrode contact points are exactly underneath the screws (which can be easily seen through the transparent silicone insulation). Meticulous positioning of both ends is mandatory to allow correct function at all four electrode contact points. The insulation sheath is then pulled over the connector and kept in place by two non-absorbable silk sutures. The flank incision is closed in layers. Care should be taken to avoid pulling out the electrode.*

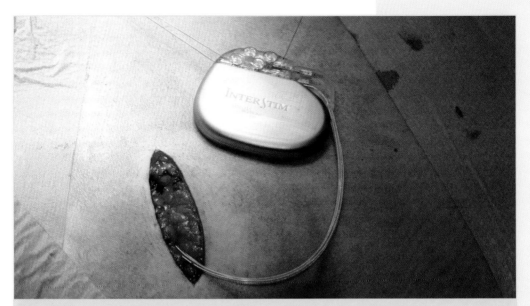

Figure 13.18 *Two non-absorbable sutures are placed in the fixation openings of the pulse generator and armed with mosquito clamps. The extension cable is inserted into the slots of the pulse generator; the four fixing screws, which establish electrical contact with the pulse generator, are tightened.*

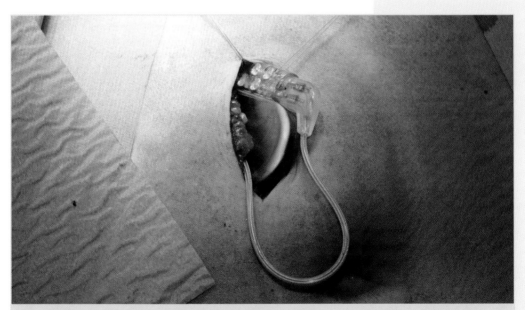

Figure 13.19 *The pulse generator is inserted into the subcutaneous pocket and fastened to the fascia, using the prepared sutures. Note that the surface of the pulse generator bearing the label should face outwards, towards the skin. Surplus extension cable is looped and tucked under the pulse generator.*

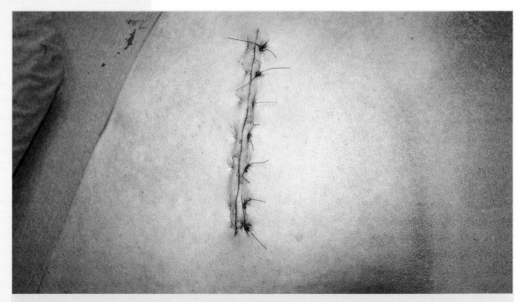

Figure 13.20 *The abdominal incision is closed in layers. The skin is closed with interrupted, non-absorbable monofilament sutures to allow drainage of fluid into the sterile dressing. No drain is placed, in order to avoid secondary infection of the alloplastic material. The implant is usually activated when postoperative pain (particularly at the abdominal incision) has ceased and the telemetrical programmer can be gently pressed over the pulse generator without causing pain.*

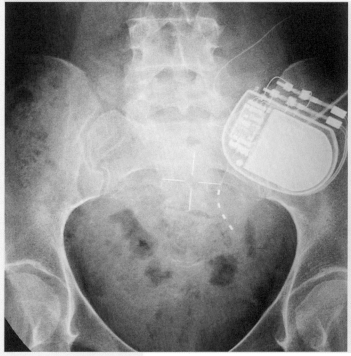

Figure 13.21 *An anterior–posterior X-ray of the sacrum and abdomen showing correct placement of all components. The electrode is located in the left S3 foramen.*

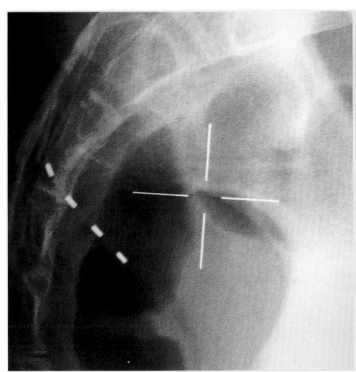

Figure 13.22 *A lateral X-ray of the sacrum with the electrode located in the left S3 foramen. X-rays in two planes should be performed the day after surgery in order to confirm correct placement of all components.*

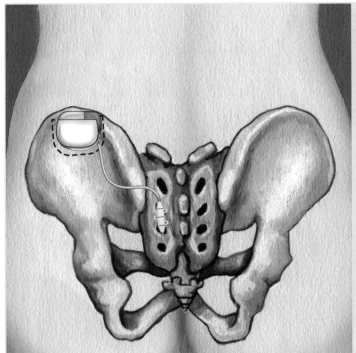

Figure 13.23 *The pulse generator can, alternatively, be placed subcutaneously above the gluteus maximus muscle fascia caudal to the rim of the iliac bone (buttock implant). This allows the entire procedure to be performed without re-positioning of the patient, and seems to cause less pain at the pulse generator implant site (see Chapter 16, page 193).*

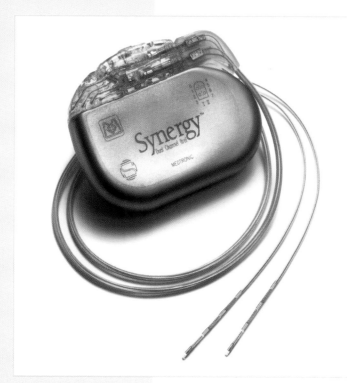

Figure 13.24 *For bilateral sacral nerve stimulation, a two-channel pulse generator (Synergy®) should be used, which allows independent stimulation of two implanted electrodes.*

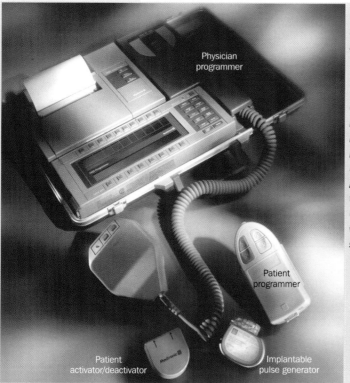

Physician programmer

Patient programmer

Patient activator/deactivator

Implantable pulse generator

Figure 13.25 *Detailed programming of the pulse generator is possible only with the telemetrical control unit used by the physician. The patient is able to use either a control magnet to activate or deactivate the implanted pulse generator (Itrel I and Itrel II pulse generators), or a specific patient programmer (Itrel III, InterStim, and Synergy pulse generators) that allows the patient to change stimulation intensity (voltage), frequency and pulse width within pre-programmed limits set by the physician.*

14 Clinical results of sacral nerve stimulation

Sacral nerve stimulation for the treatment of refractory urinary urge incontinence

R.A. Schmidt, U. Jonas and K. Oleson*

Introduction

Urinary incontinence affects 13 million Americans with an estimated 1 million new cases diagnosed each year. The total annual cost of care for patients with incontinence in the United States is estimated at US$11.2 billion in the community and US$5.2 billion in nursing homes [1]. Standard treatments, such as pelvic muscle exercises [2, 3], pharmacological therapy [4–6], and non-implantable pelvic floor stimulation [7, 8] change pelvic muscle physiology, act on the bladder directly to relax an overactive detrusor or act on the neural reflexes that influence detrusor behaviour. Urge incontinence may result from an imbalance of facilitatory and excitatory control systems causing a hyperexcitable voiding reflex [9]. Neuromodulation also acts on neural reflexes but does so internally by stimulation of the sacral nerves [10].

Sacral nerve stimulation (SNS) is based on research dedicated to the understanding of the voiding reflex as well as the role and influence of the sacral nerves on voiding behaviour [11–13]. This research led to the development of a technique to modulate dysfunctional voiding behaviour through SNS [10]. The exact mechanism by which stimulation improves urinary symptoms is not fully understood, although various hypotheses have been suggested [14–21]. It is thought that SNS induces reflex-mediated inhibitory effects on the detrusor through afferent and/or efferent stimulation of the sacral nerves. In this chapter we demonstrate the effectiveness of SNS for the treatment of urge incontinence.

Materials and methods

This prospective randomised study was conducted in accordance with regulatory requirements of the 16 contributing worldwide centres. Study candidates were recruited from the general urological population and underwent baseline screening, including medical history, urodynamic testing and quantification of voiding behaviour by means of diaries. Patients who met specific inclusion criteria and gave informed consent were entered into the study (see Appendix). Test stimulation was performed during a

> **Key Points**
> - Urinary incontinence affects 13 million people in the USA alone.
> - Each year 1 million new cases are diagnosed.
> - Care costs: US$11.2 $\times$ 10^9 (community) or US$5.2 $\times$ 10^9 (nursing homes).
> - SNS modulates dysfunctional voiding behaviour.
> - Detrusor inhibition is induced via afferent and/or efferent stimulation of sacral nerves.
> - Study candidates had baseline screens, including voiding diaries.

*With members of the Sacral Nerve Stimulation Study Group (see page 168).
Reprinted with permission from the *Journal of Urology*.

trial period of 3–7 days to assess sacral nerve integrity and to quantify the effects of trial stimulation on dysfunctional voiding behaviour [10, 22]. Patients recorded voiding behaviour in a diary during this trial period. An improvement greater than 50% in baseline voiding symptoms during test stimulation qualified a patient for surgical implantation. Qualified patients were randomly assigned to a treatment or control group. The treatment (stimulation) group underwent surgical implantation of the SNS system and received stimulation therapy according to the recommended parameters. The control (delay) group was delayed from surgical implantation for 6 months and received standard medical treatment (Fig. 14.1).

The stimulation group underwent surgery to implant a multiprogrammable neurostimulator. A subcutaneous pocket was made for the neurostimulator, typically in the lower quadrant of the abdomen, and the lead was positioned along the targeted sacral nerve and anchored in place. Follow-up evaluations were conducted 1, 3 and 6 months after implantation, and every 6 months for a mean of 14.7 (range 0.9–39.7) months. Controls were

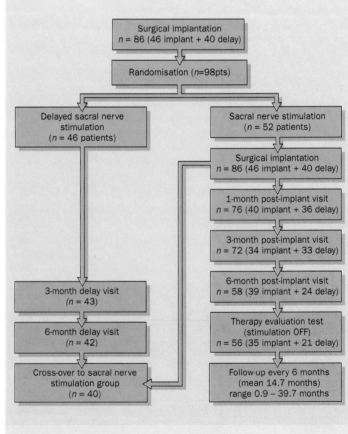

Figure 14.1 Study protocol flow chart

evaluated 3 and 6 months after randomisation, and were allowed to cross over if they remained good surgical candidates, demonstrated no change in baseline medical conditions which would make device implantation inappropriate, and consented to implantation procedures and follow-up. Efficacy of SNS was evaluated by comparing 6-month voiding diary results between the two groups. A second efficacy test (therapy evaluation test) was performed 6 months after implantation, and consisted of deactivating stimulation for a minimum of 3 days, documenting the effects of inactive stimulation on voiding behaviour for 3 days and then reactivating stimulation. In this paired comparison, patients served as their own controls and voiding behaviour with and without SNS was compared.

Voiding diaries were used to quantify the effects of SNS on urge incontinence and comprised the primary outcome measure [1, 23]. Efficacy was based on the number of daily incontinence episodes, the severity ranking of episodes and the number of absorbent pads replaced daily as a result of incontinence. To minimise bias in the collection of diary results, patients were not informed of the specific diary parameters used to evaluate urological conditions. The SF-36 Health Survey was used to measure quality of life in eight conceptual areas, to document baseline status and to characterise changes in quality of life after SNS. The eight conceptual areas provide summary measurements for two main areas of quality of life: the Standardised Physical Component Scale measures the effect of medical conditions on physical health; the Standardised Mental Component Scale measures that effect on mental health. The scores are transformed from 0 (low) to 100 (high), with higher values representing more favourable states.

Urodynamic testing was conducted at baseline to rule out treatable aetiologies, to segregate the urge incontinence population into groups with and without demonstrable detrusor instability, and to evaluate bladder function at the 6-month visit [24–27]. Interim data analysis was performed using group sequential data analysis [28]. This technique resulted in the conservative adjustment of the significance level to 0.0005 to account for those patients who did not complete the 6-month follow-up at the interim data analysis and to accommodate multiple comparisons of the three primary diary variables. Continuous study variables were compared using the two-sided Student *t*-test and dichotomous data were compared using Fisher's exact test. Efficacy was evaluated by ordered logistic regression to compare the distribution of symptom changes between the two groups.

Safety was assessed prospectively from relevant medical events, management, possible aetiology and resolution status. Common definitions for classification of adverse events were used. Events not resolved after the initial report were followed until there was complete resolution or no further clinical improvement could be expected. Results were evaluated by an independent data monitoring board comprising of experts in urology, regulatory affairs and statistics.

Key Points

- SNS efficacy was evaluated by comparing 6-month diary results in both groups.
- In a therapy evaluation test, 6 months after implant, stimulation was withheld for ≥ 3 days.
- Effects were recorded, then stimulation reactivated and effects compared.
- Voiding diaries were used to quantify SNS effects on urge incontinence.
- SF-36 Health Survey assessed QoL at baseline and QoL changes after SNS.
- Baseline urodynamic tests ruled out treatable causes.
- Such tests also delineated groups with/without detrusor instability.
- Urodynamic tests evaluated bladder function at 6 months.
- Safety was evaluated prospectively, using common classification of adverse effects.

Key Points

- SNS efficacy was based on 98 patients with successful test stimulation results.

Table 14.1 *Demographic summary of 155 patients with urge incontinence*

No. women (%)	125 (80.6)
No. men (%)	30 (19.4)
Mean age ± SD (range)	46.6 ± 13.0 (20.2 – 78.9)
Mean years urinary symptoms ± SD before enrolment (range)	9.0 ± 7.4 (0.6 – 35.4)
No. previous medical treatment for urinary problems (%)*	153 (98.7)
Pharmacological	144 (92.5)
Non-surgical	55 (35.5)
Surgical	88 (56.8)

*Medical treatment categories were not mutually exclusive

Table 14.2 *Voiding diary results at 6 months for 76 patients with urge incontinence*

Diary parameter	Stimulation group (34 patients)			Delay group (42 patients)		
	Mean baseline ± SD	Mean 6 months ± SD	P - value	Mean baseline ± SD	Mean 6 months ± SD	P - value*
Incontinent episodes/day	9.7 ± 6.3	2.6 ± 5.1	<0.0001	9.3 ± 4.8	11.3 ± 5.9	0.002
Severity rank of incontinence	2.0 ± 0.7	0.8 ± 0.9	<0.0001	1.8 ± 0.6	2.0 ± 0.6	0.006
Absorbent pads replaced daily owing to incontinence	6.2 ± 5.0	1.1 ± 2.0	<0.0001	5.0 ± 3.7	6.3 ± 3.6	0.003

Severity of incontinence was ranked on a logarithmic scale as: 1 (mild) – drops of urine; 2 (moderate) – 1 to 2 tablespoons per incontinence episode; and 3 (heavy) – soaked pad or outer clothing.

* Student's *t*-test (two-sided)

Results

From December 1993 to April 1997, 155 urge-incontinence patients were enrolled into the study (Table 14.1). A total of 914 procedures (706 non-surgical and 208 surgical) were performed for treatment of urinary problems before enrolment. Results from the baseline voiding diaries of the 155 patients documented severe, frequent episodes of urge incontinence. The mean number of daily incontinence episodes plus or minus standard deviation was 8.9±5.9, mean leak severity ranking was 1.9±0.6, and a mean of 4.8±4.8 absorbent pads were replaced daily. In the 3-day diaries at baseline, 90.3% of patients had at least one moderate or heavy incontinence episode and 74.8% had at least one.

Efficacy of SNS was based on results from the 98 randomised patients who underwent a successful test stimulation procedure. The remaining 57 patients did not demonstrate significant improvement during test stimulation and were not randomised into the study. Statistical analysis of medical history, pre-study treatments

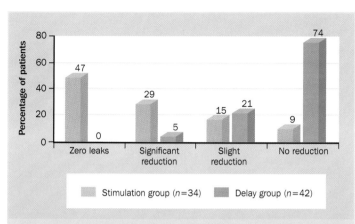

Figure 14.2 *Daily incontinence episodes at 6-month follow-up for 76 patients with urge incontinence (p<0.0001). Ordered logistic regression, adjusted significance level p = 0.0005. 'Zero leaks' was defined as no incontinence; 'significant reduction' as 50% or greater; 'slight reduction as less than 50%; 'no reduction' as no change or a slight increase.*

and baseline demographic factors indicated no concomitant factors to explain why these patients did not respond to test stimulation.

At the interim data analysis 6-month diaries were collected from 76 randomised patients (34 in the stimulation group plus 42 in the delay group). Symptoms of urge incontinence at 6 months were significantly reduced in the stimulation group (Table 14.2). The stimulation group had significantly fewer daily incontinence episodes than the delay group ($p<0.0001$, Fig. 14.2). Of the stimulation group, 47% were completely dry at 6 months. There was no reduction in incontinence episodes after 6 months of treatment in three patients. Device explantation due to pain with stimulation was performed in one of these patients, and two had increased frequency (from 16.7 to 23.8 and from 1.5 to 2.7 daily episodes).

At 6 months the average severity ranking of heavy incontinence episodes was significantly lower in the stimulation than in the delay group ($p<0.0001$, Fig. 14.3). At baseline the stimulation group documented an average of 3.4±3.8 daily heavy incontinence episodes, which decreased to 0.3±0.9 at 6 months after implantation ($p<0.0001$). The delay group had an average of 2.6±3.5 heavy episodes at baseline, which increased to 3.9±3.8 at 6 months with conservative treatment. A greater reduction in the frequency of use of absorbent pads was demonstrated by the stimulation group ($p<0.0001$, Fig. 14.4).

Voiding diary results from 52 patients indicated a return of baseline urge incontinence when stimulation was inactivated during the therapy evaluation test 6 months after implantation. When stimulation was inactivated the average frequency of daily incontinence episodes increased from 2.9 to 9.5, the average severity ranking of leaks increased from 0.8 to 1.9, and average daily absorbent pad use

Key Points

- There was no significant difference in mental health between groups.
- Stimulus group had significantly better perceptions of physical health than delay group.
- SNS gave sustained clinical benefit (>50% symptom reduction) 18 months post implant.

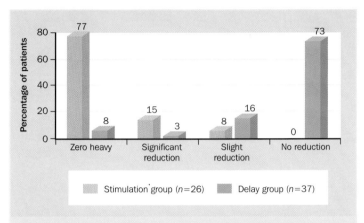

Figure 14.3 *Severity of episodes of heavy incontinence at 6-month follow-up for 76 patients with urge incontinence (p<0.0001). *Eight stimulation-group and five delay-group patients had no episodes of heavy incontinence at baseline or 6 months. 'Zero heavy' was defined as heavy incontinence at baseline and none at 6 months; 'significant reduction' as 50% or greater; 'slight reduction' as less than 50%; 'no reduction' as no reduction in heavy incontinence.*

increased from 1.2 to 5.8 (all $p<0.0001$). These data indicate that efficacy is dependent on active stimulation and that stimulation therapy is completely reversible.

There was no significant difference in the mental health component of the SF-36 Health Survey between 28 stimulation-group and 32 delay-group patients (mean score 47 versus 45). However, the stimulation group demonstrated significantly favourable perceptions of physical health status compared with the delay group (mean score 46 versus 36, $p=0.0008$). Bladder function was not adversely affected by SNS. Measurements from simple uroflowmetry and detrusor pressure/uroflow studies revealed no differences in parameters between the two groups at 6 months; no *de novo* urinary retention was reported in the stimulation group.

Water cystometry showed that bladder storage volume at the first sensation of fullness occurred at a higher average fill volume in the stimulation group (222 versus 79ml in the delay group, $p=0.017$). Bladder volume at the first unstable detrusor contraction on average occurred at a higher fill volume in the stimulation group (151 versus 70ml). A higher proportion of the stimulation group demonstrated stable detrusor function at 6 months (56% versus 16%, $p=0.014$).

Effective SNS therapy appeared to provide sustained clinical benefit, defined as a greater than 50% reduction in symptoms, 18 months after implantation (Table 14.3). The study physicians are proactively continuing their annual follow-up of the implant cohort for 5 years to determine the effects of chronic therapy.

Details of any adverse effects of SNS treatment are given in Chapter 16 of this volume.

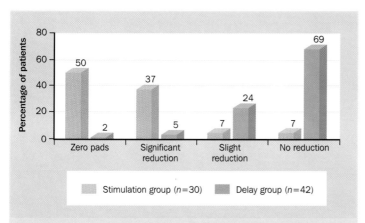

Figure 14.4 Absorbent pads replaced daily at 6-month follow-up for 76 patients with urge incontinence (p<0.0001). * Four stimulation-group patients did not replace absorbent pads at baseline or 6 months. 'Zero pads' was defined as no absorbent pads replacement; 'significant reduction' as 50% or greater; 'slight reduction' as less than 50%; 'no reduction' as no change or a slight increase.

Table 14.3 Sustained clinical benefit 18 months after implant

	Percentage of patients with clinical benefit after implant		
	At 6 months (n = 58)	At 12 months (n = 38)	At 18 months (n = 21)
Any leaking episode			
Dry	47	45	52
50% reduction or greater	28	34	24
Total clinical success	75	79	76
Heavy leaking episodes			
Eliminated	77	70	84
50% reduction or greater	13	10	0
Total clinical success	90	80	84
Absorbent pads replaced daily			
Eliminated	57	55	57
50% reduction or greater	26	21	19
Total clinical success	83	76	76

Discussion

Urinary urge incontinence remains a complex problem for patients and clinicians. Although standard treatments target the bladder as the source of the problem, 62.5% of surveyed patients with urge incontinence were 'not satisfied' with these standard treatments [29]. In selecting the most appropriate study design with regard to

Table 14.4 Revision surgery in 51 of 157 patients

Revision type (no. of adverse events)*	No. patients	No. adverse events	No. operations (status)
Permanent explant: Pain at implant site (3) Change in bowel function (1) Infection (2)	6	6	6
Temporary explant/reimplantation: Pain at implant site (1) Infection (2) Allergic reaction to implanted material (1)	4	4	8 (4 explant, 4 reimplant)
Device exchange: Technical problems (6) Lead migration (10) Change in bowel function (1) Pain at implant site (3)	14	20	19 (1 pending)
Reposition lead/extension: Pain at implant site (6) Change in bowel function (3) Lead extension/migration (3) Technical problem (4) Transient electric shock (1)	16	17	16 (1 pending)
Reposition: implantable pulse generator pain at the implantable pulse generator site (25)	23	25	22 (3 pending)
Totals	51	72	76

Categories are not mutually exclusive as several patients had more than one type of operation and several patients had more than one adverse event

Key Points

- Standard treatment did not satisfy 62.5% of patients surveyed.
- Blinding was not possible, so the delay group acted as controls.

randomisation, masking and control, a number of factors were considered, including a desire to conduct a randomised clinical trial, delivery of therapy by surgical implantation of a device, the potential for progression or spontaneous improvement of urge incontinence, and the limited medical treatment options available. Our aim was to conduct a randomised trial in an ethical manner. Neither physician nor patient could be blinded because, during the test stimulation procedure, patients were aware of the distinct sensations of SNS; it was therefore not possible to blind them to non-treatment by implanting sham devices or by providing suboptimal (low-level) stimulation. Logically, the physicians could not be blinded either; thus, we selected a delayed-treatment group as controls and a 6-month period was chosen because patients were documented to be refractory to standard medical treatment, including surgery, in more than 50%. By the time that SNS therapy was considered, the remaining treatment options were to live with urge incontinence symptoms or to choose life-altering surgery, such as augmentation cystoplasty. Because SNS therapy is serving an otherwise unmet medical need, no other therapy could have been used ethically for a control group.

Our data support the view that dynamic activity and basal tone of the pelvic floor, as well as the associated afferent signalling to the spinal cord, are fundamental elements of lower urinary tract dysfunction. Spasticity of the pelvic muscles is associated with over-facilitation of the detrusor and urge incontinence; conversely, non-relaxation of the pelvic floor can inhibit the voiding reflex and result in urinary retention; SNS modulates this aberrant neural activity. Although the precise mechanism of action is unknown, the results of our randomised study support the use of this modality for treat-ment of refractory urge incontinence.

The therapy evaluation test results also suggest that, once estab-lished, lower urinary tract dysfunction is permanent. All 52 patients who underwent inactivation of SNS 6 months after implantation had a documented return to baseline symptoms of urge inconti-nence; SNS was, therefore, continuously required to modulate the neural instability that influenced voiding behaviour; hence, patients may require lifelong SNS therapy. The compelling benefits for treat-ment of a refractory population outweigh the attendant risks. The observed revision rate of 32.5% (see Chapter 16) is expected to decrease as improved surgical techniques reduce the potential for adverse events, including pain, at the neurostimulator site.

Currently, no consistent pretreatment urodynamic findings can accurately predict which patients with incontinence will respond to medical or surgical therapy [30–32]. The voiding diary is a valuable tool, providing subjective and objective parameters that can be used to assess the effect of SNS on symptoms. Patients have the oppor-tunity to participate actively in the decision to pursue long-term SNS therapy. As such, incorporation of voiding diaries and the test stim-ulation procedure into clinical practice is integral to evaluation.

In conclusion, SNS is safe and effective in treating severe symp-toms of urinary urge incontinence in a refractory population.

Key Points

- SNS therapy serves an unmet medical need; no other therapy could be used for controls.
- Pelvic floor dynamic activity and basal tone are fundamental to LUT dysfunction.
- SNS modulates the associated afferent signalling to the spinal cord.
- Therapy evaluation test shows that, once established, LUT dysfunction is permanent.
- Patients may therefore need lifelong SNS therapy.
- The benefits outweigh the risks (which should decrease with improved surgery).
- Pretreatment urodynamic data cannot predict patient response to medical/surgical therapy.
- Voiding diaries are of prime importance.
- SNS is a safe/effective treatment of refractory urge incontinence.

Acknowledgements

Jeffrey A. Cerkvenik provided statistical analyses; Kathleen A. Herzog contributed expertise and performed extensive literature research.

Appendix

Inclusion criteria:
- age greater than 16 years;
- refractory to standard medical therapy;
- bladder capacity of 100ml with normal upper urinary tract;
- good surgical candidate;
- able to complete study documentation and return for follow-up evaluation.

Exclusion criteria:
- neurological conditions (multiple sclerosis, diabetes with peripheral nerve involvement, spinal cord injury, stroke);
- stress urinary incontinence;
- primary pelvic pain.

Key Points

- Retention is caused by a hypercontractile/acontractile detrusor or obstruction.
- Beneficial SNS probably depends on excitation of myelinated afferents.
- Integrity of peripheral somatic/autonomic motor innervation is also important.
- Study patients with idiopathic urinary retention had either complete or partial retention due to hypocontractile or acontractile detrusor, or functional outlet obstruction for urethral overactivity.

Efficacy of sacral nerve stimulation for urinary retention: results up to 18 months after implantation

U. Jonas, C. J. Fowler and V. Grünewald*

Introduction

Retention can be caused by a hypocontractile or acontractile detrusor (weak or no bladder muscle contraction), obstruction due to urethral overactivity or mechanical outlet obstruction of the urethra, such as strictures, cancer or benign prostatic hyperplasia. The inability to empty the bladder can, with time, result in secondary health consequences, such as reflux, upper urinary tract damage, urinary tract infection and overflow incontinence. Patients mostly depend on instrumental drainage of the bladder, such as timed self-catheterisation or suprapubic catheters.

In 1981, Tanagho and Schmidt successfully introduced chronic electrical stimulation of the sacral nerves using a surgically implanted sacral foramen electrode and a battery-powered pulse generator for treatment of different kinds of neurogenic and non-neurogenic lower urinary tract dysfunction, refractory to conservative treatment [10, 33, 34]. In several retrospective studies it was demonstrated that electrical stimulation of the sacral spinal nerves could restore coordinated voiding [16, 19, 35]. The precise pathophysiology causing urinary retention and the mechanism of action of sacral electrical stimulation remain unknown. However, clinical and animal experimental studies suggest that the stimulation effect depends primarily on excitation of myelinated afferent nerve fibres as well as the integrity of the peripheral somatic and autonomic motor innervation [36]. We investigate, in a prospective, randomised multicentre trial, the efficacy of sacral neurostimulation in patients with idiopathic urinary retention.

Study design and methods

A prospective randomised study was conducted in accordance with regulatory requirements of the countries where data were collected, including provisions for protection of human subjects and the Declaration of Helsinki. The study was performed at 13 worldwide centres that recruited patients from the general urological population between 12 December 1993 and 1 June 1998. Patients with idiopathic urinary retention enrolled in the study had either complete retention (inability to initiate voiding) or partial retention (residual urine remains post-voiding). They presented with hypocontractile or acontractile detrusor, or functional outlet obstruction due to urethral overactivity.

Based on initial test results, including medical history, urodynamic testing, and quantification of baseline voiding behaviour in diaries, a total of 177 retention cases meeting the specific criteria were enrolled in the study (Table 14.5). A percutaneous test stimulation

*With members of the Sacral Nerve Stimulation Study Group (see page 168). Reprinted with permission from the *Journal of Urology*.

Table 14.5 Inclusion and exclusion criteria

Inclusion criteria	Exclusion criteria
Age older than 16 years	Neurological condition including multiple
Refractory to standard medical therapy	sclerosis, diabetes with peripheral
Minimum 100ml bladder capacity with	nerve involvement, spinal cord injury
normal upper urinary tract	and stroke
Good surgical candidate	Stress urinary incontinence
Able to complete study documentation	Primary pelvic pain
and return for follow-up evaluation	

Key Points

- \>50% improvement in baseline voiding symptoms indicated suitability for implantation.
- Treatment-group patients had early implant of the SNS system.
- Control-group patients (implant delayed for 6 months) had standard medical treatment.
- Residual volume was the primary diary variable for assessment of treatment efficacy.

procedure was performed in all 177 patients for 3–7 days to assess the integrity of the sacral nerves and quantify the effects of trial sacral nerve stimulation (SNS) on dysfunctional voiding behaviour; 68 (38.4%) qualified for implantation.

SNS therapy is delivered as test stimulation and surgical implantation. Test stimulation is performed as an outpatient procedure, and is used to locate and assist the integrity of S3-derived nerves which, when stimulated, produce levator ani contraction and great-toe movement. Stimulation of these sacral nerves demonstrates possible efficacy of intervention on symptoms and allows the patient to experience the sensation of stimulation during various activities. Greater than 50% improvement in baseline voiding symptoms during test stimulation qualified a patient for surgical implantation of an InterStim system. Details of the technique of test stimulation and surgical implantation have been published previously [19, 34, 37].

Of the 68 patients who qualified for implantation, 37 were randomly assigned to a treatment and 31 to a control group. Patients in the treatment group underwent early surgical implantation of the SNS system, while implantation was delayed in the control group for 6 months and standard medical treatment was given. Follow-up evaluations for the treatment group were conducted at 1, 3, 6, 12 and 18 months after implant. Control-group patients were followed at 3 and 6 months and, if device implant remained medically indicated, they were crossed over to the treatment group.

Efficacy

Voiding diaries used to quantify the effects of SNS on urinary retention were the primary outcome measure of the study. Efficacy of SNS was based on analysis of a 3-day voiding diary, which generated 16 diary variables reported as averages during 24 hours, with an overall diary average provided as well. Voiding diary variables were evaluated from diary data collected at baseline during test stimulation and throughout study follow-up. The post-void catheterised volume per catheterisation (residual volume) was used as the primary diary variable for assessment of treatment efficacy in retention cases.

Efficacy was evaluated by comparing the baseline with the 6-month voiding diary results of the treatment and control groups, and by comparing the baseline with the 18-month voiding diary results for all patients with implants. A second efficacy test (called the therapy evaluation test) was performed 6 months after implant, and consisted of deactivating stimulation for a minimum of 3 days before reactivation and documenting the effects of inactive stimulation on voiding behaviour for 3 days, with patients serving as their own control.

Statistical analysis

Data were analysed using group sequential data analysis [28], and ordered logistic regression was used to compare distribution of symptom changes between the two groups. Continuous study variables were compared using a two-sided Student t-test.

Results

Demographics

A total of 177 patients with retention were enrolled in the study, of whom 74% were female and 26% were male. Mean age plus or minus standard deviation (SD) at test stimulation was 42.9±12.7 years (range 17.4–81.0) and symptom duration before study enrolment was 7.1±8.5 years (range 0.0–43.2). On average, patients catheterised 4.6±2.9 times daily with an average of 335±186 ml per catheterisation. The total daily catheterised volume was 1,447±976 ml and the total daily voided volume was 614±921 ml. Of the 177 patients, 153 (86%) had received pharmacological treatment, including α-blockers, β-blockers and antibiotics; 62 (35%) had undergone a total of 271 non-surgical interventions, including biofeedback, urethral dilatations, psychological counselling and timed voiding; and 83 (47%) had undergone a total of 239 surgical interventions, including hysterectomy, prostate surgery, cystocele repair, and bladder neck suspension for treatment of voiding disorders before the study.

Test stimulation outcome

A total of 98 test stimulation procedures (1–5 tests) were conducted on the 68 patients. The voiding diary results obtained during test stimulation are summarised in Table 14.6. All voiding and retention parameters improved clinically and were statistically significant. All 68 patients returned to baseline retention status with either low or 0 voided volumes after test stimulation was completed. The remaining 109 retention study patients (61.6%) did not qualify for device implantation because they did not achieve a more than 50% improvement in the primary voiding diary parameter.

Implant outcome
Efficacy at 6 months
Results at 6 months were available in 29 treatment and 22 control group patients. Of the remaining patients, six were not yet

Table 14.6 *Voiding diary results at baseline versus test stimulation*

Diary variables	Mean baseline ± SD	Mean test stimulation ± SD	P-value*
Primary diary variable: catheter vol/ catheterisation (ml)	333 ± 164	109 ± 143	<0.0001
Catheterisation variables			
No. cathetersations/day	4.9 ± 2.7	2.7 ± 2.8	<0.0001
Total catheter vol/day (ml)	1577 ± 1041	243 ± 316	<0.0001
Max. catheter vol (ml)	573 ± 374	203 ± 226	<0.0001
Voiding variables			
No. voids/day	3.6 ± 4.4	6.5 ± 2.4	<0.0001
Total vol voided/day (ml)	698 ± 1051	1912 ± 883	<0.0001

*Paired t-test for test stimulation versus baseline with $p = 0.05$ considered statistically significant

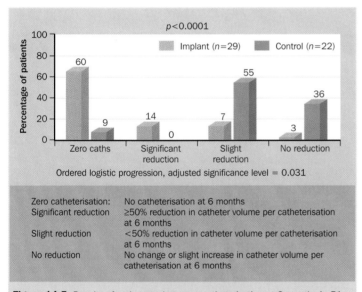

Ordered logistic progression, adjusted significance level = 0.031

Zero catheterisation:	No catheterisation at 6 months
Significant reduction	≥50% reduction in catheter volume per catheterisation at 6 months
Slight reduction	<50% reduction in catheter volume per catheterisation at 6 months
No reduction	No change or slight increase in catheter volume per catheterisation at 6 months

Figure 14.5 *Results of catheter volume per catheterisation at 6 months in 51 randomised patients.*

enrolled for 6 months, three had been lost to follow-up and eight were in the study but did not turn in a voiding diary. Statistical analysis of the primary diary variable demonstrated that the treatment group had significant reduction in residual volumes ($p<0.0001$) compared to the control group at 6 months (Fig. 14.5). Table 14.7 summarises the results of the voiding diary analysis for both groups at baseline and 6 months, and indicates a highly significant improvement in voiding and bladder evacuation in the treatment compared with the control group.

Table 14.7 Voiding diary results at baseline versus 6 months

Diary variables	Av control ± SD (22 patients)		Av implants ± SD (29 patients)		P value*
	Baseline	6 months	Baseline	6 months	
Primary diary variable: catheter vol/catheterisation (ml)	350 ± 152	319 ± 195	339 ± 176	49 ± 106	<0.0001
Catheterisation variables					
No. catheterisations/day	4.0 ± 1.7	3.9 ± 2.2	5.7 ± 3.1	1.4 ± 2.6	<0.0001
Total catheter vol/day (ml)	1379 ± 845	1305 ± 890	1744 ± 1047	237 ± 564	<0.0001
Max catheter vol (ml)	563 ± 276	484 ± 292	613 ± 461	72 ± 145	<0.0001
Voiding variables					
No. voids/day	3.2 ± 4.1	2.9 ± 4.3	4.0 ± 4.9	6.5 ± 3.1	0.002
Total vol voided/day (ml)	560 ± 769	488 ± 730	722 ± 1036	1808 ± 879	<0.0001

*Two sample t-tests comparing mean differences with p = 0.05 considered statistically significant.

Therapy evaluation test

A total of 34 patients from the treatment and control groups after crossover completed the therapy evaluation test, and nine additional patients refused the test because of medical and emotional concerns with returning to baseline retention. As documented in the voiding diary analysis results, the 34 patients had a statistically significant increase in residual urine (p<0.0001) and decrease in voided volumes (p<0.0002) when stimulation therapy was inactivated (Fig. 14.6 and Table 14.8). This result was completely reversible after reactivation of stimulation.

Efficacy at 18 months after implant

Voiding diaries were available for 21 patients at 18 months. Three patients withdrew from the study before the 18-month visit owing to lack of efficacy in two and an adverse event in one. However, these patients were included in the statistical analysis. Therefore, efficacy of SNS at 18 months was evaluated with data from a total of 24 retention cases.

Compared with baseline, the 24 patients who received implants for retention had significant improvement in voiding function through 18 months. Improved ability to empty the bladder was documented in the voiding diaries, which indicated a decrease in average catheter volume per catheterisation (range 305–74ml, p<0.0001), number of catheterisations daily (range 6.1 to 2.9ml, p<0.0001), total catheter volume daily (range 1560–343ml, p<0.0001), and maximum voided volume (range 323–488ml, p=0.02). Catheterisation was completely eliminated in 14 (58%) of the 24 implanted patients.

The therapeutic effect of SNS had a significant, positive impact on patient ability to empty at 18 months. Patients were considered to have a successful outcome if they either eliminated catheterisation or significantly reduced residual volumes by 50% or more. Based on these criteria, 71% of implanted cases were treated successfully with SNS (Fig. 14.7). Following implantation, the InterStim system can be reprogrammed to find optimal levels of stimulation for individual

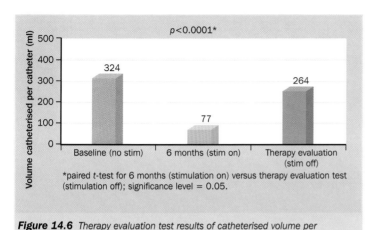

Figure 14.6 *Therapy evaluation test results of catheterised volume per catheterisation in 34 patients with retention.*

Table 14.8 *Therapy evaluation results*

Diary variables	No. patients	Av 6 months ± SD (stimulation on)	Av therapy evaluation ± SD (stimulation off)	p - value*
Primary diary variable: catheter vol/catheterisation (ml)	34	77 ± 137	264 ± 153	<0.0001
Catheterisation variables:				
No. catheterisations/day	34	1.5 ± 2.5	4.6 ± 2.9	<0.0001
Total catheter vol/day (ml)	34	259 ± 554	1360 ± 984	<0.0001
Max catheter vol (ml)	34	112 ± 191	374 ± 224	<0.0001
Voiding variables:				
No. voids/day	34	6.8 ± 3.1	4.2 ± 5.6	0.003
Vol voided/void (ml)	19†	242 ± 92	138 ± 85	0.0002
Total vol voided day (ml)	34	1767 ± 800	648 ± 889	<0.0001

*Paired t-test comparing 6 months (on) with the therapy evaluation test (off) with $p = 0.05$ considered statistically significant.
†Includes only patients who voided at both times.

patients. A total of 48 patients had 6 months of data after implant related to reprogramming of the neurostimulator and averaged 3.9 reprogrammings during that time (range 1–14).

Urodynamic tests were conducted at a baseline and 6 months after implant to rule out treatable aetiologies at baseline. No deterioration in urodynamic function was seen during this period, and at 6 months after implant the number of patients able to void 100ml or more increased significantly (p=0.03) compared with baseline. Also, patients reported an increase in peak flow rate during a detrusor pressure study that averaged 8.7ml and peak flow rates in the control group decreased by an average of 1.3mls daily (p=0.04).

Key Points
- Urodynamic tests at 6 months showed the benefit of SNS.

Implant safety

Details of complications associated with implantation are given in Chapter 16 of this volume.

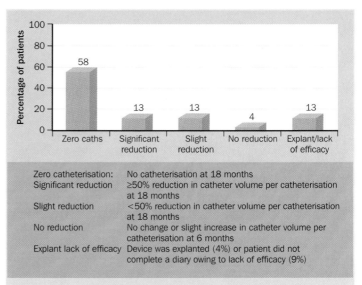

Figure 14.7 *Results of catheter volume per catheterisation at 18 months in 24 patients who received implants for retention.*

Discussion

There have been several reports on the positive results of SNS for the treatment of non-obstructive urinary retention [14, 38–40]. However, to our knowledge, we report the first prospective randomised study that provides evidence in a sufficient number of select patients known to be refractory to standard medical treatments — including pharmacological approaches, non-surgical and other surgical interventions — in whom SNS was effective in restoring voiding function. Our results show that, compared with a control group, patients implanted with the InterStim system had significant reductions in residual urine volume per catheterisation at 6 months ($p<0.0001$). Results from the control group of patients at 6 months demonstrated that significant improvement in retention with time is not likely to occur. Clinical improvement was maintained throughout the 18-month follow-up. Of the 24 patients with implants, 14 (58%) no longer needed catheterisation and three (13%) had a 50% or greater reduction in volume per catheterisation at 18 months.

To our knowledge, how an intervention known to be effective for the treatment of frequency, urgency and urge incontinence can also restore voiding in some patients remains unknown. However, our study highlights some observations that require an explanation beyond hypothesis. Inactivation of SNS therapy during the therapy evaluation test resulted in a significant increase in residual volumes ($p<0.0001$), demonstrating that clinical benefit of SNS is solely attributable to stimulation. Also, comparison of the therapy evaluation test results (stimulation off) with the voiding diary results collected at baseline (no stimulation) indicated that symptoms of retention observed when stimulation was inactivated were similar to those observed at baseline. Thus, SNS therapy did not cure the underlying mechanism of urinary retention but, rather, modulated aberrant dysfunctional reflexes causing voiding dysfunction [41]. Nonetheless, the clinical effect is maintained by the chronic implant, and all patients with retention who completed the therapy evaluation test requested that stimulation therapy be resumed.

It seems likely that neuromodulation by foraminal stimulation of the sacral nerve depends on electrical stimulation of afferent axons that modulate sensory processing of the voiding reflex pathways of the central nervous system [19, 42–44]. Although several reflex mechanisms are known to be involved in neuromodulation to suppress bladder hyperactivity, how sacral somatic afferent activation promotes voiding is less clear. Some forms of urinary retention may be due to inappropriate activation of the 'guarding reflex', which is the spinally mediated reflex whereby the urinary sphincter contracts to prevent urinary incontinence on sudden increase in intravesical pressure. Brain pathways are necessary to turn off urethral guarding reflexes and allow efficient bladder emptying, and so sphincter dyssynergia results after spinal cord injury, because of loss of descending brain mechanisms. However, spinal cord disease that produces dyssynergia is almost inevitably accompanied by other neurological deficits, such as spasticity and weakness of the lower limbs [45]. Since an exclusion criterion for entering this study was evidence of neurological disease, retention due to spinal cord disease is unlikely to have been a factor for these patients.

Before development of brain control of voiding, at least in animals, stimulation of somatic afferent pathways passing through the pudendal nerve to the perineum can initiate voiding by activating bladder efferent pathways and turning off the excitatory pathways to the urethral outlet [46, 47]. Furthermore, because sphincter activity can generate afferent input to the spinal cord that can inhibit reflex bladder activity, suppression of sphincter reflexes would facilitate bladder activity. It is proposed that SNS turns off excitatory outflow to the urethral outlet and so promotes bladder emptying, although the underlying cause of development of the abnormal reflex resulting in retention is unknown in most cases.

As with neuromodulation in other patient groups, there are two fundamental problems that may result in treatment failure. The first problem relates to the responsiveness of the underlying condition, since there are many different causes of urinary retention, some of which might not be expected to respond to neuromodulation. In our study only, 68 of 177 (38.4%) patients with retention had a successful stimulation test, which contrasts with the 68% success rate seen in a highly select group of young women who had urinary retention and abnormal electromyogram activity in the striated urethral sphincter (Fowler's syndrome). Of those women, ten were included in our series, and it appears that they responded particularly well to neuromodulation [40]. It is hypothesised that a primary abnormality of the striated muscle of the urethral sphincter causes abnormal persistence of the guarding reflex. No diagnosis or pathophysiological explanation for urinary retention was available for the remaining 37 patients who underwent implant of a permanent stimulator. Technical failure

Key Points

- SNS did not *cure* the mechanisms of urinary retention.
- However, it modulated dysfunctional reflexes that caused voiding dysfunction.
- The clinical effect is maintained by the chronic implant.
- How sacral somatic afferent activation promotes voiding is not clear.
- SNS may turn off excitatory outflow to the urethral outlet, promoting bladder emptying.
- Treatment failure may follow lack of response of condition, or technical failure.

Key Points

- Bilateral stimulation needs careful evaluation as it is more invasive.
- SNS effectively treats severe refractory voiding dysfunction or urinary retention.

of the test stimulation may also be a factor for a patient who has a condition that is expected to respond. It is currently impossible to differentiate between these two alternative explanations for non-response to test stimulation, and further study of the mechanism underlying response to test stimulation is warranted. However, since dislocation of the lead is a frequent problem during test stimulation, it is likely that it failed in a proportion of patients for this reason.

Another problem that may adversely affect outcome is technical failure during implantation of the permanent stimulator. Of the patients who had successful test stimulation, 17% did not improve to the same extent with the surgical implant, which implies that there was a problem with appropriate lead placement for achieving a favourable clinical result. The possibility of neurophysiological monitoring to achieve optimum electrode placement is now being investigated. In addition, alternative surgical procedures are being considered, such as bilateral electrodes or even more invasive techniques of implantation to place the electrode in closer vicinity to the nerve — that is, sacral laminectomy and placement of cuff electrodes [48].

Although there is some evidence from animal experimental studies [41] and limited first clinical experiences in humans [49] that bilateral stimulation might increase treatment efficacy, this approach needs further careful evaluation because a surgical procedure that is substantially more invasive is being performed in patients without obvious neurological deficit. As a result of the recent multicentre study [37, 50], a new test stimulation lead has been designed to improve the outcome of test stimulation. Another way to circumvent the problem of test stimulation lead dislocation is a two-stage implant, with surgical implantation of the lead electrode only at stage 1 and of the pulse generator at stage 2 in case of a positive test stimulation procedure. So far there is limited experience with this approach [51], but such a procedure would obviously alter the current minimal invasiveness of test stimulation.

Conclusions

Results of our prospective, randomised, clinical study demonstrate that SNS is effective for treating severe voiding dysfunction or urinary retention in a refractory population. The test stimulation procedure is an important diagnostic tool that allows the patient and physician to have the clinical effect of stimulation and make an informed choice about pursuing chronic implantable therapy. This procedure offers a clinical advantage, as there are currently no consistent pretreatment factors that can accurately predict which patients will respond to therapy.

Acknowledgement

Jeffrey A. Cerkvenik provided statistical assistance.

Sacral neuromodulation in the treatment of urgency–frequency symptoms: a multicentre study on efficacy and safety

M.M. Hassouna, S.W. Siegel and A.A.B. Lycklama à Nijeholt*

Introduction

Refractory urinary urgency–frequency symptoms remain an enigma, as few effective treatments are available for this condition. Urgency–frequency is characterised by the uncontrollable urge to void, resulting in frequent, small-volume voids.

We report 6-month and long-term treatment outcomes with the use of sacral nerve stimulation (SNS) in a prospective, randomised multicentre study. SNS or neuromodulation of the micturition reflex, is an accepted concept for the management of refractory urinary symptoms through the stimulation of the afferent nerves of the pelvic floor [40, 52].

Materials and methods

A total of 51 patients presenting with refractory symptoms of urinary urgency–frequency were prospectively enrolled into the clinical study and had completed a 6-month diary at the time of administrative database closure on 1 June 1998. Patient enrolment was generated from the urological population at 12 worldwide (eight North American and four European) centres under an identical protocol approved by institutional health ethics committees with written voluntary patient informed consent.

Study candidates older than 16 years, and who were refractory to standard medical therapies, underwent baseline evaluation to rule out treatable aetiologies. Prestudy evaluation included medical and urological history, physical evaluation, urodynamic testing and completion of two 3-day voiding diaries. Patients with a bladder capacity of at least 100ml and normal upper tracts were enrolled into the study. Exclusion criteria included neurological conditions, primary stress incontinence, and primary pelvic pain symptoms.

Standardised voiding diaries translated into various local languages, were used by patients to record void, catheter or leaking episodes. Patients collected and measured urine volumes using cups provided by the investigator. Key voiding-diary variables for the urgency–frequency population included the number of voids daily, volume voided per void and degree of urgency before void. The degree of urgency before void, as well as pelvic/bladder discomfort, were ranked by patients as 0 (none), 1 (mild), 2 (moderate) or 3 (severe).

All 51 patients subsequently underwent trial test stimulation of the sacral nerves. This office-based procedure assesses nerve integrity

Key Points
- SNS effects on urgency–frequency were recorded in a prospective, randomised study.
- Patients with bladder capacity ≥ 100ml and normal UUT were enrolled.

*With members of the Sacral Nerve Stimulation Study Group (see page 168).
Reprinted with permission from the *Journal of Urology*.

through percutaneous transforaminal stimulation of the S3 or S4 sacral nerve. Patients who responded favourably to the office procedure completed trial stimulation therapy at home for 3–7 days and documented the effects of stimulation on urgency–frequency behaviour in a voiding diary. Reduction in primary voiding diary parameters of 50% or more during the trial phase qualified patients for surgical implantation of the InterStim System device and they were randomised into the study. The subcutaneously implanted devices include a neurostimulator, a lead placed adjacent to the targeted sacral nerve and an extension that connects these two devices. Of the 51 patients, 25 who received the device were randomly assigned to the stimulation group (treatment arm of the study) and the remaining 26 who received standard medical treatment for 6 months were assigned to the control group (control arm of the study).

At initial evaluation of efficacy, 6 months after therapy, voiding-diary data were compared between the stimulation group and control group (stimulation versus no stimulation). Control-group patients were given the opportunity to cross over to the stimulation group after completion of the 6-month waiting period. Efficacy of SNS therapy was further evaluated in the stimulation group by assessment of urinary symptoms after stimulation therapy was temporarily inactivated after 6 months of therapy (stimulation on versus off). Long-term efficacy was evaluated at 12 and 24 months in all patients with devices.

Urodynamic testing was conducted at baseline and at 6 months of follow-up in both groups, and was used as a secondary study parameter. Urodynamic testing involved simple uroflowmetry with residual determination, water cystometry and a detrusor pressure/uroflow study. Water cystometry parameters were obtained with the subject sitting or supine, fill rate of 50ml/min, and with the temperature of the filling medium at 37°C. Cystometry measurements were obtained at first sensation of fullness, at first uninhibited detrusor contraction and at maximum fill before void.

The SF-36 Health Survey was used as a secondary study endpoint to assess eight conceptual areas of physical and mental health at baseline and at 6 months. An additional question on general health status documented patient perceptions about the transition of their health status over time. Demographic and baseline diary parameters were analysed to validate global data pools. Statistical analysis of the study results was accomplished using group sequential data analysis [28]. This method allowed interim analysis of the study results at specified intervals during the study. To account for the population sample size at the time of analysis and the potential for multiplicity bias, the significance level was conservatively adjusted down to 0.01 for the primary diary variables at 6 months, and was established at 0.05 for the remaining non-primary diary variables and secondary study variables. Ordered logistic regression was used to compare diary results of the stimulation group and control groups at 6 months. Comparison of treatment group averages was accomplished with a two-sided Student t-test and comparison of proportions was completed using Fisher's exact test. Commercial software was used for all analyses.

Results

Baseline information for the 51 randomised urgency–frequency cases is summarised in Table 14.9. In reviewing the history of all medical interventions used to treat symptoms of the study population, pharmacotherapy failed in 94% of the patients within 2 years before study enrolment. A total of 229 non-surgical and 125 surgical interventions had been performed on the study population before study enrolment. Non-surgical interventions included external stimulation (transcutaneous electric nerve stimulation), biofeedback, urethral dilatation, pain management, cones/timed voiding and psychological counselling. The 125 surgical interventions included hydrodistention (76), bladder/sphincter surgery (13), prostate surgery (1), urethral stricture repair (1), suspension/sling (6), denervation (4), cystocele repair (2) and other procedures such as hysterectomy and laparoscopy (22).

Treatment versus control at six months

Compared with the control group, in the stimulation group the daily number of voids was significantly reduced from 16.9±9.7 to 9.3±5.1 at 6 months ($p<0.0001$). In contrast, the daily number of voids did not change for the control group at 6 months (baseline 15.2±6.6; 6 months, 15.7±7.6). Patients whose baseline frequency was more than seven voids daily were considered to have a successful clinical outcome if they voided within the normal range of four to seven times daily or reduced the number of voids by at least 50%.

The distribution of improvement rankings for the 51 randomised patients who completed 6 months of follow-up is shown in Figure 14.8. Of the 25 patients in the stimulation group, 14 (56%) demonstrated 50% reduction or greater in the number of voids at 6 months after implant and/or achieved the normal range of 4 to 7 voids per day. Two stimulation-group patients (8%) demonstrated no reduction or a slight increase in the number of voids daily at 6 months. The clinical outcome of these patients had improved by 12 months, as evidenced by voiding-diary results. One stimulation-group

Table 14.9 *Demographic summary*

Female patients (%)	90
Male patients (%)	10
Age in years at test stimulation (mean ± SD)	39.0 ± 11.8
Duration (years)before study of urinary symptoms enrolment	8.1 ± 9.2 years
No. of voids/day (mean ± SD)	16.0 ± 8.2
Volume (ml) voided per void (mean ± SD)	121 ± 70
Maximum voiding volume (ml) (mean ± SD)	288 ± 156
Total voided volume (ml/day) (mean ± SD)	1693 ± 866
Percentage who felt empty (mean ± SD)	44 ± 39
Pelvic/bladder discomfort (0, none–3, severe)	2.1 ± 0.8
(0 none – 3 severe)	

Key Points

- Average volume voided/per void statistically significantly increased in the stimulation group.
- Average degree of urgency statistically significantly decreased in the stimulation group.
- SNS goal was to enable patients to sense urgency at a more appropriate urine volume.

patient (4%) underwent device explantation before 6 months owing to therapy-related bowel dysfunction and was conservatively considered to have treatment failure. Stimulation-group patients demonstrated statistically significant increases ($p<0.0001$) with respect to average voided volume per void, compared with the control group, at 6 months (Table 14.9). The stimulation group also had statistically significant reductions in the average degree of urgency before voiding compared with the control group at 6 months (Table 14.10).

Changes in the degree of urgency were compared with changes in voided volumes to define the impact of SNS on urgency–frequency behaviour. The goal of SNS was to enable patients to sense urinary urgency at a more appropriate volume of urine (as opposed to eliminating urgency completely). Therefore, the criteria for clinical success with respect to degree of urgency included increased voided volumes with either the same or a reduced degree of urgency. Under this definition, 88% (22) of the stimulation group and 32% (8) of the control group patients demonstrated a successful clinical outcome with respect to degree of urgency. A comparison of the ratio of clinical successes and clinical failures in the stimulation group and control groups indicated a statistically significant improvement in favour of the stimulation group ($p=0.0001$), suggesting that the improvement was also perceived by the patients.

Stimulation on versus off

After 6 months of receiving SNS therapy, 22 of the 25 patients had the stimulators inactivated by the study physicians. One patient underwent device explant before 6 months and two patients refused to complete the test owing to strong concerns with the

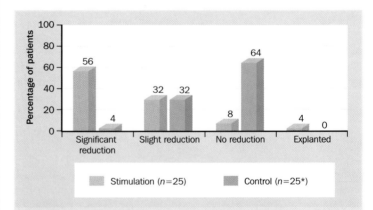

Figure 14.8 *Average number of voids daily at 6 months (p<0.0001). *One control patient had 4–7 voids at baseline and 6 months and, therefore, was not included in the study. Results obtained using ordered logistic regression with adjusted significance at 0.01. Reduction in number of voids daily is defined as significant (>50% reduction in number of voids daily at 6 months and/or normal range of 4–7 voids daily), slight (<50%), or no (no change or slight increase). 'Explanted' describes a case in which the device was removed before 6 months.*

Table 14.10 *Volume voided per void and degree of urgency before voiding*

Patient group	No. of Patients	(mean ± SD)	
		Baseline	6 months
Average volume (ml) voided per void			
Stimulation	25	118 ± 74	226 ± 124*
Control	26	124 ± 66	123 ± 75
Degree of urgency before voiding			
Stimulation	25	2.2 ± 0.6	1.6 ± 0.9
Control	25	2.4 ± 0.5	2.3 ± 0.5

* $p<0.0001$

Key Points

• After 6 months, inactivation of SNS led to a statistically significant symptom increase.

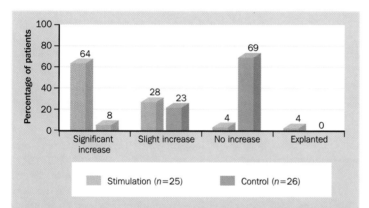

Figure 14.9 *Average volume voided per void (p<0.0001). Results obtained using ordered logistic regression with adjusted significance at 0.010. Increase in volume voided per void is defined as significant (>50% increase in volume), slight (<50% increase), or no (no increase or slight decrease). 'Explanted' describes a case in which the device was removed before 6 months.*

potential return of baseline symptoms. With respect to the three primary diary variables for urgency–frequency, patients demonstrated statistically significant increases (i.e. worsening) in symptoms when stimulation was off. The average number of voids per day increased from 8.6 to 13.9 ($p=0.0003$), voided volume per void decreased from 242 to 144 ml ($p<0.0001$), and the degree of urgency prior to void increased from a ranking of 1.5 to 2.1 ($p=0.0003$). These results demonstrate that the effectiveness of the therapy was dependent upon the presence of active stimulation. Additional statistical comparisons revealed the reversibility of SNS therapy. Diary results obtained with stimulation inactivated were statistically and/or clinically equivalent to the voiding diary results collected at baseline (no stimulation).

At the time of database closure, 15 control-group patients crossed over to the stimulation arm of the study, completed 6 months of post-implant follow-up and completed the on/off test.

Key Points

- SF-36 Health Survey showed a positive impact of therapy on QoL at 6 months.
- By this criterion, 88% of stimulation vs 32% of control group had a good clinical result.
- Comparison with baseline urgency–frequency status showed sustained clinical benefit.
- These improvements occurred without significant change in diurnal output.
- SNS has no negative effect on voiding function.

The remaining 11 control-group patients were not expected to have completed the 6-month evaluation at the time of database closure. Test results for the implanted control-group patients were similar in profile to those noted for the stimulation-group patients. All 37 patients requested reactivation of stimulation therapy at the conclusion of the test.

Urodynamic testing and quality of life

Urodynamic tests conducted at 6 months post-implant indicated no negative effect of SNS on the ability to void. Compared with the control group, statistically significant differences in favour of the stimulation-group patients were documented during the water cystometry test, indicating increased bladder storage at first sensation of fullness and bladder capacity (Table 14.11)

Results from the SF-36 Health Survey showed the positive impact of the therapy. Compared with the control group, the stimulation group demonstrated statistically significant improvements in various aspects of quality of life, including physical functioning ($p<0.0001$), role physical ($p=0.01$), bodily pain ($p=0.01$), general health ($p=0.003$), vitality ($p=0.01$), social function ($p=0.002$), and mental health ($p=0.01$).

Patients treated with SNS on average reported fewer limitations in physical activities, less bodily pain and less health-associated difficulty with work or other daily activities than did those who did not receive an implant. The findings related to physical function, role physical, and bodily pain are similar to those of other clinical studies examining the merits of surgical procedures to alleviate physical conditions such as knee replacement, hip replacement and heart-valve surgeries [53–55]. The stimulation group reported higher levels of energy and less nervousness and depression than did the control group. In addition, patients with an implant reported an improved ability to perform normal social activities without interference due to physical or emotional problems (Fig. 14.10). At 6 months' follow-up, the stimulation group perceived a statistically significantly greater degree of improvement in their general health status than did the control group without the device implant ($p<0.0001$).

Information on implantation safety can be found in Chapter 16.

Sustained clinical benefit

Comparison with baseline urgency–frequency status showed that clinical benefit was sustained through 12 months (Table 14.12).

These results indicate that patients with urgency–frequency treated with SNS have significantly improved efficiency in bladder storage and emptying and reduced pelvic/bladder discomfort at 12 months compared with baseline. These favourable changes in bladder function occurred without a significant change in diurnal output from baseline to 12 months ($p = 0.80$). No negative changes were noted with respect to any voiding diary parameter, suggesting that SNS does not negatively affect voiding function. Concomitant variables such as gender, age, and implant foramen location did not statistically influence clinical outcome with respect

Table 14.11 Results of water cystometry, baseline through 6 months

Test variable	n	Control (mean ± SD) Average at baseline	Average at 6 months	n	Stimulation (mean ± SD) Average at baseline	Average at 6 months	P value*
At first sensation of fullness							
Bladder volume (ml)	25	104 ± 77	92 ± 69	23	107 ± 97	161 ± 119	0.01
Detrusor pressure (cmH$_2$O)	24	4.0 ± 4.1	4.5 ± 5.2	23	7.9 ± 7.5	4.6 ± 4.9	0.098
At maximum fill volume or just before void							
Bladder volume (ml)	25	253 ± 93	227 ± 104	24	234 ± 128	325 ± 185	0.008
Detrusor pressure (cmH$_2$O)	24	5.5 ± 6.7	7.0 ± 8.1	23	15.4 ± 15.2	11.8 ± 17.2	0.10
Peak detrusor pressure during cystometry (cmH$_2$O)	23	7.3 ± 4.9	9.8 ± 10.2	22	27.4 ± 28.6	16.5 ± 21.8	0.01
Volume at peak detrusor pressure (ml)	24	205 ± 107	212 ± 114	21	218 ± 119	302 ± 165	0.099

Only patients who demonstrated uninhibited detrusor contractions during cystometry at baseline and at 6 months were included in the analysis.

*Wilcoxon rank-sum test comparing baseline with 6-month difference with significance at 0.05.

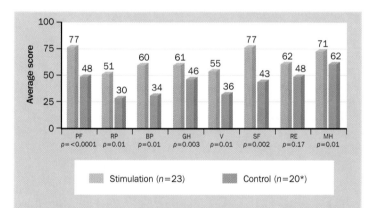

Key Points

- By this criterion, 88% of stimulation vs 32% of control group had a good clinical result.
- Clinical benefit was sustained in 21 patients followed up for 2 years.

Figure 14.10 SF-36 scores of all randomised patients at 6 months. *Some patients did not complete all responses at each visit, and so sample sizes actually range from 20 to 23 in the stimulation group and from 18 to 20 in the control group. p-values are derived from repeated-measures analysis of variance comparing means at baseline, 3 months and 6 months with significance at 0.05. PF, physical function; RP, role physical; BP, bodily pain; GH, general health; V, vitality; SF, social function; RE, role emotional; MH, mental health.

to the three primary diary parameters for urgency–frequency symptoms (all $p > 0.05$).

More recent analysis of the long-term results demonstrated sustained clinical benefit in the 21 treated patients who were followed up through 2 years post-implantation. The percentage of patients with documented clinical success remained uniform with respect to the primary voiding-diary parameters (Table 14.13).

Table 14.12 Results at 12 months

		n*	Average at baseline	Average at 12 months	P-value*
Primary	No. of voids/day	33	16.6 ± 8.5	9.0 ± 4.5	<0.0001
diary	Volume voided/void (ml)	33	132 ± 89	233 ± 141	<0.0001
variables†	Degree of urgency (0, none–3, severe)	33	2.2 ± 0.6	1.8 ± 0.8	0.005
Other	Total volume voided/day (ml)	27	1834 ± 1072	1792 ± 927	0.80
voiding	Max voided volume (ml)	27	334 ± 223	440 ± 231	0.001
variables	Percentage who felt empty	27	44 ± 43	81 ± 33	0.0002
	Pelvic/bladder discomfort (0, none–3 severe)	26	2.0 ± 1.0	0.9 ± 1.0	<0.0001
	Force of urine stream (1, strong–4, poor)	27	2.7 ± 0.8	1.9 ± 0.9	0.0005

*Paired t-test, significance level = 0.05.

†For the primary variables, 3 patients who left the study were conservatively included as treatment failures.

Key Points
- Conservative treatment has given only 44% subjective, no objective, improvement.

Table 14.13 Clinical success of primary diary variables 6 months through 2 years*

	Percentage of patients		
Diary variable	6 months (n = 56)	12 months (n = 46)	2 years (n = 21)
Number of voids/day†	46	54	43
Volume voided/void‡	53	57	62
Degree of urgency before void§	84	80	81

*Revised database closure in June 1999.

†Number of voids daily reduced 50% or greater, or the normal range of 4–7 voids daily achieved by patients with a baseline frequency of >7 voids per day.

‡Increase in volume voided per void of 50% or greater.

§Increased voided volumes with the same or reduced degree of urgency.

Discussion

Etiology and impact of urgency–frequency symptoms

The aetiology of irritative voiding symptoms such as urgency–frequency remains unknown. Research to determine the genesis of, and potential treatments for, this condition has included investigation of viral infection, bacteria, retained bacterial DNA in bladder tissue after infection, damage to the bladder mucosa or glycosaminoglycan protective layer, neurally mediated inflammation and/or ischaemia and autoimmune disease [56]. Until recently, refractory urinary urgency–frequency syndromes presented a dilemma for clinicians, owing to the complexity of symptoms and lack of effective treatment. It has been estimated that pharmacotherapy and other conservative forms of treatment have provided only 44% subjective improvement and no significant objective improvement [1]. Patients who do not achieve a satisfactory response with these standard forms of treatment are left with drastic, more morbid, options, including urinary diversion.

Chronic symptoms of urgency–frequency dramatically affect patient quality of life. Our baseline study results obtained with the SF-36 Health Survey demonstrated that our patients overall reported significantly lower scores ($p<0.0001$) than published United States norms with respect to the eight conceptual areas measured for quality of life. Results for the physical function scale of the SF-36 suggest that the effect of urgency–frequency on limitations in physical activities due to health is similar to that of other complicated chronic medical conditions, including congestive heart failure, hypotension and musculoskeletal conditions such as osteoarthritis and rheumatoid arthritis [57].

Patients suffering from refractory urgency–frequency often resort to extreme compensating measures to help manage the symptoms, which result in concomitant problems in the gastrointestinal system (such as constipation). Baseline voiding diaries indicated that 81% of the study patients voided with significantly higher frequency and lower volumes than did the general population. Investigator review of the diary data confirmed that these patients decreased daily fluid intake as compensating behaviour to reduce symptoms of urgency–frequency. Average diurnal output in this group of 42 patients was 1162ml (normal 2000±1000ml). Poor fluid management can exacerbate or contribute to the high associated rates of irritable bowel syndrome and gastroparesis in patients presenting with voiding problems [58–60].

Visceral pain symptoms

Because the study investigators chose to evaluate urinary symptoms (urgency and frequency) rather than specific diagnoses, they did not specifically focus on the population with interstitial cystitis. The hallmark symptoms of interstitial cystitis typically include urinary frequency, urgency, nocturia, pain on bladder filling (typically relieved by voiding) and suprapubic pain [56]. More than 77% of the study patients complained of associated pelvic/bladder discomfort at baseline. Compared with the control group, the stimulation group had a statistically significant reduction in the average degree of pelvic/bladder discomfort as documented by a voiding-diary ranking of 2.0 (moderate) down to 0.6 (less than mild) at 6 months ($p<0.0001$). Additionally, as measured by the SF-36 Health Survey, the stimulation group reported significantly fewer limitations due to bodily pain than did the control group ($p=0.01$).

These observations can be explained by the gate-control theory first proposed by Melzack [20]. He proposed that pain perceived from a visceral origin could be blocked by converging impulses arising from somatic origin and supplied by the same dermatome. Reduction in pain symptoms can also be explained by the recent results of a double-blind animal study which demonstrated that SNS reduces c-*fos* gene expression [61]. As c-*fos* genes become activated only when sensory cells are exposed to noxious input from the afferent C fibres, the demonstration that neuromodulation can block these fibres suggests a potential mode of action for pain symptoms. Further study on the possible implications of the relief of associated pain symptoms in this patient group is warranted.

Key Points

- Patients with urgency–frequency often restrict fluid intake, causing irritable bowel syndrome and gastroparesis.
- Pelvic/bladder pain was significantly reduced in stimulation vs control group.
- This may be explicable in terms of Melzack's gate-control theory.
- SNS also reduces c-*fos* expression, i.e. blocks noxious input from afferent C fibres.

Mechanism of action

SNS for the treatment of voiding dysfunction was introduced into modern urology practice after the pioneering work of Tanagho *et al.* [62]. The mechanism by which SNS affects dysfunctional bladder behaviour is not fully understood. The activation of spinal inhibitory pathways through stimulation of the afferent input in the S3 nerve can provide a partial explanation in patients with urgency and incontinence [49, 63]. However, stimulation of large sensory afferents running from the pelvic floor may also produce inhibition of the detrusor motor neurons, either directly at a spinal level or via other neural pathways [64].

Current theory suggests that dysfunction and anatomical change result when an unnatural bias develops between inhibitory and facilitatory neural activity in the pelvic floor. For example, overfacilitation of the detrusor can result in symptoms of urgency–frequency and urge incontinence. SNS is believed to have a conditioning effect on neural excitability and can restore neural equilibrium [65]. In consideration of these theories, SNS has been demonstrated to effectively relieve severe symptoms of urinary urge incontinence and now provides clinicians with an important new option in treating patients with significant symptoms of urgency–frequency.

Conclusions

SNS is an effective, safe, and reversible therapy for the treatment of significant symptoms of urinary urgency–frequency. Compared with a concurrent control group at 6 months, the group of patients receiving SNS demonstrated statistically significant improvement in urinary frequency, voided volumes, and degree of urgency before voiding (all $p<0.0001$). Statistically significant improvement in various aspects of the SF-36 Health Survey and water cystometry confirmed the effectiveness of SNS. Sustained clinical benefit with respect to the primary voiding-diary parameters was documented through 18 and 24 months after implantation.

Appendix

The three sections of this chapter have been reprinted with permission from the *Journal of Urology*.

Schmidt RA, Jonas U, Oleson K. Sacral nerve stimulation for the treatment of refractory urinary urge incontinence. *J Urol* 1999; 162: 352–57.

Jonas U, Fowler CJ, Grünewald V. Efficacy of sacral nerve stimulation for urinary retention; results up to 18 months after implantation. *J Urol* 2001; 165: 15–19.

Hassouna MM, Siegel SW, Lycklama à Nijeholt AAB. Sacral neuromodulation in the treatment of urgency–frequency symptoms: a multicentre study on efficacy and safety. *J Urol* 2000; 163: 1849–54.

The Sacral Nerve Stimulation Study Group comprises the following teams:

The USA

Boone, T., MD, Baylor College of Medicine, Houston, TX; Chancellor, M.B., MD, University of Pittsburgh School of Medicine, PA; Das, A., MD, Albany Medical College, Albany, NY; Kaplan, S., MD, Columbia University, New York, NY; Milarn, D., MD, Vanderbilt University, Nashville, TN; Rivas, D., MD, Thomas Jefferson University Medical College, Philadelphia, PA; Schmidt, R.A., MD, University of Colorado Health Science Center and Fitzsimons Army Medical Center, Denver, CO; Siegel, S., MD, Metropolitan Urologic Specialists, St Paul, MN; Stone, A., MD, University of California Davis Medical Center, Sacramento, CA; Tutrone, R., MD, Greater Baltimore Medical Center, Baltimore, MD.

Canada

Elhliali, M., MD and Corcos, J., MD, Royal Victoria Hospital, Montreal, Quebec; Gajewski, J., MD, QEII Health Science Center, Halifax, Nova Scotia; Hassouna, M.M., MD, University of Toronto, Ontario.

Europe

Bemelmans, B., MD and Meuleman, E., MD, Academisch Zeikenhuis, Radbound HB Nijmegen, The Netherlands; Cantanzaro, F., MD, Azienda USSI, Desio, Italy; Dijkema, H., MD, Twenteborg Ziekenhuis, Almelo, The Netherlands; Fall, M., MD, Sahlgrenska Hospital, University of Gothenborg, Gothenborg, Sweden; Fowler, C.J., MD, The National Hospital for Neurology and Neurosurgery, London, United Kingdom; Jonas, U., MD and Grünewald, V., MD, Klinik für Urologie, Hannover Medical School, Hannover, Germany; van Kerrebroeck, P.E.V., MD and Janknegt, R.A., MD, Academisch Seikenhuis, Maastricht, The Netherlands; Lycklama à Nijeholt, A.A.B., MD, Leiden University Medical Centre, The Netherlands; Madersbacher, H., MD, University Hospital Innsbruck, Innsbruck, Austria.

References

1. United States Department of Health and Human Services. *Urinary incontinence in adults: acute and chronic management. AHCPR Publication No. 96–0682.* Public Health Service, Agency for Health Care Policy and Research. March 1996.
2. Benvenuti F, Caputo OM, Bandinelli S et al. Reeducative treatment of female genuine stress incontinence. *Am J Phys Med Rehabil* 1987; 66: 155.
3. Dougherty M, Bishop K, Mooney R et al. Graded pelvic muscle exercise. Effect on stress urinary incontinence. *J Reprod Med* 1993; 38: 684.
4. Holmes DM, Montz FJ, Stanton SL. Oxybutynin versus propantheline in the management of detrusor instability. A patient-regulated variable dose trial. *Br J Obstet Gynaecol* 1989; 96: 607.
5. Moore KH, Hay DM, Imrie AE et al. Oxybutynin hydrochloride (3 mg) in the treatment of women with idiopathic detrusor instability. *Br J Urol* 1990; 66: 479.
6. Appell RA. Clinical efficacy and safety of tolterodine in the treatment of overactive bladder: a pooled analysis. *Urology* 1997; Suppl. 50: 90.
7. Vodušek DB, Plevnik S, Vrtacnik P, Janez J. Detrusor inhibition on selective pudendal nerve stimulation in the perineum. *Neurourol Urodyn* 1988; 6: 389.

8. Bergmann S, Eriksen BC. Anal electrostimulation in urinary incontinence. Technical description of a new device. *Urol Int* 1986; 41: 411.

9 Fall M, Lindström S. Electrical stimulation. A physiologic approach to the treatment of urinary incontinence. *Urol Clin North Am* 1991; 18: 393.

10. Schmidt, RA, Senn E, Tanagho EA. Functional evaluation of sacral nerve root integrity. Report of a technique. *Urology* 1990; 35: 388–92.

11 Bradley WE, Timm GW, Chou SN. A decade of experience with electronic stimulation of the micturition reflex. *Urol Int* 1971; 26: 283.

12 Jünemann KP, Lue TF, Schmidt R A, Tanagho EA. Clinical significance of sacral and pudendal nerve anatomy. *J Urol* 1988; 139: 74.

13. Tanagho EA, Schmidt RA, de Araujo CO. Urinary striated sphincter: what is its nerve supply? *Urology* 1982; 20:415.

14. Elabbady AA, Hassouna MM, Elhilali MM. Neural stimulation for chronic voiding dysfunctions. *J Urol* 1994; 152: 2076–80.

15. Dijkema HE, Weil EH J, Mijs PT, Janknegt RA. Neuromodulation of sacral nerves for incontinence and voiding dysfunctions. Clinical results and complications. *Eur Urol* 1993; 24: 72.

16. Vapnek JM, Schmidt RA. Restoration of voiding in chronic urinary retention using the neuroprosthesis. *World J Urol* 1991; 9: 142–4.

17. Bosch JLHR, Groen J. Effects of sacral segmental nerve stimulation on urethral resistance and bladder contractility: how does neuromodulation work in urge incontinence patients? *Neurourol Urodyn* 1995; 14: 502.

18. Koldewijn E L, Fosier PRWM, Meuleman EJH *et al*. Predictors of success with neuromodulation in lower urinary tract dysfunction: results of trial stimulation in 100 patients. *J Urol* 1994; 152: 2071.

19. Thon WF, Baskin LS, Jonas U, Tanagho EA, Schmidt RA. Neuromodulation of voiding dysfunction and pelvic pain. *World J Urol* 1991; 9: 138–41.

20. Melzack R. Folk medicine and the sensory modulation of pain. In: PD Wall and R Melzack (eds); *Textbook of Pain*. London: Churchill Livingstone, 1994; 1191.

21. Collins JJ, Imhoff TT, Grigg P. Noise-enhanced information transmission in rat SAI cutaneous mechanoreceptors via aperiodic stochastic resonance. *J Neurophys* 1996; 76: 642.

22. Siegel SW. Management of voiding dysfunction with an implantable neuroprosthesis. *Urol Clin North Am* 1992; 19: 163.

23. Elser DM, Fantl, JA, McClish DK. and the Continence Program for Women Research Group. Comparison of 'subjective' and 'objective' measures of severity of urinary incontinence in women. *Neurourol Urodyn* 1995; 14: 311,

24. Blaivas JG. Techniques of Evaluation. In: SV Yalla, E J McGuire, A Elbadawi. JG Blaivas (eds) *Neurourology and Urodynamics: Principles and Practice*. New York: Macmillan Publishing Co., 1988; 155.

25 Tapp AJS, Cardozo LD, Versi E, Cooper, D. The treatment of detrusor instability in post-menopausal women with oxybutynin chloride: a double blind placebo controlled study. *Bri J Obstet Gynaecol* 1990; 97: 521.

26. Elia G, Bergman A. Pelvic muscle exercises: when do they work? *Obstet Gynecol* 1993; 81: 283.

27. Nygaard IE, Kreder KJ, Lepic MM *et al*. Efficacy of pelvic floor muscle exercise in women with stress, urge and mixed urinary incontinence. *Am J Obstet Gynecol* 1996; 174: 120.

28. O'Brien PC, Fleming TR. A multiple testing procedure for clinical trials. *Biometrics* 1979; 35: 549–53.

29. National Association for Continence (NAFC). *Consumer focus 96: a survey of community dwelling incontinent people*. 1996.

30. Diokno A C. Epidemiology and psychosocial aspects of incontinence. *Urol Clin North Am* 1995; 22: 481.

31. Stein M, Discippio W, Davia M, Taub H. Biofeedback for the treatment of stress and urge incontinence. *J Urol* 1995; 153: 641.

32. Karram MM, Bhatia NN. Management of coexistent stress and urge urinary incontinence. *Obstet Gynecol* 1989; 73: 4.

33. Tanagho, EA, Schmidt RA. Electrical stimulation in the clinical management of neurogenic bladder. *J Urol* 1988; 140: 1331–9.

34. Schmidt, RA. Advances in genitourinary neurostimulation. *Neurosurgery* 1986; 19: 1041–4.

35. Grünewald V, Höfner K, Thon, WF *et al*. Sacral electrical neuromodulation as an alternative treatment option for lower urinary tract dysfunction. *Rest Neurol Neurosci* 1999; 3: 189–93.

36. Lindström S, Fall M, Carlsson CA *et al*. The neurophysiological basis of bladder inhibition in response to intravaginal electrical stimulation. *J Urol* 1983; 129: 405–10.

37. Schmidt RA, Jonas U, Oleson KA *et al*. Sacral nerve stimulation for treatment of refractory urinary urge incontinence. *J Urol* 1999; 162: 352–7.
38. Shaker HS, Hassouna MM. Sacral root neuromodulation in the treatment of various voiding and storage problems. *Int Urogynecol J Pelvic Floor Dysfunct* 1999; 10: 336–43.
39. Everaert K, Plancke H, Lefevere F *et al*. The urodynamic evaluation of neuromodulation in patients with voiding dysfunction. *Br J Urol* 1997; 79: 702–7.
40. Swinn MJ, Kitchen N, Goodwin RJ *et al*. Sacral neuromodulation for women with Fowler's syndrome. *Eur Urol*, 2000; 38: 439–43
41. Schultz-Lampel D, Jiang C, Lindstrom S *et al*. Experimental results on mechanisms of action of electrical neuromodulation in chronic urinary retention. *World J Urol* 1998; 16: 301–4.
42. Chancellor MB, Chartier-Kastler EJ. Principles of sacral nerve stimulation (SNS) for the treatment of bladder and urethral sphincter dysfunctions. *Neuromodulation* 2000; 3: 15–26.
43. Fowler CJ, Swinn MJ, Goodwin RJ *et al*. Studies of the latency of pelvic floor contraction during peripheral nerve evaluation show that the muscle response is reflexly mediated. *J Urol* 2000; 163: 881–3.
44. Vodušek DB, Light KJ, Libby JM. Detrusor inhibition induced by stimulation of pudendal nerve afferents. *Neurourol Urodyn* 1986; 5: 381–9.
45. Fowler CJ. Neurological disorders of micturition and their treatment. *Brain* 1999; 122: 1213–31.
46. Yoshimura N, de Groat WC. Increased excitability of afferent neurons innervating rat urinary bladder after chronic bladder inflammation. *J Neurosci* 1999; 19: 4644–53.
47. Kruse MN, de Groat WC. Spinal pathways mediate coordinated bladder/urethral sphincter activity during reflex micturition in decerebrate and spinalized neonatal rats. *Neurosci Lett* 1993; 152: 141–4.
48. Hohenfellner M, Schultz-Lampel D, Dahms S *et al*. Bilateral chronic sacral neuromodulation for treatment of lower urinary tract dysfunction. *J Urol* 1998; 160: 821–4.
49. Braun PM, Boschert J, Bross S *et al*. Tailored laminectomy: a new technique for neuromodulator implantation. *J Urol* 1999; 162: 1607–9.
50. Hassouna MM, Siegel SW, Lycklama à Nijeholt AAB *et al*. Sacral neuromodulation in the treatment of urgency–frequency symptoms: a multicenter study on efficacy and safety. *J Uro* 2000; 163: 1849–54.
51. Janknegt RA, Weil EH, Eerdmans PH. Improving neuromodulation technique for refractory voiding dysfunctions: two-stage implant. *Urology* 1997; 49: 358–62.
52. Bosch JLHR, Groen J. Sacral (S3) segmental nerve stimulation as a treatment for urge incontinence in patients with detrusor instability: results of chronic electrical stimulation using an implantable neural prosthesis. *J Urol* 1995; 154: 504.
53. Katz JN, Larson MG, Phillips CB *et al*. Comparative measurement sensitivity of short and longer health status instruments. *Med Care* 1992; 30: 917.
54. Lansky D, Butler JBV, and Waller FT. Using health status measures in the hospital setting: from acute care to outcomes management. *Med Care* 1992; 30: MS57.
55. Phillips RC, Lansky D. Outcomes management in heart valve replacement surgery: early experience. *J Heart Valve Dis* 1992; 1: 42–50.
56. Jones CA, Nyberg L. Epidemiology of interstitial cystitis. *Urology* 1997; 49(Suppl 5A): 2.
57. McHorney CA, Ware JE, Raczek AE. The MOS 36-Item Short-Form Health Survey (SF-36): II Psychometric and clinical tests of validity in measuring physical and mental health constructs. *Med Care* 1993; 31: 247.
58. Alagiri M, Chottiner S, Ratner V *et al*. Interstitial cystitis: unexplained associations with other chronic disease and pain syndromes. *Urology* 1997; 49 (Suppl 5A): 52.
59. Lemieux MC, Kamm MA, Fowler CJ. Bowel dysfunction in young women with urinary retention. *Gut* 1993; 34: 1397.
60. Goldman HB, Dmochowski RR. Lower urinary tract dysfunction in patients with gastroparesis. *J Urol* 1997; 157: 1823.
61. Wang Y, Tsang C, Hassouna MM. Neuromodulation reduced c-*fos* gene expression in spinalized rats: a double-blind randomized study. *J Urol* 1999; 275 (abstr 1065).
62. Tanagho EA, Schmidt RA, Orvis BR. Neural stimulation for control of voiding dysfunction: a preliminary report in 22 patients with serious neuropathic voiding disorders. *J Urol* 1989; 142: 340,
63. Ohlsson BL, Fall M, Frankeberg-Sommar S. Effects of external and direct pudendal nerve maximal electrical stimulation in the treatment of the uninhibited overactive bladder. *Br J Urol* 1989; 64: 374.
64. Wheeler JS, Walter JS, Zaszczurynski PJ. Bladder inhibition by penile nerve stimulation in spinal cord injury patients. *J Urol* 1992; 147: 100.
65. Schmidt RA, Doggweiler R. Neurostimulation and neuromodulation: a guide to selecting the right urologic patient. *Eur Urol* 1998; 34 (Suppl 1):23.

15 Additional tools for patient selection and outcome evaluation in sacral nerve modulation

Psychometric test evaluation in urinary retention

M. Spinelli, D. Molho, C. Morganti and G. Giardiello*

Introduction

Changes in the lower urinary tract associated with both disorders of bladder emptying (complete or partial retention) and those of micturition frequency with sensorimotor urgency associated to a greater or lesser extent with incontinence, are important issues in functional urology. All who have attempted to classify these disorders have reported that, in both retention and frequency disorders, in addition to the various possible types of dysfunction of the central or peripheral nervous system controlling the bladder/urethra and pelvic floor, there is always a pathogenic component linked to behavioural disorders. So far, however, there have been very few (if any) documented, controlled studies of a possible psychological trait associated with urological disorders. In clinical practice there is a wide variation in the methods of evaluation and treatment of the patients involved, most of whom are female. Their disorders are either immediately classified as psychosomatic or, at the other extreme, they are treated, by invasive techniques, as simple, organic disturbances.

Clinical experience has shown that, whereas a certain number of patients exhibiting some of the above-cited pathologies can be successfully treated by sacral neuromodulation (SNM), others derive no benefit from the various therapies adopted in urology. In particular, the progress of the symptoms, together with some of the behavioural reactions of the patients examined, has led us to believe that the symptoms could be a somatic expression of internal psychological conflict. We have seen that, in the first stages of treatment and in particular during the trial percutaneous nerve evaluation (PNE) test, these patients respond well to therapy; however, following definitive implant of the sacral nerve stimulation (SNS) system, the previous symptoms reappear for no apparent reason.

We have attempted to verify the hypothesis that these disorders, in some cases, could have a psychological aetiology and so belong to that category of disorders defined in the *Diagnostic and Statistical Manual of Mental Disorders* (DSM-IV) of the American Psychiatric Association as somatoform disorders [1]. This category includes a

Key Points
- In both retention and frequency a pathogenic component is linked to behavioural disorder.
- Few/no controlled studies exist of psychological trait(s) linked to urological disorders.
- There is wide variation in clinical examination/treatment methods of such patients.
- Some patients do not benefit from sacral neuromodulation.
- These patients' symptoms may be somatic expression of internal psychological conflict.
- Such patients respond well to PNE but their symptoms return after SNS system implant.
- Could these disorders be somatoform (DSM-IV)?

*With members of the GINS Group (see page 181).

variety of disorders (such as psychosomatic and conversion disorders, hypochondria, somatoform pain disorders) having in common the physical expression of anxiety, emotional conflict, and other psychological problems. Such a diagnostic category of psychiatric disorder implies that any general medical condition is ruled out; it also means that increased understanding of the pathophysiology of the symptoms could change the significance of the potential psychological causes.

Hitherto, no studies have assessed and analysed the possible psychological factors connected with urinary retention, even though, in the psychiatric literature, there are reports of this symptom within a general picture of somatic conversion disorders and, in particular, in relation to visceral manifestations [2]. In effect, any connection between urological disorders and conversion is immediately detectable, in view of the chronic and monosymptomatic nature of this urological condition together with the fact that it nearly always affects women between the ages of 20 and 30 years.

Study of patients with urinary retention

Our initial study involved 15 female patients (mean age 33, range 19–56 years), with bladder-emptying disorders associated with complete or partial chronic urinary retention, who were treated in Fornaroli Hospital, Magenta, Italy, between January and December 1998 (Table 15.1). In 12 cases retention was the only urological symptom; in the remaining three cases it was associated with disorders of micturition frequency or was accompanied by various forms of bladder instability. Some patients had not been seen previously by us; others were in the intermediate or final stages of their treatment or were being followed up. The psychological examination involved the Minnesota Multiphase Personality Inventory (MMPI 2) together with an interview conducted by the psychologist attached to the Department of Urology. The MMPI 2 is the most used and most versatile personality-assessment tool and is suitable for populations both with and without psychiatric disorders. Its numerous clinical scales can provide evidence of neurotic and psychotic profiles and of any predisposition towards somatoform disorders. The tests were administered and elaborated by the psychologist of the Spinal Unit of Magenta Hospital, within the Division of Urology. In order to make the psychological examination as objective as possible, the psychologist was blind to patients' urological disorders and to their course of treatment.

Assessment of the psychological diagnoses by means of the two instruments (MMPI 2 and

Table 15.1 Characteristics of female patients with urinary retention

Age	
Mean	33.5
Range	19–56
Distribution	
19–40 years	8
41–60 years	7
Marital status	
Single	7
Married	8
Divorced	0
Widowed	0
Education	
Middle school	5
Training college	5
High school	4
University	1
Occupation	
Unemployed	6
Teacher	2
Nurse	2
Housewife	4
Office worker	1

interview) was such that any conditioning that one instrument might have on the results of the other was minimised. Indeed, the psychologist analysed the results (through informed scoring) only after having completed both the test and the interview. The urologist, for his part, continued his normal course of treatment and was not informed of the results of the psychological evaluation.

The results of the MMPI 2 are first presented separately and then considered in relation to the global profile of each patient. Table 15.2 shows the distribution of patients according to the parameters of the DSM-IV table: nearly half of the patients were diagnosed as having 'undifferentiated somatoform disorders'. This diagnosis includes all those patients with one or more symptoms that cannot be directly explained by a general medical condition (urinary retention is very common among these) or in whom, if there is a general medical condition, the global impairment exceeds that expected and persists for at least 6 months. However, this category (which, in fact, can be deducted from the case history) is inadequate for differentiation of the psychological and somatic causes of urinary retention. The diagnosis of pain disorder (three patients) is undoubtedly more significant. Such patients complain of pain in various parts of the body but it is not clear as to whether the cause was due to a disease, a syndrome or a general medical condition. The diagnosis of 'unspecified somatoform disorder' in two patients is also insufficiently convincing as this is a residual category to classify those patients who cannot be categorised elsewhere.

The results obtained from the MMPI and the psychological interview were more significant. Some patients displayed a pattern of symptoms

Key Points

- Diagnosis for 7/15 patients was 'undifferentiated somatoform disorder'.
- This category is inadequate for differentiation between psychological/somatic retention.
- Diagnosis of pain disorder (3 patients) is more significant.
- Psychometry revealed symptoms of conversion disorder in some patients as hypothesised.

Table 15.2 Distribution of female patients according to the parameters of the DSM-IV

Diagnosis (Type of conversion/somatisation disorder)	No. of patients
Undifferentiated somatoform disorder	7
Hypochondriasis	0
Pain disorder	3
Somatoform disorder not otherwise specified	2
Body dysmorphic disorder	0
No somatoform disorder	3
Total	15

Table 15.3 Diagnostic criteria for F44, conversion disorder (300.11)

A One or more symptoms or deficits affecting voluntary motor or sensory function that suggest a neurological or other general medical condition.

B Psychological factors are judged to be associated with the symptom or deficit because the initiation or exacerbation of the symptom or deficit is preceded by conflicts or other stressors.

C The symptom or deficit is not intentionally produced or feigned (as in fictitious disorders or malingering).

D The symptom or deficit cannot, after appropriate investigation, be fully explained by a general medical condition or by the direct effect of a substance, or as a culturally sanctioned behaviour or experience.

E The symptom or deficit causes clinically significant distress or impairment in social, occupational, or other important areas of functioning, or warrants medical evaluation.

F The symptom or deficit is not limited to pain or sexual dysfunction, does not occur exclusively during the course of somatisation disorder, and is not better accounted for by another mental disorder.

(DSM-IV)

that conformed to all the diagnostic criteria for conversion disorders (as defined by the DSM-IV and shown in Table 15.3), thus confirming one of the hypotheses of the study. In some patients the psychological evaluation revealed a neurotic personality, which approached what has been defined in the psychiatric literature as an hysterical personality. The traits observed in some of our patients can be summarised as follows:

1. *affective traits* — pronounced immaturity, expressed as excessive dependence on the parental figure and with low tolerance to frustration; marked attention-seeking and accentuated egocentricity, together with conflicts of impulse (see later);
2. *cognitive traits* — imaginative, very impressionable, false idea of self, as if the patient has to hide behind a fictitious character in whom any relational or intrapsychic conflict is removed; in some cases, this develops into frank mythomania;
3. *real events* — a direct correlation between the onset or the exacerbation of the symptoms and 'stressful events', which are, in most cases, sexual experiences described by the patient as traumatic.

According to psychoanalytical theory, conversion results from the removal of an unconscious intrapsychic conflict and from the conversion of the anxiety into a physical symptom. Conflict takes place between an instinctive impulse (sexual in our study) and prohibition of its expression. Unlike other somatoform disorders, the conversion symptom has a symbolic relation with the psychological conflict in the patient. It is therefore clear that, in causing the urinogenital system to become disrupted, the patient expresses herself (or himself) through what is termed as 'the language of the organs'. In using the organic symptom for expression, the patient has the double advantage of (a) removing the psychological conflict from the conscious mind (principal advantage) and (b) avoiding unwelcome responsibility or commitments, or gaining attention or particular consideration from the surrounding environment (secondary advantage). Naturally, although the patient gains certain 'advantages' from the conversion symptoms, the entire process takes place outside the consciousness of the individual, thus ruling out any possibility that the symptom can be produced intentionally.

Another characteristic described in the psychiatric literature, is that of 'belle indifference', which refers to the incongruous attitude of insouciance shown by the patient in relation to her own symptoms. We observed how some patients were not at all worried by (or were, indeed, indifferent to) the possibility of their having a significant disability or needing prolonged hospitalisation.

Results of analysis

The results of psychological evaluation in 22 patients on the Italian register were classified according to the degree of pathology revealed and, particularly, with regard to the possible cor-

Table 15.4 *Results of SNS therapy compared with psychological profile*

Results of implantation	MMPI 2 profile*			
	0	1	2	nv †
Positive	6	3	2	1
Intermediate	0	2	0	0
Negative	0	0	7	1

*0, normal; 1, symptoms as reactions to the organic disease; 2, clinical results indicating psychosis, including symptoms of hysteria, and/or hypochondria.

†nv, test invalid

Key Points

- Of 8 patients with SNS failure, 7 had clinical results indicating psychosis.
- Of 12 patients with effective SNS, only 2 had clinical results indicating psychosis.
- In most cases there was good agreement between interview/MMPI results.

relation with the urological symptom. Thus, the psychologist interpreted the test results according to three categories: these were scored as 0 (normal), 1 (symptoms as reactions to the organic disease) or 2 (clinical results indicating psychosis). According to these definitions, the results of the psychological evaluation showed that six patients fell into category 0, five into category 1, and nine into category 2; in the remaining two the test was invalid (Table 15.4). Of the eight patients who experienced failure of SNS therapy, seven fell into category 2 and in one the test was invalid. Two patients with intermediate results of implantation were category 1. Of the 12 patients in whom SNS therapy was effective, the psychological profile of six was category 0, of three was category 1, of two was category 2, and in one patient the test was invalid. The statistical analysis showed a correlation between the psychological profile and the clinical outcome ($p<0.004$, χ^2 test).

With regard to the final diagnosis of psychological pathology (category 2[+]) in nine patients, in two cases (A and B) there is a clear lack of congruence between the two evaluations: whereas, in patient A, the results of the psychological interview are normal (or near normal) with a pathological MMPI, in patient B the reverse is true, the MMPI result being normal whereas the results of the psychological interview show a clearly hysterical personality. The reason for this variance lies in the fact that, for both profiles, (MMPI and interview), the patient can adopt such a defensive attitude as to falsify the results of the tests, totally or partially. However, generally in the MMPI it is possible to see when, and to what degree, the patient has attempted to distort the answers. In this way the test results can either be invalidated or validated, using appropriate correctors to compensate for the defensive behaviour of the patient, with the result that a more accurate symptomatic picture can be produced.

However, with regard to the non-pathological profiles (final diagnostic categories 0 and 1), agreement between the results is undoubtedly more pronounced if a variation of 0–1 between the test score results and those of the interview is regarded as completely normal.

Key Points

- These psychometric tests may help determine patient eligibility for permanent implant.
- Urge incontinence strongly affects patients' QoL.
- SNM is effective in urge incontinence but few studies exist of QoL after implant.
- Impact of SNM on QoL of patients with detrusor hyperactivity was studied.
- Importance of QoL evaluation in defining SNS success was assessed.
- Correlation between QoL-I and voiding diary parameters was analysed.

Conclusions

After a preliminary assessment in the pilot centre and subsequent extension to the other centres associated with the Italian Group of Sacral Neuromodulation, we are able to state that these evaluations can be usefully implemented in the diagnostic phase in order to determine patient eligibility for permanent implantation for SNS therapy.

Quality–of–life evaluation in incontinent patients

F. Cappellano, P. Bertapelle, M. Spinelli and G. Giardiello*

Introduction

Urinary urge incontinence is an important health issue that strongly affects patients' quality of life (QoL). Current treatments of urge incontinence are limited and do not consistently provide satisfactory results. As noted in the literature, patients suffering from urge incontinence often experience loss of self-esteem, symptoms of depression, embarrassment and poor QoL [3–6]. Sacral neuromodulation (SNM) has been effective in the treatment of symptoms of urinary urge incontinence [6,7]; however, whereas there have been several reports of clinical effectiveness, only three [7–9] have investigated changes in the QoL of patients after implantation.

Over the past ten years, evaluation of QoL has introduced a new target into analysis of the results by taking into account the personal opinions of the patients, by means of a general questionnaire or with specific tools for assessing the impact of a specific disease on QoL.

The aim of the study reported here was to investigate the impact of SNM on QoL and to assess the importance of this evaluation in defining the success of SNM in patients suffering from detrusor hyperactivity (detrusor instability and detrusor hyperreflexia). Data analysis has investigated the correlation between the quality-of-life index (QoL-I) and parameters noted in a voiding diary.

Patients and methods

From May 1998 to December 2000, 113 patients (82 female, 31 male, mean age 51.1 years, range 17–79 years) who underwent implantation of an SNM system were enrolled in a national prospective registry. Patients suffering from urge incontinence due to detrusor instability (44 patients: 11 male, 33 female) or hyperreflexia (16 patients; 7 male, 9 female, whose urological condition was attributable to multiple sclerosis (5), trauma (2 L1, 1 C6), herniated disc at level L4–L5 (1), myelitis (5), Parkinson's disease (1),

*With members of the GINS Group (see page 181).
Reprinted with permission from the *Journal of Urology*.

and cerebral ischaemia (1)) were asked to complete a QoL questionnaire (© Eli Lilly & Co., 1994, developed by the University of Washington Cost and Outcomes Assessment Team; used by permission; Italian translation edited by Wagner *et al.* [10]). The questionnaire was modified by the addition of two questions: (1) 'Would you have the implant done again?'; (2) 'Would you recommend it to a friend or a relative?' The questionnaire is a 22-item, domain-specific, validated and self-reported test shown to be sensitive to the detection of any change in self-perceived severity of incontinence. Data analysis considered the original 22 items together; the answers to the two additional questions were analysed separately. The QoL-I is expressed as a score ranging from 0 (poor self-perceived QoL due to incontinence) to 100 (incontinence did not negatively affect QoL). Healthy people obtained a score of 100.

The questionnaire and voiding diary were completed before the implantation procedure and at 3, 6, 9, 12, 18, 24 and 36 months after implantation. The questionnaire score and voiding diary were analysed to investigate the correlation between the clinical outcome and QoL-I.

> **Key Points**
> - QoL was assessed by a (modified) previously developed, validated questionnaire.
> - QoL improved after implant.
> - Most patients were glad to have received the implant and would recommend it.
> - Strong correlation was found between number of incontinence episodes and QoL-I.

Results

The QoL improved after implantation of an SNM system. For the group with detrusor instability, the QoL-I increased from 34.4±22.8 to 76.3±21.8 at 3 months' follow-up ($p<0.001$), to 83.6±17.3 at 6 months' follow-up ($p<0.001$), to 74.9±25.4 at 9 months' follow-up ($p<0.01$), to 72.7±28.8 ($p<0.01$), and to 83.8±16.6 ($p<0.01$) at 12 and 18 months' follow-up repectively. With regard to the clinical effect of SNM, the average number of incontinent episodes per day decreased from 5.8±4.2 to 0.6±1.0 at 3 months' follow-up ($p<0.01$), to 1.1±2.1 at 6 months after implantation ($p<0.01$), to 0.8±1.2 at 9 months' follow-up, to 0.9±1.5 at 12 months' follow-up ($p<0.01$), and to 1.2±1.5 at 18 months after implant (Fig.15.1). When patients were asked, at 3 months' follow-up, if, with hindsight, they would have the implant done again, 93% of patients responded in the affirmative, and 96% said that they would recommend it to a relative or a friend. At 18 months' follow-up, 90% of patients responded in the affirmative to question 1, and 100% in the affirmative to question 2.

In the group of hyperreflexic patients, an increase in QoL-I was noted from 37.3±16.6 at baseline to 65.9±6.8 at 3 months' follow-up ($p<0.01$), to 67.6±4.0 at 6 months after implant, and 62.9±10.8 at 9 months' follow-up. Analysis of the voiding diaries revealed a decrease in the number of incontinent episodes per day from 6.3±6.9 to 0.9±1.6 at 3 months' follow-up ($p<0.01$), to 1.5±0.5 at 6 months after implant ($p<0.01$), and to 1.2±1.6 at 9 months' follow-up.

Data analysis demonstrated a strong correlation between the number of episodes of incontinence and the QoL-I (Spearman ρ, -0.761; $p<0.001$; Fig. 15.2).

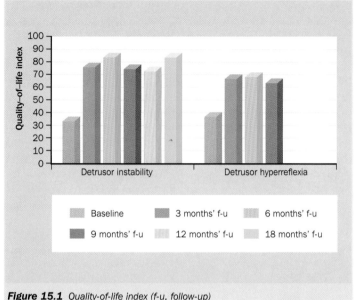

Figure 15.1 Quality-of-life index (f-u, follow-up)

Discussion

The QoL questionnaire used in our study is domain-specific for incontinence and the results show a marked improvement in QoL after SNM, as agreed by all patients who were asked to complete the questionnaire. The average time used to complete the questionnaire was 5–10 minutes; even the most elderly patients were able to understand and complete the questionnaire.

Previous reports have documented how QoL evaluation, using the SF-36 Health Survey, has demonstrated an improvement in patients' perception of physical health status after implantation of the SNS system [7] and in their physical functioning, physical and emotional role, pain and mental health [8]. A third publication has reported a significant improvement in physical functioning and standardised physical component scale [9]. These data are in agreement with the improvement in QoL-I reported here and confirm that implantation of the SNM system can benefit patients' QoL.

In the current literature, the results of SNM are usually expressed as the percentage of improvement of the main symptom versus the baseline calculated on the basis of a voiding diary; however, these data do not reflect personal satisfaction of the patients. We believe that analysis of QoL could add an additional dimension to evaluation of the effectiveness of

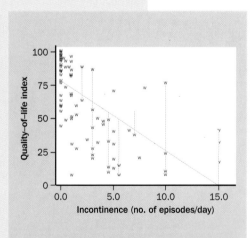

Figure 15.2 Regression analysis, quality-of-life index vs number of episodes of incontinence per day ($R^2 = 0.43$)

SNM and would provide in-depth understanding of the impact of the therapy on the patient's life.

Significant improvement of QoL is detectable at the first follow-up at 3 months after implant and is maintained throughout subsequent recorded assessments. Furthermore, a strong correlation can be traced between the QoL-I and the number of episodes of incontinence; QoL-I score correlates with a reduction in the number of episodes of leakage.

Our study has demonstrated a strong relationship between the improvement in the QoL and the clinical success of the therapy; the QoL-I, therefore, represents an additional and useful tool for the evaluation of the outcome of SNM in patients with urge incontinence and its impact on their lives. This additional evaluation should be extended to the whole field of functional surgery, with more emphasis being given to the effect of therapy on patients' QoL and to the integration of clinical and objective data.

> **Key Points**
> - QoL-I improvement also reflects clinical success.
> - QoL-I analysis should be used to evaluate outcome in all types of functional surgery.

Conclusions

This study has confirmed that sacral neuromodulation is an effective therapy for urge incontinence and that it can have a positive effect on a patient's quality of life.

Acknowledgement

The authors are grateful to Tiziana De Santo for her statistical expertise.

Appendix

The second section of this chapter was reprinted with permission from the *Journal of Urology*:

Cappellano F, Bertapelle P, Spinelli M et al. Quality of life assessment in patients who undergo sacral neuromodulation implantation for urge incontinence: an additional tool for evaluating outcome. *J Urol* 2001; 166: 2277–80.

As at December 2000, the Italian Group of Sacral Neuromodulation (GINS Group) comprises the following teams: Andretta, E. and Signorelli, G., Osp. Civile, Dolo; Bertapelle, P. and Carone, R., CTO-CRF-MA, Torino; Bonini, R. and Spreafico, L., Osp. E. Franchini, Montecchio E.; Cappellano, F. and Catanzaro, F., Multimedica, Sesto S. Giovanni; Centemero, A. and Guazzoni, C., Osp. Ville Turro, Milano; Cisternino, A. and Pagano, F., Osp. Clin. Iniversitario, Padova; D'Amico, A. and Curti, P., Pol. G.B. Rossi, Verona; De Marco, A. and Quattrone, P., CTO, Napoli; Gianneo, E. and Comeri, G., Osp. S. Anna, Como; Giocoli Nacci, G. and Pagliarulo, A., Policlinico G. di Bari; Kocjancic, E. and Frea, B., Osp. Maggiore, Novara; La Pira, G. and De Grande, G., Osp. Umberto I, Siracusa; Levorato, C.A. and Lembo, A., Osp. Riuniti,

Bergamo; Lombardi, G. and Del Popolo, G., Osp. Careggi, Firenze; Minardi, D. and Muzzonigro, G., Pol. Umberto I, Ancona; Natale, F. and Cervigni, M., Osp. S. Carlo di Nancy, Roma; Ostardo, E. and Garbeglio, A., Osp. S.M. degli Angeli, Pordenone; Pastorello, M. and Molon, A., Osp. SacroCuore, Negrar; Pistolesi, D. and Selli, C., Spedali Riuniti di S. Chiara, Pisa; Schettini, M., Osp. S. Giovanni di Dio e Ruggi D'Aragona, Salerno; Simeone, C. and Cosciani, S., Spedali Civili, Brescia; Spinelli, M. and Zanollo, A., Osp. Fornaroli, Magenta; Tuccitto, G. and Anselmo, G., Osp. Cà Foncello, Treviso; Vallone, R. and Cruciani, E., Osp. Generale S.G. Calibita Fatebenefratelli, Roma.

References

1. American Psychiatric Association. *Diagnostic and Statistical Manual of Mental Disorders* (DSM-IV) Washington DC: APA, 1994.
2. Bass C (ed.). *Somatization: Physical Symptoms and Psychological Illness.* Oxford: Blackwell Scientific Publications, 1990.
3. *Urinary incontinence in adults: clinical practice guideline.* Urinary Incontinence Guideline Panel. AHPCR Pub. No. 96 – 0682. Rockville, Maryland: Agency for Health Care Policy and Research, Public Health Service, United States Department of Health and Human Services, 1996.
4. Thiede HA. The prevalence of gynecologic disorders. *Obstet Gynecol Clin North Am* 1989; 16: 709–16.
5. Ory MG, Wyman JF, Yu L. Psychological factors in urinary incontinence. *Geriatr Med* 1986; 2: 657–71.
6. Janknegt RA, Hassouna MM, Siegel SW *et al*. Long term effectiveness of sacral nerve stimulation for refractory urge incontinence. *Eur Urol* 2001; 39: 101–6.
7. Schmidt RA, Jonas U, Oleson KA *et al*. for the Sacral Nerve Stimulation Study Group. Sacral nerve stimulation for the treatment of refractory urinary urge incontinence. *J Urol* 1999; 162: 352–7.
8. Shaker HS, Hassouna MM. Sacral nerve root neuromodulation: an effective treatment for refractory urge incontinence. *J Urol* 1998; 159: 1516–19.
9. Weil EH, Ruiz-Cerdá JL, Eerdmans PH *et al*. Sacral root neuromodulation in the treatment of refractory urinary urge incontinence: a prospective randomized clinical trial. *Eur Urol* 2000; 37: 161–71.
10. Wagner TH, Patrick DL, Bavendam TG *et al*. Quality of life of persons with urinary incontinence: development of a new measure. *Urology* 1996; 47: 67–72.

16 Complications of sacral nerve stimulation

U. Jonas and U. van den Hombergh

Introduction

In order to investigate the use of sacral nerve stimulation (SNS) therapy for the treatment of urinary voiding dysfunction, Medtronic Inc. (Minneapolis, MN, USA) decided to conduct a randomised prospective study for which the investigational device exemption (IDE) approval from the US FDA was received on 10 December 1993. Since the first publication on SNS therapy [1], many studies have been performed and quite extensive data on the efficacy and safety of SNS reported in the literature. However, most of these were retrospective, single-centre studies reporting complication rates of 22–43% [2–6]. The reported rate of re-operation varied widely and ranged from 6–50% [5, 7, 8].

This chapter gives an overview of the adverse events experienced in the first prospective, randomised multicentre trial. This chapter will also disclose how these events were managed, their possible aetiology and resolution status. Justification for the pooling of safety data for patients with different voiding difficulty indications is also provided. A total of 633 patients (210 with urge incontinence, 194 with retention, and 229 with urgency–frequency) from 14 North American and nine European centres were enrolled into this study until September 1999. FDA clearance to market the InterStim System for the indication of urge incontinence was granted on 29 September 1997. The additional indications of retention and urgency–frequency were approved on 15 April 1999.

The investigators that contributed patients to this study are listed in Chapter 14, page 168.

Safety experience

The Medtronic (MDT-103) study included 633 patients categorised into three diagnostic groups for urinary voiding dysfunction, namely (1) urinary urge incontinence, (2) retention, and (3) urgency–frequency. The safety of the test stimulation procedure and the permanent implantation in the treatment of urinary voiding dysfunction is described on the basis of the results collected up to June 1998 (test stimulation) and September 1999 (implant procedure), respectively. After the first FDA approval, the test stimulation data, including adverse events related to the test, were not collected. For this reason, the sample sizes of the safety analysis for the test stimulation differ from those for the permanent implant.

Key Points
- MDT-103 is the first prospective, randomised, multicentre trial on treatment of voiding dysfunction by SNS.
- It involved a total of 633 patients with different types of voiding dysfunctions: urge incontinence 210; urinary retention 194; urgency–frequency 229.

Justification for pooling data

A total of 633 patients from all three patient diagnostic categories were enrolled in the MDT-103 study, to be assessed by the test stimulation procedure. Of these 633 patients, 250 had been implanted with the SNS system by the end of the reporting period. The rationale for the use of combined data from all patient groups to demonstrate the safety of the test stimulation hardware and the permanently implanted hardware is based upon a review of current theories on the mechanism of action (see Chapter 3).

A general hypothesis for the mechanism of action is that SNS modulates neural reflexes, thus enabling a return to, or reassertion of, normal micturition patterns. Although it is not yet completely understood how this effect is achieved, this hypothesis supports the use of identical methods in the application of SNS to patients presenting with a variety of types of voiding dysfunction.

In addition, the protocol was identical for all patients enrolled in the study. Thus, (a) baseline testing and qualification for study participation via the inclusion/exclusion criteria, (b) application of SNS through the use of test stimulation hardware and permanently implanted hardware, and (c) follow-up procedures and the method for setting stimulation programme parameters were identical for all study patients, regardless of patient diagnostic category.

The therapy- and device-related complications reported in the study were compared by patient category to justify pooling the experience of the three groups for the purpose of demonstrating the safety of the SNS system. Analysis using Fisher's exact test showed no significant differences between the patient categories. This justifies the use of combined data from patients undergoing test stimulation as well as from those undergoing permanent implantation for demonstration of safety of the test stimulation and implant hardware.

Baseline characteristics

The baseline characteristics of all enrolled study patients can be found in Chapter 14. They were reported in three major publications related to each patient group involved in this multicentre study [9–11]. The overall proportions of men and women enrolled into the study were 20.7% and 79.3%, respectively. Patients first noted voiding dysfunction symptoms, on average, 8 years prior to enrolment into the study.

Test stimulation

A total of 914 test stimulation procedures were conducted on the 581 patients enrolled in the study until 1998. The number of test stimulation procedures performed per patient is shown in Table 16.1. Test stimulation data of the remaining 52 patients (633 minus 581) have not been collected and therefore are not available.

Test stimulation leads

Two temporary, percutaneous leads were available for use in the study: (a) the Medtronic test stimulation lead with discrete electrode,

Table 16.1 Number of test stimulation procedures performed per patient

Patient group	No. of patients	1	2	3	4	5	6	7	Total
		\multicolumn{8}{No. of procedures}							
Urge incontinence	184	115	46	12	9	1	1	0	290
Voiding difficulty	177	120	38	14	3	2	0	0	260
Urgency–frequency	220	126	61	22	8	1	1	1	364
Total	581	361	145	48	20	4	2	1	914

Table 16.2 Test stimulation leads

Device	No. of test stimulation procedures*
Medtronic temporary test stimulation lead with discrete electrode (i.e. Medtronic model 3065U test stimulation kit or bulk accessory)	567 (62.0)
Non-Medtronic multifilament test stimulation lead (i.e. Flexon Wire)	295 (32.3)
Medtronic model 3080 lead used as test stimulation lead**	1 (0.1)
Unknown (not documented)	51 (5.6)
Total test stimulation leads used in 581 patients	914

*Percentages in parentheses
**In one case, the investigator used the model 3080 lead during test stimulation procedure instead of either of the test stimulation leads.

Key Points

- Adverse events (a.e.) during test stimulation were recorded up to first FDA approval.
- Of 581 patients with 914 tests, 76.8% had no a.e.
- 180 a.e. required no (92) or non-surgical (88) intervention; 1 required surgery.
- On database closure all 181 a.e. were fully resolved.
- Most a.e. involved suspected migration of the test lead.

and (b) a non-Medtronic multifilament lead. A summary of the number of procedures performed with each type of lead used is provided in Table 16.2.

Test stimulation events

Events occurring during test stimulation were recorded until the first FDA approval was obtained. There were 914 test stimulation procedures conducted on the 581 patients enrolled in the study: 446 patients (76.8%) experienced no adverse events; the remaining 135 (23.2%) experienced a total of 181 adverse events, reported in 166 (18.2%) of the test procedures. Of these 181 events, 92 (50.8%) required no intervention, 88 (48.6%) required non-surgical intervention, and one (0.6%) required hospitalisation or surgical intervention (Fig. 16.1). At the time of database closure, 100% of the 181 reported adverse events were fully resolved.

The reported test stimulation events associated with the devices or use of stimulation, are summarised in Table 16.3. Suspected migration of the test stimulation lead comprised the majority 108 (59.7%) of adverse events associated with the 914 test stimulation procedures. This adverse event was not unexpected, because the temporary lead electrode did not provide an active fixation mechanism. The second

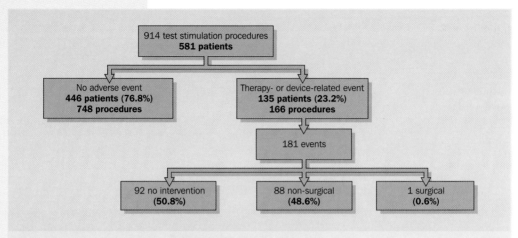

Figure 16.1 *Therapy-related adverse event flowchart for test stimulation.*

Table 16.3 *Test stimulation adverse events*

Test stimulation adverse event	No. of events	Incidence (%)/914
Suspected lead migration	108	11.8
Technical problem	24	2.6
New pain	19	2.1
Suspected device problem	10	1.1
Persistent skin irritation	6	0.7
Change in bowel function	4	0.4
Infection at test stimulation lead site	3	0.3
Change in voiding function	3	0.3
Other	3	0.3
Transient electric shock	1	0.1
Total	181	19.8

most frequent event, 'technical problem', was documented in 24 (2.6%) of the 914 test stimulation procedures (there were two procedures that had two technical problems each). Technical problems were primarily attributed to external device handling issues, including the following:

- disconnection of external cable;
- loss of ground pad contact with the skin;
- inadequately adjusted 9V battery required by the external test stimulator device;
- suspected device problem (patient dropped the test stimulator into the toilet).

Test stimulation events requiring surgical intervention

In the 914 test stimulation procedures conducted during the study, one adverse event necessitated surgical intervention. The overall surgical revision rate associated with the test stimulation procedure was 0.1% (one of 914 procedures). The test stimulation lead distal electrode detached during the test stimulation procedure in two patients; in both cases, radiography demonstrated that the electrode was cut off above the surface of the sacrum; the electrode was surgically removed in one case, and examination of the detached electrode indicated that the lead body had been sheared off proximal to the electrode by the insertion of the foramen needle. The design of the test stimulation lead has been modified to address this adverse event: the new model 3057 test stimulation lead has a non-discrete electrode design, in which the electrode is formed by removing the insulation from the distal portion of the lead body (see Chapter 8). The original design (model 041830) utilised a discrete component crimped onto the distal end of the lead body. Animal studies conducted with the model 3057 test stimulation lead showed no detachment of the electrode; handling studies conducted outside the USA have confirmed this finding. This modified lead design is approved by the FDA for use as part of the InterStim Continence Control System.

Test stimulation events requiring non-surgical intervention

Of the 181 adverse events associated with the test stimulation procedure, 88 (48.6%) required non-surgical intervention (Table 16.4). At the time of database closure, 100% of the 88 reported events were fully resolved.

The leading event, suspected lead migration of the test stimulation lead, was reported in 44 incidents (35 patients); these were resolved with non-surgical intervention. At the discretion of the investigator, the test stimulation lead was either exchanged to allow continuation of test stimulation, or removed. Migration of the test stimulation lead was an expected event in the study, because the test stimulation lead electrode employs passive fixation rather than an active fixation mechanism. Analysis of the patient demographic data revealed no concomitant factors that predicted the potential for migration of the test stimulation lead.

Technical problems requiring non-surgical intervention were reported 15 times; these consisted of disconnection of the external cable connections or poor contact with the ground pad, resulting in loss of stimulation.

New pain was reported in 11 cases, requiring non-surgical intervention. Six patients reported leg pain during the test stimulation procedure. This was resolved by either discontinuation of the stimulation, adjustment of the lead or reduction of the amplitude output of the external test stimulator. Three patients reported tailbone or

> **Key Points**
> • Out of 914 test stimulation procedures, only one required surgical intervention.

Table 16.4 Adverse events related to test stimulation: non-surgical intervention

Adverse events	No. of events
Suspected lead migration	44
Technical problem	15
New pain	11
Suspected device problem	5
Persistent skin irritation	4
Infection at test stimulation lead site	3
Change in bowel function	2
Change in voiding	2
Other	2
Total	88

lower back pain in four events while one remaining patient reported pain in the left buttock, hip and groin, and numbness with stimulation. This patient reduced the stimulation amplitude; this resolved the problem within a day.

Suspected device problems requiring non-surgical intervention were reported in five patients and were all related to difficulties with the connection between the test stimulation lead and the external test stimulation cable.

Persistent skin irritation requiring non-surgical intervention was documented in three patients (four events). There was redness without infection at the test stimulation lead site in two patients and irritation at the ground pad site in one. Analgesics or hydrocortisone solved the problem in each case; topical ointment was used to treat the irritation.

Infection at the test stimulation lead site was reported in three patients. As a precaution, the test stimulation lead was removed and antibiotic treatment was prescribed.

An adverse change in bowel function, described as constipation, was documented in two patients; this stopped on cessation of trial stimulation. In fact, neither patient qualified for device implantation on the basis of the results of test stimulation and they were excluded from the study.

An adverse change in voiding function was documented in two patients, but this was ceased when trial stimulation was stopped. Neither patient qualified for device implantation and they were excluded from the study.

Test stimulation events requiring no intervention

Of the 181 adverse events associated with the test stimulation procedure, 92 (50.8%) reported events were resolved without medical intervention (Table 16.5). The most frequent event, suspected lead migration of the test stimulation lead, was reported in 64 cases. No medical intervention was reported to treat this event. Patients reporting a loss of stimulation sensation were instructed either to increase the amplitude of the external test stimulator, or to return to the investigator's office for the scheduled removal of the test stimulation lead.

As previously stated, migration of the test stimulation lead was anticipated, because the lead electrode does not provide active fixation.

The suspected device problems reported in four patients were: (a) dislodgment of the distal electrode; (b) difficulty with the connection; (c) obstructed foramen needle (product analysis of the returned foramen needle revealed that foreign material was introduced into the needle after the physician removed the preloaded needle stylet); and (d) inability to pass the test stimulation lead through the foramen needle. In the case of this fourth problem, the test stimulation lead was returned to Medtronic for product analysis, which indicated that the outer diameter of the test stimulation electrode

Table 16.5 *Adverse events related to test stimulation: no intervention*

Adverse events	No of events
Suspected lead migration	64
Technical problem	9
New pain	8
Suspected device problem	4
Change in bowel function	2
Persistent skin irritation	2
Transient electric shock	1
Change in voiding function	1
Other	1
Total	92

exceeded the inner diameter of the foramen needle. As a corrective action, Medtronic processed an engineering change order to specify tighter tolerance limits on the outer diameter of the test stimulation electrode during manufacturing. No new reports of this event have been received since this action was taken and no adverse outcome to the patient was reported.

Transient electric shock was reported in one patient; this did not require medical intervention. Syncope (fainting) was reported for one patient during the office phase of the test stimulation procedure; however, when the test stimulation procedure was stopped the patient recovered without further incident.

Post-implant events

A total of 250 patients enrolled in the study were implanted with a SNS system, representing 6,506 months of device experience. Of the 250 implanted patients, 157 (62.8%) experienced a total of 368 adverse events associated with the device or use of stimulation therapy. Probability of the first and every additional therapy-related event occurring over time has been shown in Figure 16.2. Of the reported 368 events, 56 (15.2%) required no intervention, 151 (41.0%) required non-surgical intervention, and 161 (43.8%) required surgical intervention (Table 16.6). Overall, 89.4% (329) of the 368 events were fully resolved. The data from previous analyses indicated that the revision rate has not significantly changed over time.

> **Key Points**
> - Post-implant events (368) occurred in 157/250 patients; most needed surgical intervention.
> - 329/368 events had been resolved at database closure.

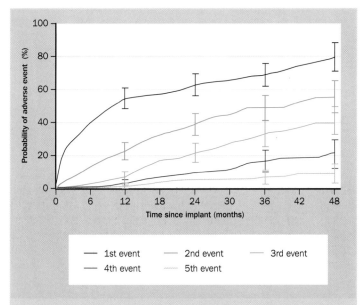

Figure 16.2 *Probability of therapy-related adverse events associated with the implanted InterStim system up to 48 months after implantation.*

Table 16.6 Post-Implant events in 157 of 250 patients receiving implants grouped according to subsequent intervention

Adverse event	No. of events	Subsequent intervention		
		None	Non-surgical	Surgical
Pain at IPG site	60	4	13	43
New pain	50	13	25	12
Suspected lead migration	39	4	7	28
Infection	28	3	9	16
Pain at lead site	18	7	4	7
Transient electric shock	23	5	15	3
Suspected device problem	28	4	9	15
Change in bowel function	12	2	4	6
Technical problem	10	2	0	8
Persistent skin irritation	3	0	3	0
Change in menstrual cycle	2	1	1	0
Suspected nerve injury	1	0	1	0
Device rejection	2	0	0	2
Other (number of events)	92	11	60	21
Lack of efficacy (13)				
Undesirable change in sensation of stimulation (13)				
Change in sensation of stimulus (12)				
Foot or leg movement (8)				
Worsening of baseline symptoms (5)				
Haematoma or seroma (4)				
IPG turns on/off (4)				
Numbness or tingling (3)				
Unable to perceive stimulus (3)				
Chronic buttock/lumbar pain (2)				
Chronic pelvic pain (2)				
Fever (2)				
Possible skin perforation at IPG (2)				
Urinary hesitancy (2)				
Vaginal cramps (2)				
IPG turns over when patient bends (2)				
Asthma, dyspnoea, rash, hives (1)				
Black stool (1)				
Fell, bladder spasms, increased frequency (1)				
Grand mal (1)				
Irritative complaint upon defecation (1)				
Lack of orgasm (1)				
Replacement of IPG due to end of life (1)				
Stimulus causing chest pain (1)				
Stress UI (1)				
Strong anal sensation (1)				
Superficial connection (1)				
Swollen feeling in abdomen (1)				
Interference with ECG (1)				
Total	368	56	151	161

ECG, electrocardiograph; IPG, implantable pulse generator

In the 250 implanted patients, post-implant adverse events associated with the devices or use of stimulation include the following (with the probability of an event at 12 months calculated using life-table analysis, indicated in parentheses):

- pain at IPG site (14.2%)
- new pain (10.8%)
- suspected lead migration (9.1%)
- infection (7.0%)
- pain at lead site (5.5%)
- transient electric shock (5.6%)
- suspected device problem (2.2%)
- adverse change in bowel function (3.0%)
- technical problem (3.9%)
- persistent skin irritation (0.8%)
- change in menstrual cycle (0.9%)
- suspected nerve injury (0.4%)
- device rejection (0.4%)
- other (14.1%).

There were no statistical differences in the safety profile of the InterStim System with respect to the three indications (urge incontinence, retention, and urgency–frequency).

All post-implant events (n=368) and those events that required surgery at (a) 12 and (b) 24 months are summarised in Figure 16.3.

Post-implant events requiring surgical intervention

Of the 368 post-implant adverse events attributed to the devices or use of stimulation therapy, 161 (43.8%) required surgical intervention. There were no reports of serious adverse device effects or permanent injury associated with the devices or with the SNS procedure. Event resolution was documented for 150 (93.2%) of the 161 reported events; the remaining events were still being actively followed.

The 161 adverse events requiring surgical intervention were reported in 96 (38.4%) of the 250 patients receiving implants. Of the 250 implanted patients, the probability of one adverse event resulting in surgical intervention during the clinical study was 29.6% at 12 months.

The event rate appeared to drop in the next 12 months, as the probability of one adverse event resulting in surgical intervention at 24 months was 39.9%. The probability of an adverse event requiring a second surgical intervention was 8.7% at 12 months and 16.1% at 24 months (Fig. 16.4).

Repositioning of the lead/extension was the most frequent surgical treatment, comprising 24.2% of the 161 events. Repositioning was performed to address such problems as implant site complaints, lack of efficacy and bowel dysfunction. Surgical repositioning of the IPG was the next most frequent surgical treatment, resulting in 21.1%, or 34 of the 161 revision events. Surgical repositioning of the IPG is considered a minor surgical procedure and is commonly performed under local anaesthesia.

Key Points

- Repositioning of lead/extension was the most frequent surgical treatment (24.2%).
- Next was surgical repositioning of IPG (21.1%).

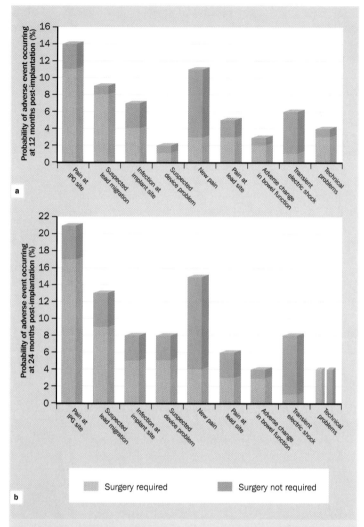

Figure 16.3 *Probability of various types of adverse events after implantation requiring (or not requiring) surgery at (a) 12 months or (b) 24 months.*

Although sample sizes were small, it appeared that surgical revision in the first year after implantation reduced the probability of achieving a successful clinical outcome. Thus, of those patients with urge incontinence who experienced an adverse event requiring surgery within a year of implantation, 15/26 (58%) achieved a successful clinical result (≥50% reduction in leaks per day). Of the 51 patients who did not require surgery, 41 (80%) had a successful clinical outcome. Similarly, whereas 9/17 (53%) of those patients with retention who required surgery in the first year after implantation achieved a successful clinical result (≥50% reduction in catheterised volume per catheterisation), the clinical outcome was

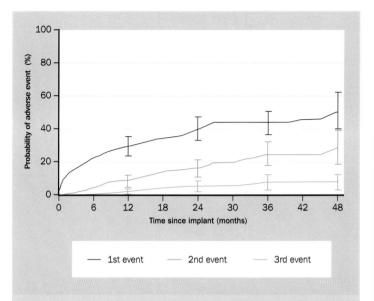

Figure 16.4 *All therapy- or device-related post-implant adverse events requiring surgery up to 48 months after implantation. Error bars represent 95% confidence intervals.*

successful in 24/27 (89%) of those patients who did not require surgery. Finally, of those patients with urgency–frequency who required surgery within a year of implantation, 7/17 (41%) achieved a successful result (≥50% reduction in voids per day or reduction to normal level); however, the clinical outcome was successful in 18/34 (53%) of those patients who did not require surgery.

Buttock placement

Buttock placement has become an alternative site for implantation of the IPG, which is typically implanted in the upper buttock. Physicians favour this procedure because the length of surgery is usually reduced: during lead placement, the patient is in the prone position; positioning the neurostimulator in the upper buttock means the patient does not have to be turned, and a new sterile field established over the abdomen.

In the latest post-approval study annual report, buttock placement data has been collected in 31 patients up to September 2000. Probabilities of therapy or device related post-implant events requiring IPG revision or explant surgery are shown in Figure 16.5. At 12 months follow-up, there is a 7.9% probability that buttock placement patients will require neurostimulator revision surgery, compared to a 19.8% probability for patients with other neurostimulator placement.

As shown in Figure 16.6, the probability of a patient having an adverse event requiring surgery in buttock placement patients is 15% compared to 30% in patients with other neurostimulator implants. In

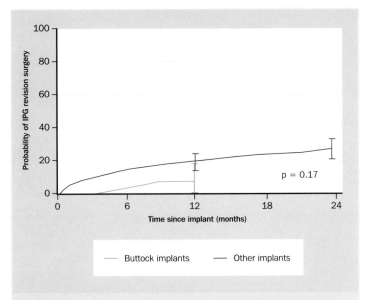

Figure 16.5 *Probability of neurostimulator revision surgery: buttock vs other neurostimulator placement. Error bars represent 95% confidence intervals.*

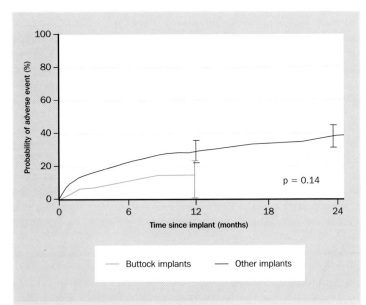

Figure 16.6 *Probability of adverse event requiring surgery: buttock vs other neurostimulator placement.*

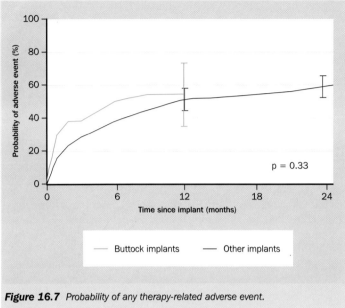

Figure 16.7 *Probability of any therapy-related adverse event.*

other words, adverse events requiring surgery is about half in buttock placement patients in comparison to other patients. In Figure 16.7, the probability of any therapy- or device-related adverse event is approximately the same for buttock placement and other placement of the neurostimulator (54% and 51.9%, respectively).

Common types of surgical intervention
1. *Repositioning of the lead/extension* — due to suspected lead migration, a change in bowel function, foot or leg movement, new pain, lack of efficacy, pain at the lead site, a technical problem, a change in stimulation sensation, transient electric shock, strong anal sensation, urinary hesitancy or numbness or tingling.
2. *Temporary explant/reimplantation* — due to suspected lead migration, a suspected device problem, infection, chronic pelvic pain, device rejection, lack of efficacy, end of battery life, technical problems, IPG movement or a change in bowel sensation.
3. *Repositioning of the IPG* — due to pain at the IPG site, new pain or a superficial connection.
4. *Device exchange* — due to suspected lead migration, a suspected device problem, technical problems, lack of efficacy, pain at the IPG and lead site, new pain, transient electric shock or infection.

5. *Permanent explant* — due to infection, pain at the IPG/implant site, device rejection, new pain or a change in bowel function.
6. *Other* — it has been reported that surgery was performed to rectify a suspected device problem, new pain and chronic pain.

Medtronic Inc. now provides training/labelling to minimise the necessity for surgical revision in future patients receiving implants.

Conclusions

Data regarding the safety of SNS for various types of urinary voiding dysfunction (including urge incontinence, retention, and urgency–frequency) have been assembled from 633 patients undergoing 914 test stimulation procedures and 250 patients implanted with the InterStim System. At of the end of the study reporting period, no patient had experienced permanent injury resulting from SNS.

In 6,506 months of device experience for the 250 implanted patients, there were no reported unanticipated device effects associated with the InterStim System. A total of 368 post-implantation events associated with the devices or use of SNS were documented in 157 of the 250 implanted patients. Overall, 89.4% (329) of the 368 events were resolved at the time of database closure.

References

1. Tanagho EA and Schmidt RA. Electrical stimulation in the clinical management of the neurogenic bladder. *J Urol* 1988; 140: 1331–9.
2. Dijkema HE, Weil EH, Mijs PT, Janknegt RA. Neuromodulation of sacral nerves for incontinence and voiding dysfunctions. Clinical results and complications. *Eur Urol* 1993; 24: 72–6.
3. Shaker HS, Hassouna M. Sacral nerve root neuromodulation in idiopathic nonobstructive chronic urinary retention. *J Urol* 1998; 159: 1516–9.
4. Shaker HS, Hassouna M. Sacral root neuromodulation in idiopathic nonobstructive chronic urinary retention. *J Urol* 1998; 159: 1476–8.
5. Bosch R, Groen J. Sacral (S3) segmental nerve stimulation as a treatment for urge incontinence in patients with detrusor instability: results of chronic electrical stimulation using an implantable neural prosthesis. *J Urol* 1995; 154: 504–7.
6. Grünewald V, Höfner K, Thon WF, Kuczyk M, Jonas U. Sacral electrical neuromodulation as an alternative treatment option for lower urinary tract dysfunction. *Restor Neurol Neurosci* 1999; 14: 189–93.
7. Elabbady A, Hassouna MM, Elhilali M. Neural stimulation for chronic voiding dysfunctions. *J Med* 1994; 152: 2076–80.
8. Koldewijn EL, Meuleman EJ, Bemelmans BLH, van Kerrebroeck P, Debruyne F. Neuromodulation effective in voiding dysfunction despite high reoperation rate. *J Urol* 1999; 255 (Abstract 984).
9. Schmidt RA, Jonas U, Oleson KA et al. Sacral nerve stimulation for treatment of refractory urinary urge incontinence. Sacral Nerve Stimulation Study Group. *J Urol* 1999; 163: 352–7.
10. Hassouna MM, Siegel SW, Lycklama à Nijeholt AAB. Sacral neuromodulation in the treatment of urgency–frequency symptoms: a multicenter study on efficacy and safety. *J Urol* 2000; 163: 1849–54.
11. Jonas U, Fowler CJ, Chancellor MB et al. Efficacy of sacral nerve stimulation for urinary retention: results 18 months after implantation. *J Urol* 2001; 165: 15–19.

17 Bilateral sacral neurostimulation

General introduction

D. Schultz-Lampel, M. Hohenfellner, J.W. Thüroff,
P-M. Braun and K-P. Jünemann

Key Points
- Follow-up results showed that the clinical benefits of unilateral SNS are significant, but could be improved.
- This prompted an evaluation of surgical techniques and stimulation parameters for the treatment of bladder dsyfunctions.
- Possible improvement may follow bilateral stimulation.

Sacral nerve stimulation (SNS), using the technique of Tanagho and Schmidt, (with an electrode slipped into the S3 foramen), has become a treatment option for many types of voiding dysfunction [1]. As reported in Chapter 14, the follow-up results obtained 18 months after unilateral stimulation showed clinical benefit in 76% of urge incontinent patients and in 71% of patients with urinary retention (Fig. 14.7). On the basis of this data, it seemed of interest to evaluate several modifications in surgical technique and stimulation parameters, in order to improve the results of sacral neuromodulation for the treatment of bladder dysfunction.

In neurophysiological studies, the effects of unilateral and bilateral stimulation were compared, indicating the use of bilateral as preferable to unilateral stimulation. At the same time, the standard technique of sacral neuromodulation has already been modified in the clinical setting. This involves not only the bilateral insertion of quad electrodes at the S3 level, using the traditional technique of Tanagho and Schmidt, but also the investigation of new approaches that achieve closer contact with the nerves. These techniques include access to the nerves via laminectomy, or 'tailored laminectomy' (see page 209) using the standard quad electrodes. Cuff electrodes (a modified design of electrodes which surround the nerves in close contact) have been developed in order to improve not only the short-term but also the long-term results of sacral neuromodulation (see page 207).

The following chapter describes the scientific basis of bilateral sacral nerve stimulation and the first clinical results using two different techniques of bilateral sacral neuromodulation.

The scientific basis of bilateral sacral neurostimulation

D. Schultz-Lampel and J. W. Thüroff

Introduction

SNS has become a treatment option for several types of voiding dysfunction [2–13]. In order to improve long-term results [14, 15], several technical modifications were introduced in the treatment of bladder

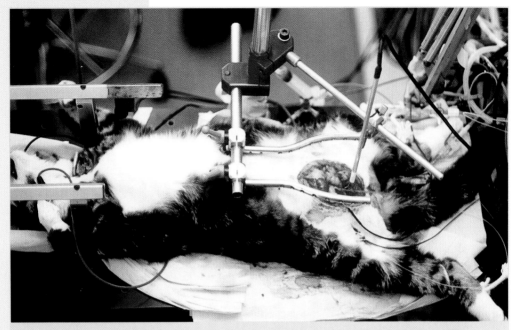

Figure 17.1(a) *Experimental set-up (dorsal view): cat with laminectomy L6–S3, stimulation electrode at S2.*

Key Points

• Animal experiments
  investigated the scientific
  basis of bilateral stimulation.

dysfunction. Because one such modification may be the bilateral introduction of electrodes at the S3 foramina, neurophysiological studies were performed to compare the efficacy of unilateral and bilateral SNS and to ascertain a scientific basis for the application of bilateral neurostimulation in the clinical setting [15, 16].

Sacral neurostimulation in the experimental set-up

Clinical sacral foramen stimulation was experimentally reproduced in isolated S2 SNS in ten chloralose-anaesthetised cats. In five cats and 105 stimulation sequences, unilateral stimulation of the right and left S2 nerves was compared with bilateral S2 stimulation. Stimulation was performed with a custom-made stimulator. Most experiments used monopolar cathodal stimulation with square angular impulses of pulse width 200ms. Stimulation intensities ranged between 1μA and 2mA and were reported as multiples of the threshold of those intensities inducing striated muscle contractions (M response of α-motor axons to foot, pelvic floor, or tail). Stimulation frequencies ranged between 1 and 100Hz; stimulation time varied between 5 seconds and 3 minutes. Stimulation responses were recorded from the bladder (isovolumetric changes in bladder pressure), peripheral nerves (compound action potentials of the pudendal nerve and branches and of the pelvic nerve and branches), and striated muscles of the foot, anus, and pelvic floor (foot EMG, anal EMG, pelvic floor EMG) and displayed on a four-channel chart recorder (Figs. 17.1a and 17.1b).

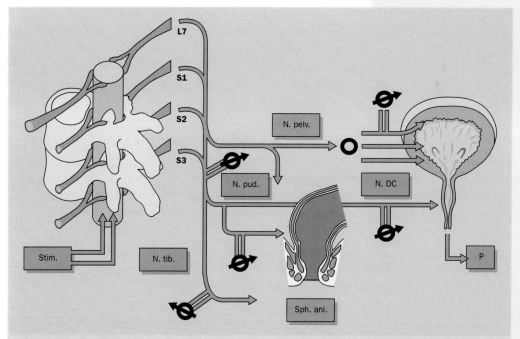

Figure 17.1(b) *S2 stimulation and recording of responses from the bladder, peripheral nerves (pudendal nerve and branches, pelvic nerve and branches), and pelvic floor and foot EMG (stim., stimulation; Ø, recording; P, bladder pressure; pelv. n., pelvic nerve; pud. n., pudendal nerve; tib. n., tibial nerve; dors. clit. n., dorsal clitoris nerve; sph. ani, anal sphincter).*

Effect of unilateral and bilateral sacral neurostimulation

Isolated SNS had both excitatory and inhibitory effects on the bladder (Fig. 17.2); both effects were consistently dependent on stimulation frequency and intensity. Bladder excitation and inhibition were identified as reflex responses, as they were abolished after transection of the dorsal roots (Fig. 17.3).

In unilateral stimulation, excitation was best at low stimulation frequencies (2–5Hz) and low intensities (0.8–1.4 × threshold). Inhibition was the dominating effect at higher frequencies (7–10 Hz) and higher intensities (1.4–2 × threshold).

In all experiments, bladder excitation occurred at 0.8–1.0 × threshold of α motor axons with a maximum at 1.2 × threshold. At 1.0–1.2 × threshold, bladder inhibition occurred after cessation of stimulation ('off-inhibition'), whereas bladder inhibition during stimulation started at 1.4 × threshold and increased with increasing intensities ('on'-inhibition), which also provoked strong striated muscle contractions (Figs. 17.4a and 17.4b).

Lower frequencies (1–5Hz) induced significant increase of bladder pressure with 'off'-inhibition after cessation of the stimulation; 10Hz stimulation resulted in only marginal bladder excitation but complete bladder inhibition during the stimulation ('on'-inhibition)

Key Points
- Bilateral (vs unilateral) stimulation did not increase excitatory response but did increase bladder inhibition.

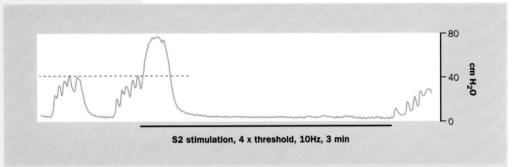

S2 stimulation, 4 x threshold, 10Hz, 3 min

Figure 17.2 *Effect of isolated S2 stimulation on bladder contractility (n=490 stimulation sequences). Recording of bladder pressure at stimulation intensities exceeding the threshold of ∞-motor axons (M response) with spontaneous contractions of the bladder occurring at bladder volume of 30ml. Application of the stimulus (4 x threshold, 10Hz, 3 min) during a spontaneous contraction induces a dual effect on the bladder — an initial increase of contraction amplitude from 40 to 70cmH$_2$0, representing bladder excitation, followed by a decrease in contraction amplitude to zero, corresponding with complete bladder inhibition, that persists to the end of stimulation.*

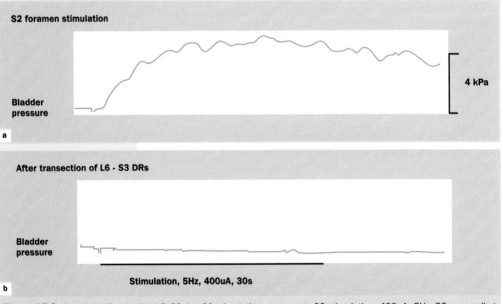

Figure 17.3 *Sacral deafferentation L7–S3 (n=20 stimulation sequences; S2 stimulation, 400μA, 5Hz, 30s, recording of bladder pressure): (a) induction of a bladder contraction before transection of the dorsal roots; (b) bladder contraction is completely abolished after transection of the dorsal roots.*

Key Points

- Bilateral stimulation at the same level led to marked summation of two unilateral stimuli.

(Figs. 17.5a and 17.5b). Bilateral stimulation at the same segmental level induced effective bladder inhibition, even at subthreshold intensities (0.8–1.0×M response) (Fig. 17.6a). On unilateral stimulation, bladder contractility initially increased by 12(±2)% (S2 stimulation left) and 13(±1.2)% (S2 stimulation right), respectively. This was followed by a slight decrease of bladder pressure in

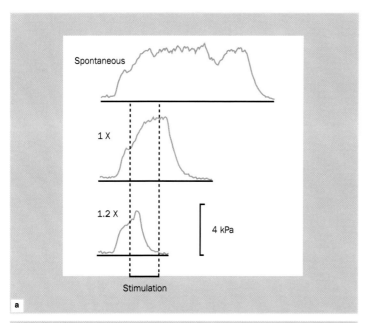

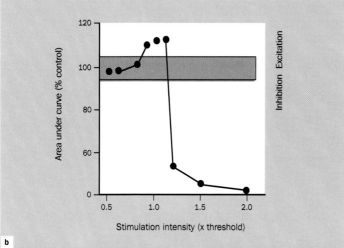

Figure 17.4 *Dependency of bladder response on stimulation intensity: (a) isolated S2 stimulation, stimulation time 15 s, recording of bladder pressure, stimulation intensity measured as x-times threshold of the M response; (b) excitatory and inhibitory activity as a percentage of the spontaneous bladder contraction depending on stimulation intensity (area under the curve): bladder excitation dominating at 0.8–1.2 × threshold; bladder inhibition dominating at 1.4–2 × threshold.*

17(±1) % (S2 stimulation left) and 13(±4)% (S2 stimulation right), respectively, indicating the onset of bladder inhibition.

Compared with unilateral stimulation, bilateral stimulation did not increase the excitatory response (increase of bladder pressure in 2±0.5%), but did cause a significant increase in bladder inhibition (decrease of bladder pressure in 33+4%, p<0.0001) (Fig. 17.6b).

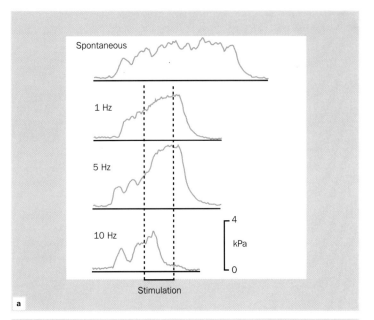

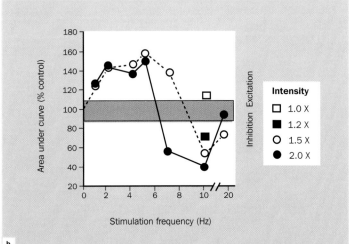

Figure 17.5 *Dependency of bladder response on stimulation frequency: (a) isolated S2 stimulation, stimulation time 15s, recording of bladder pressure, stimulation intensity measured as x-times threshold of the M response, stimulation frequency 1, 5, and 10Hz; (b) excitatory and inhibitory activity as a percentage of the spontaneous bladder contraction depending on stimulation frequency (area under the curve): bladder excitation dominating at 2–5Hz; bladder inhibition dominating at 7–10Hz.*

This confirmed that bilateral stimulation at the same level produced a pronounced summation effect of two unilateral stimulations. In contrast, simultaneous stimulation of several ipsilateral segments at different levels (for example, stimulation at S2 and S3 right side) did not increase bladder inhibition.

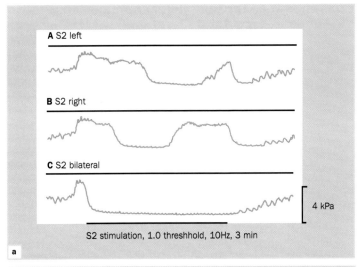

A S2 left

B S2 right

C S2 bilateral

4 kPa

S2 stimulation, 1.0 threshhold, 10Hz, 3 min

a

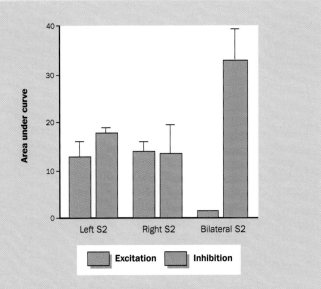

b

Figure 17.6 *Comparison of unilateral and bilateral stimulation (n=105 stimulation sequences in five cats; S2 stimulation left, right, and bilateral, 1 x threshold, 10Hz, 3 min, recording of bladder pressure): (a). A: unilateral stimulation S2 left does not result in bladder inhibition; B: unilateral stimulation S2 right does not result in bladder inhibition; C: bilateral stimulation S2 results in obvious bladder inhibition; (b) excitatory and inhibitory efficacy of unilateral and bilateral stimulation, expressed as percentage of the spontaneous contractions recorded in controls (area under the curve): increase of bladder contractility (excitation) of 12±2% and 13±1.5%, respectively, followed by decrease of bladder contractility (inhibition) of 17±1% and 13±4%, respectively in unilateral S2 stimulation, left and right; bilateral S2 stimulation increases bladder pressure in only 2±0.5%, but causes a significant increase of bladder inhibition (decrease of bladder pressure in 33±4%, p<0.0001).*

Consequences for the clinical application of sacral neuromodulation

The experimental findings demonstrate that, as far as bladder inhibition is concerned, unilateral sacral neuromodulation can be applied only at suboptimal stimulation parameters because uncomfortable skeletal muscle contractions limit stimulation at optimal inhibitory intensities. However, bilateral SNS is able to achieve effective bladder inhibition at intensities below the muscle-twitch threshold without producing disruptive side effects. Therefore, bilateral sacral neuromodulation may be more effective at even lower stimulation intensities, thus reducing unhelpful side effects, potential nerve damage and possibly increasing the life of the stimulator battery.

These experimental findings have already influenced the clinical application of SNS. Since 1994, several investigators have used bilateral sacral neuromodulation in the clinical setting [17–20]; the initial clinical results have confirmed the experimental findings of the improved efficacy of bilateral compared with unilateral stimulation. However, long-term studies are needed to confirm the persistence of this improvement. Finally, further studies must also determine the technique that is most effective and least invasive.

Bilateral sacral neuromodulation: cuff electrodes placed via a sacral laminectomy

M. Hohenfellner, S. Dahms, C. Hampel, K.E. Matzel and J.W. Thüroff

Introduction

Evaluations in single and multicentre trials have confirmed that chronic sacral neuromodulation, based on unilateral sacral foramen electrode implantation, exerts statistically significant therapeutic effects compared with controls in series of patients with urgency syndromes [21–23] and failure to empty [24, 25]. However, individual cases show greater variation: some centres have reported a near-perfect efficacy of chronic sacral neuromodulation [11, 12, 26–28], whereas other groups experienced therapeutic failure rates of 20–51% during chronic sacral neuromodulation although all of their implanted patients had responded successfully to the previous test trials [5, 9, 29, 30]. These failures could not be attributed to a specific indication but affect cases of storage failure as well as of failure to empty and painful conditions, the latter cases being the most likely to experience failure. Only psychological disorders, already present at the time of implantation, could be identified as a factor that significantly increases the risk of implant failure [31].

The precise causes of these unexpected failures of chronic sacral neuromodulation have not yet been elucidated, although several possible explanations have been debated. These include the observation that each half of the bladder has its own seperate innervation [32–34]; low-pressure compression trauma of the spinal nerve resulting in a conduction block due to nutritional impairment [35]; fibrosis between electrode and target nerve; electrode dislocation; and the nervous system's natural plasticity [36] leading to reactivation of pathological reflex arcs.

Rationale of modified sacral neuromodulation

In order to improve the reliability of chronic sacral neuromodulation on the basis of the above-mentioned hypotheses, the technique for sacral neuromodulation was modified [19]. In view of the bilateral innervation of the bladder, a technique for bilateral electrostimulation was developed. To increase stimulation efficacy by rendering the electrode–nerve interaction more precise and confining the stimulation current to the target nerve, the position and design of the electrode were altered. In the original procedure, a quad electrode was slipped blindly into the sacral canal via a sacral foramen, and its position was confirmed solely by functional stimulation responses. In the modified technique, the spinal nerves are exposed via a small sacral laminectomy that permits the electrodes to be attached directly to the target nerve. To minimise the spread of current to the neighbouring spinal nerves, the electrodes have three contacts (the so-called 'guarded bipolar' configuration). In this set-up, current flow is from a central cathode to two cuff anodes [37, 38]. The rationale of this approach was also to minimise trauma to the nerves, by exposing them instead of approaching them blindly, and to prevent the growth of fibrotic tissue between nerve and electrode, as far as possible.

Technique of modified bilateral sacral neuromodulation

Between test stimulation and implantation, an interval of at least 2 weeks is stipulated to reduce the risk of implant infection. Further precautions include swabbing the patient's skin in the surgical area with disinfectant twice daily for three days preoperatively; for peri- and postoperative prophylaxis, an appropriate antibiotic is administered for 10 days. For implantation of the stimulation system, the sacral spinal nerves S2–3 and S4 are exposed by sacral laminectomy. With the patient under general anaesthesia without muscle relaxants, a median skin incision from S2 to S4 exposes the thoracolumbar fascia. Median incision of this fascia permits cleaning of the spinous processes and vertebral arches from fascia and paravertebral muscles. At this stage it is important to keep the instruments in a cleavage plane

Key Points

- To improve SNS reliability, a modified technique was developed.
- The position and design of the electrode were altered.
- In the modified technique, sacral laminectomy enabled direct attachment of electrodes to the target nerve.
- The 'guarded bipolar' electrode configuration minimised current spread.
- The technique of modified bilateral SNS is described.

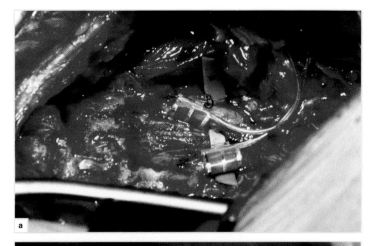

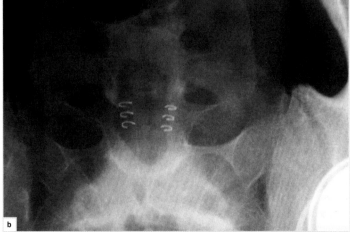

Figure 17.7 *Intraoperative (a) and radiological (b) view of bilateral guarded bipolar electrodes.*

between the bone and the periosteum to ensure haemostasis. A small piece of bone area, approximately 4×2cm, is then removed using rongeurs or a bone drill. The sacral spinal nerves are identified, and cleaned from their bed of fatty tissue with cotton pads and nerve hooks. Intraoperative electrostimulation confirms the level of the anatomical segment of the target root (usually S3). Both S3 spinal nerves are fitted with electrodes, each of which has three symmetrically arranged contacts (Fig. 17.7a). At each electrode the outer two contacts are connected to one channel and the inner contact to another (the 'guarded bipolar' design mentioned earlier). In the original technique, the electrodes were tunnelled through to a telemetrically programmable four-channel neurostimulator (Iitrel II/III, Medtronic) that was implanted into the hypogastric area of choice. However, in our last patient the buttock implantation technique was used to reduce bending of the electrodes as far as possible (Fig. 17.7b). This implantation site also appears to be more comfortable for patients. Another recent development is neurostimulators that allow independent stimulation of the left and right electrodes (Synergy, Medtronic), thus obviating the effects of different impedance on the two sides. The connectors of the electrodes are designed to allow both electrodes to be connected to the same neurostimulator. Standard stimulation parameters are used to power the outer two contacts as anodes and the inner one as a cathode (pulse width 210μs, frequency 10–15Hz).

Complications and results of modified bilateral sacral neuromodulation

Since 1994, 17 patients have been implanted with cuff electrodes attached to the sacral spinal nerves through a small sacral laminectomy. Fifteen patients (13 female, 2 male) aged between 21 and 70 years underwent surgery for treatment of lower urinary tract dysfunction; of these, seven had bladder-emptying problems and eight had storage failure. Two patients underwent surgery for treatment of anal incontinence. No intraoperative complications were encountered. The predominant postoperative complication was wound infection (n=6), which was superficial, and endangered the implant in only one patient. In one patient a functional implant had to be removed for psychological reasons (development of a conversion neurosis). In three patients, revision surgery was necessary to rectify the breakage of the wires connecting the electrodes to the neurostimulator. One patient still experiences moderate but tolerable pain in the area of surgery while seated.

In our first series, with a mean follow-up of 11 (range 9–28) months and repeated urodynamic investigations, no treatment failure was encountered (Fig. 17.8). Approximately 50% of the 11 patients experienced significant relief of their symptoms (with an alleviation of 50% or more) and the remainder had complete relief of their symptoms. The mean impedance was 1246 (746–2000)Ω with over 2000Ω measured in one patient when a wire had broken. The mean voltage was 1.5(0.7–1.5)V. In the second series, treatment of six patients was reported as successful after a follow-up of 3–22(13.6) months; however, treatment is reported to have failed in one patient with the necessary evaluation still outstanding

Outside the range of urological indications, two patients received bilateral cuff electrodes for treatment of colorectal diseases [39]. Both patients were suffering from faecal incontinence due to reduced or absent voluntary sphincteric function: in one patient this followed the Delorme procedure for rectal prolapse and sphincter repair; in the other patient this was due to the cauda syndrome secondary to fracture of the lumbar spine at level 5. In both cases, therapeutic success was achieved during a follow-up period of 32 or 26 months: the mean frequency of involuntary voiding of stool during a one-week period decreased from an average of 7 and 16 to 0 and 1, respectively.

Key Points

- Since 1994, in 17 patients, no intraoperative complications have been encountered.
- Postoperative wound infection was usually superficial.
- Other complications were psychological (1), wire breakage (3), or moderate pain (1).
- Treatment was significantly or completely successful in all but one patient.
- In two patients with colorectal disease, treatment with bilateral cuff electrodes was ultimately successful.

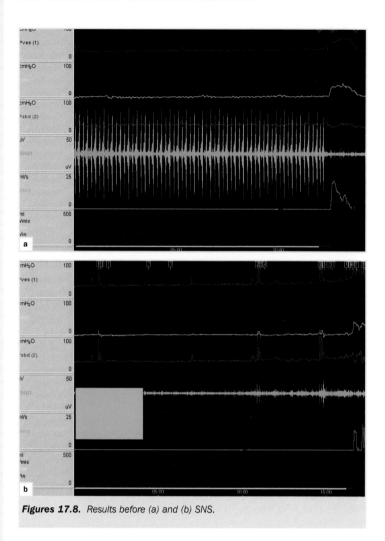

Key Points

- SNS, with sacral laminectomy and bilateral electrodes, is effective but invasive.

Figures 17.8. Results before (a) and (b) SNS.

Future perspectives

This modified technique of sacral neuromodulation makes the surgical procedure rather more sophisticated, but invasive, and a challenge for any well-trained urologist. A possible drawback is that the total stimulation system becomes more expensive because two electrodes instead of one are required. However, the direct method of electrode attachment reduces stimulation thresholds, thus reducing stimulator output and consequently prolonging battery life.

The advantage of modified sacral neuromodulation is the predicted increased efficacy. All of our patients implanted to date have experienced significant relief of their symptoms. Especially noteworthy in this respect is the patient in whom a sacral foramen electrode had given poor results but in whom sacral neuromodulation became successful when the quad electrode was exchanged for a direct nerve implant.

Tailored laminectomy for bilateral sacral nerve stimulation

P-M. Braun and K-P. Jünemann

Introduction

According to the original technique of chronic sacral neuromodulation, as described by Tanagho and Schmidt [1], the electrode is inserted unilaterally into the sacral canal via the sacral foramen (S3) without exposing this nerve. As described earlier (see page 197), modified implantation techniques, including sacral laminectomy and bilateral electrode placement, were introduced to improve SNS treatment results [19, 40–42]. However, although this procedure seemed to be more effective, it is still rather invasive. Tailored laminectomy for bilateral neuromodulator electrode implantation was developed in an attempt to minimise surgical trauma and to reduce such postoperative complications as electrode dislocation and fibrosis [20].

Technique of tailored laminectomy

The patients were placed in the prone position. After surgical cleansing and draping of the skin, the intended level of electrode implantation — generally S3 — was established by percutaneous stimulation of the sacral nerves through the dorsal sacral foramina, in a manner similar to the peripheral nerve evaluation test. This level was then marked on the skin. A midline skin incision (6–10cm) was then made two-thirds cranial to the skin mark. The subcutaneous tissue and sacral fascia were opened longitudinally along the midline parallel to the skin incision. The sacral roof was exposed by scraping off the muscles with a raspatorium within the medial rim of the dorsal sacral foramina (Fig. 17.9). The dorsal face of the os sacrum was perforated on both sides using a Rosen burr drill (Fig. 17.10). These primary perforations were enlarged with a Kerrison rongeur tailored to the electrode fixation shoes (Fig. 17.11). The nerve channels were pretunnelled with a blunt probe with a diameter equal to that of the electrodes to be implanted. Epidural fat was not removed, coagulated or even dissected. After pretunnelling, the electrodes (InterStim quadripolar electrodes, model 3886) slipped easily into the nerve channels on both sides. The correct position and level of the electrodes was reconfirmed by electrical stimulation through the actual leads. In a manner similar to that for tack-up sutures in craniotomies, a small hole was drilled with a spiral burr drill at the lateral edge of the bone window on each side; the electrodes were then fixed through this hole using non-absorbable suture material (silk 0) (Figs. 17.12 and 17.13). Via subcutaneous tunnelling, the cables and extension leads (model 7495) were then brought to the patient's flank on one side, where a second small

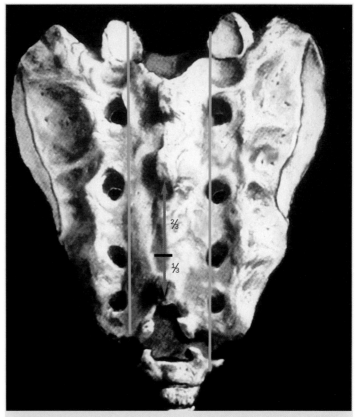

Figure 17.9 Approach to the sacral roof. Red double arrow: skin incision. Green lines: medial borderlines of the dorsal sacral foramina.

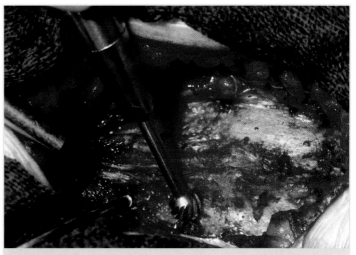

Figure 17.10 The dorsal face of the os sacrum was perforated on both sides using a Rosen burr drill.

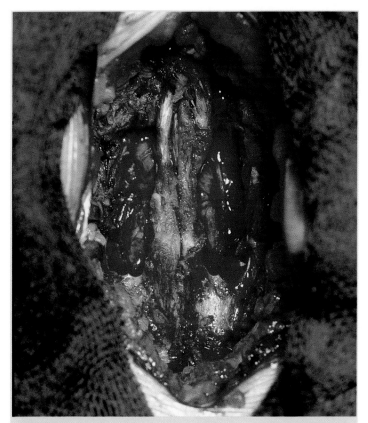

Figure 17.11 *The primary perforations were enlarged with a Kerrison rongeur tailored to the electrode fixation shoes.*

incision was made; the wounds were closed in layers. The InterStim generator (model 3023) was placed in a subcutaneous pouch on one side of the lower abdominal wall (right for right-handed, left for left-handed patients) by a standard method (Fig. 17.14).

Complications and results of tailored laminectomy and bilateral stimulation

Following urodynamic examination and previous successful percutaneous test neuromodulation, 20 patients with urge incontinence (*n*=14) or urinary retention (*n*=6) were selected for neuromodulator implantation by tailored laminectomy.

The average overall implantation time (i.e. from the first skin incision up to the last skin suture, including turnover and redraping procedures) was 2 hours 15 minutes (range 2–3 hours).

No problems with regard to wound healing and electrode dislocation were encountered. Postoperatively, one patient developed a seroma in the vicinity of the impulse generator. One system failed

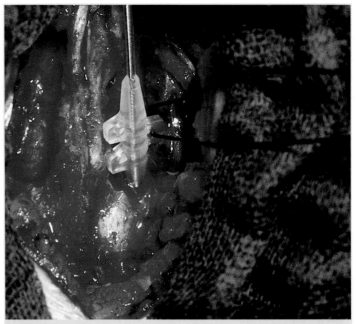

Figure 17.12 *The electrodes were fixed using non-absorbable suture material.*

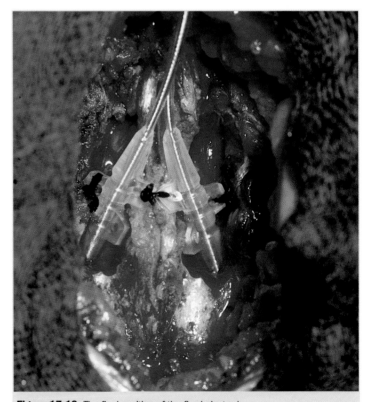

Figure 17.13 *The final position of the fixed electrodes.*

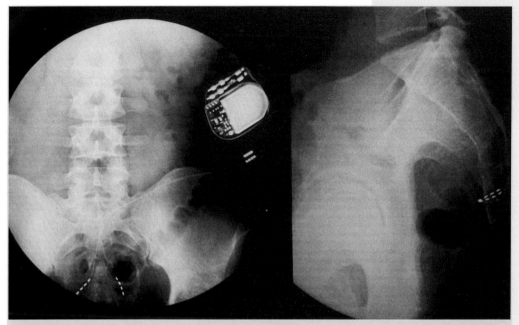

Figure 17.14 *Anterior–posterior and lateral radiographic views of an implanted system.*

owing to disrupted connection leads; correct functioning was restored by exchanging these leads while the electrodes remained in place. The impulse generator was activated on the first postoperative day. The average stimulation current required for the therapeutic effect achieved was 1.7 (range 0.5–2.5V). Frequency was 15–20Hz and pulse width 180–280µs.

In patients with urge incontinence, the number of leakages decreased from seven to one per day. The number of pads per 24 hours decreased from four to one. The functional bladder capacity increased from 198 to 352ml. Compliance increased from 15 to 31ml/cmH$_2$O. In patients with urinary retention, maximum detrusor pressure increased from initially 12cmH$_2$O to 34cmH$_2$O. The post-voiding residual urine decreased from 350 to 58ml (Table 17.1 and Fig. 17.15).

Future perspectives

The tailored sacral approach is an interesting method of sacral neuromodulation as it is a rapid, safe and easily-learned modification of the standard procedure. It ensures excellent electrode fixation combined with minimum surgical trauma (compared to conventional laminectomy), as the bone is tailored according to the shape and dimensions of the electrodes and bone removal is consequently reduced to a minimum. This minimised 'bone work' reduces not only preparation time but also the risk of postoperative complications such as infection, pain, and implant removal. Limiting the soft-tissue

Key Points

- Problems were encountered in 10% of patients with urge incontinence or urinary retention.
- In urge-incontinent patients, leakage and pad use decreased; bladder capacity and compliance increased.
- In patients with urinary retention, detrusor pressure increased and post-void urine decreased.
- Tailored laminectomy is a rapid, safe, easily-learned modification of SNS.

Key Points
- Risk of complications is minimised.

Table 17.1 *Results of tailored laminectomy and bilateral stimulation*

Disorder		Initial	Implant	Percentage change
Urge incontinence	Follow-up 14.5 (7–18) months			
	Leakages/24 h	7±3	1±0.3*	-86
	Pads/24 h	4±2	1±0.3*	-75
	Bladder capacity (ml)	198±52	352±49*	+78
	Bladder compliance (ml/cmH$_2$0)	15±4	31±8*	+107
Urinary retention	Follow-up 12.5 (6–20) months (6–20)		•	
	Maximum detrusor pressure during voiding (cmH$_2$0)	12±5	34±14*	+183
	Post-void residual (ml)	350±49	58±33*	-83

* Difference statistically significant (p <0.05).

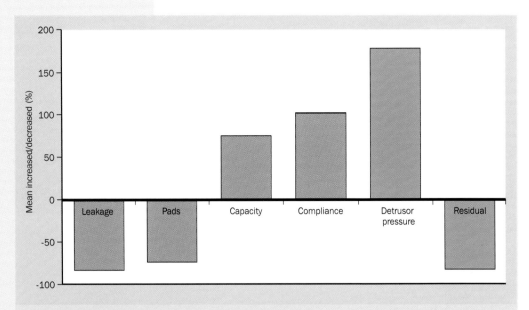

Figure 17.15 *Results for neuromodulation with tailored laminectomy.*

approach to the area between the medial borders of the dorsal sacral foramina on both sides (i.e. without opening the foramina) leaves the dorsal branches of the sacral nerves undisturbed. The tight, stable fixation of the electrodes, achieved by anchoring them to the bone with non-absorbable stitches, reduces electrode dislocation rates to an absolute minimum. This technique probably reduces peridural fibrosis, so that the stimulation current can be kept low for a longer period [43, 44].

Together with bilateral electrode implantation, neuromodulation will be possible at optimal conditions, resulting in an improvement of success rates [45]. However, further studies with a larger number of patients will be necessary to show whether the improvement attendant on this modification is confirmed by improvement in long-term follow-up.

Key Points

- Optimal conditions for SNS improve success rates.
- Long-term studies are needed for confirmation.

References

1. Tanagho EA, Schmidt RA. Electrical stimulation in the clinical management of the neurogenic bladder. *J. Urol* 1988; 140: 1331–9.
2. Schmidt RA. Applications of neurostimulation in Urology. *Neurourol Urodyn* 1988; 7: 585.
3. Bosch JLHR, Groen J. Effects of sacral segmental nerve stimulation on urethral resistance and bladder contractility: how does neuromodulation work in urge incontinence patients? *Neurourol Urodyn* 1996; 15: 502–504.
4. De Ridder D, Van Poppel H, Baert L. Sacral nerve stimulation is a successful treatment for the Fowler Syndrome. *Neurourol Urodynam* 1996; 15: 120.
5. Dijkema HE, Weil EHJ, Mijs PT, Janknegt RA. Neuromodulation of sacral nerves for incontinence and voiding dysfunction. 1993; *Eur Urol* 24: 72–6.
6. Elabbady AA, Hassouna MM, Elhilali MM. Neural stimulation for chronic voiding dysfunctions. 1994; *J Urol* 152: 2076–80.
7. Hassouna MM, Siegel SW, Lycklama à Nijeholt AAB, *et al.* Sacral neuromodulation in the treatment of urgency–frequency syndrome: a multicentre study on efficacy and safety. *J Urol* 2000; 163: 1849–54.
8. Hohenfellner M, Dahms SE, Matzel K, Thüroff JW. Sakrale Neuromodulation der Harnblase. *Urologe* [A] 2000; 39: 55-63.
9. Weil EH, Ruiz-Cerdá JL, Eerdmans PH *et al.* Clinical results of sacral neuromodulation for chronic voiding dysfunction using unilateral sacral foramen electrodes. *World J Urol* 1998; 16: 313–21.
10. Weil EH, Ruiz-Cerdá JL, Eerdmans PH. Sacral root neuromodulation in the treatment of refractory urinary urge incontinence: a prospective randomized clinical trial. *Eur Urol* 2000; 37: 161–171.
11. Shaker HS, Hassouna MM. Sacral nerve root neuromodulation in idiopathic nonobstructive chronic urinary retention. *J Urol* 1998; 159: 1476.
12. Shaker HS, Hassouna MM. Sacral nerve root neuromodulation: an effective treatment for refractory urge incontinence. *J Urol* 1998; 159: 1516.
13. Shaker HS, Hassouna MM. Sacral root neuromodulation in the treatment of various voiding and storage problems. *Int Urogynecol J Pelvic Floor Dysfunct* 1999; 10: 336–43.
14. Grünewald V, Höfner K, Becker A *et al.* Clinical results and complications of chronic sacral neuromodulation after four years of application. *Neurourol Urodyn* 1996; 15: 116.
15. Schultz-Lampel D, Jiang C, Lindström S, Thüroff JW. Neurophysiologische Effekte unilateraler und bilateraler sakraler Neuromodulation. *Aktuel Urol* 1998; 29: 354–60.
16. Schultz-Lampel D, Jiang C, Lindström S, Thüroff J W. Experimental results on mechanisms of action of electrical neuromodulation in chronic urinary retention. *World J Urol* 1998; 16: 301–4.
17. Sauerwein D, Kutzenberger B and Domurath B. Bilateraler sakraler Zugang nach Laminektomie zur permanenten Neuromodulation durch veränderte Operationstechnik und modifizierte Elektroden. *Urologe* [A] (Suppl.) 1997; 36: 57.
18. Schultz-Lampel D. *Neurophysiologische Grundlagen und klinische Anwendung der sakralen Neuromodulation zur Therapie von Blasenfunktionsstörngen.* Habilitationsschrift, Klinik für Urologie und Kinderurologie, Klinikum Wuppertal, Universität Wtten, Herdecke, 1997.
19. Hohenfellner M, Schultz-Lampel D, Dahms S *et al.* Bilateral chronic sacral neuromodulation for treatment of lower urinary tract dysfunction. *J Urol* 1998; 160: 821–4.
20. Braun PM, Boschert J, Bross S *et al.* The tailored laminectomy — new technique for neuromodulator implantation. *J Urol* 1999; 162: 1607–9
21. Bosch JLHR, Groen J. Sacral (S3) segmental nerve stimulation as a treatment for urge incontinence in patients with dètrusor instability: results of chronic electrical stimulation using an implantable neuroprosthesis. *J Urol* 1995; 154: 504–7.

22. Janknegt R, Van Kerrebroeck P, Lycklama à Nijeholt AAB *et al.* Sacral nerve modulation for urge incontinence: a multinational, multicenter randomized study. *J Urol* 1997; 157 (Suppl.): 317.

23. Schmidt RA, Gajewski J, Hassouna MM *et al.* Management of refractory urge frequency syndromes using an implantable neuroprosthesis: a North American multicenter study. *J Urol* 1997; 157 (Suppl.): 317.

24. Jonas U, Grünewald V, Group M-MS. Sacral electrical nerve stimulation for treatment of severe voiding dysfunction. *Eur Urol* 1999; 35 (S2): 66.

25. Jonas U, Fowler C, Chancellor M, *et al.* Efficacy of sacral nerve stimulation for urinary retention: results 18 months after implantation. *J Urol* 2001; 165: 15–19.

26. Groen J, Bosch JLHR, and Schröder FH. Neuromodulation (sacral segmental nerve stimulation) as treatment for urge incontinence in patients with bladder instability. *J Urol* 1993; 149.

27. Vapnek JM, and Schmidt RA. Restoration of voiding in chronic urinary retention using the neuroprosthesis. *World J Urol* 1991; 9: 142-144.

28. Siegel SW. Management of voiding dysfunction with an implantable neuroprosthesis. *Urol Clin North Am* 1992; 19: 163–70.

29. Schmidt RA. Treatment of pelvic pain with neuroprostheses. *J Urol* 1988; 139: 277A.

30. Hohenfellner M, Schultz-Lampel D, Lampel A *et al.* Functional rehabilitation of the neurogenic bladder by chronic sacral neuromodulation. *Aktuel Urol* 27 (Supplement): 1996; 89–91.

31. Weil EH, Eerdmans HP, Ruiz-Cerdá JL *et al.* Long term follow-up of patients with voiding dysfunction treated by neuromodulation. *Eur Urol* 1999; 35 (S2): 18.

32. Diokno A, Davis R, Lapides J. The effect of pelvic nerve stimulation on detrusor contraction. *Invest Urol* 1973; 11: 178–81.

33. Griffiths J. Observations on the urinary bladder and urethra. *J Anat Physiol* 1894; 29: 61–83.

34. Ingersoll E, Jones L, Hegre E. Effect on urinary bladder of unilateral stimulation of pelvic nerves in the dog. *Am J Physiol* 1957; 189: 167–72.

35. Thon WF, Baskin LS, Jonas U *et al.* Surgical principles of sacral foramen electrode implantation. *World J Urol* 1991; 9: 133–7.

36. Zvara P, Sah S, Hassouna MM. An animal model for the neuromodulation of neurogenic bladder dysfunction. *Br J Urol* 1998; 82: 267–71.

37. Brindley GS, Craggs MD. A technique for anodally blocking large nerve fibres through chronically implanted electrodes. *J Neurol Neurosurg Psychiatry* 1980; 43: 1083–90.

38. Garten S. Elektroden für besondere Zwecke. Leipzig, Verlag von S Hirzel, 1911, 339–40.

39. Matzel KE, Stadelmaier U, Hohenfellner M *et al.* Chronic sacral spinal nerve stimulation for fecal incontinence: long term results with foramen and cuff electrode. *Dis Colon Rectum* 2001; 44: 59–66.

40. Bosch JLHR, Groen J. Treatment of refractory urge incontinence with sacral spinal nerve stimulation in multiple sclerosis patients. *Lancet* 1996; 348: 717.

41. Thon WF, Baskin LS, Jonas U *et al.* Neuromodulation of voiding dysfunction and pelvic pain. *World J Urol* 1991; 9: 138.

42. Sauerwein D, Kutzenberger B, Domurath B. Bilateraler sakraler Zugang nach Laminektomie zur permanenten Neuromodulation durch veränderte Operationstechnik und modifizierte Elektroden. *Urologe* [A] (Suppl.) 1997; 36: 57.

43. Sakas DE, Booth AE. Postlaminectomy peridural fibrosis. *J Neurosurg* 1994; 80: 1130.

44. Robertson JT. Role of peridural fibrosis in the failed back: a review. *Eur Spine J* 1996; (Suppl. 1) 5:2.

45. Schultz-Lampel D, Chonghe J, Sivert L, Türhoff JW. Summation effect of bilateral sacral nerve stimulation. *Eur Urol* 1998; (Suppl. 1) 33: 61.

18 Evolution of a minimally-invasive procedure for sacral neuromodulation

M. Spinelli, G.A. Mamo, A. Arduini,

M. Gerber and G. Giardiello

Introduction

Bladder and sphincter function can be altered by electrostimulation, a therapeutic technique that has been in use for many years. The great interest in this field is well documented in the numerous publications which discuss methodology, regulated and unregulated indications, long-term results and possible explanations from a neurophysiological point of view.

There has been an increased awareness and use of this therapeutic approach in recent years as a result of the clinical outcomes achieved in situations where the only alternative treatment was major surgery. In terms of the patient's functional abilities, results in such cases have not matched expectations.

Historically, as the efficacy of a therapy is established, physicians focus on improving the administration of the therapy and developing less invasive techniques. Thus minimally-invasive techniques of electrostimulation have begun to supplant the original techniques, and are likely to improve as physicians gain experience in the administration of the therapy.

Direct stimulation versus modulation

Electrostimulation is used in a variety of ways to re-establish effective urine storage and voiding. Each method seeks to stimulate the neurological control systems by applying an electric current. Direct stimulation for complete spinal cord injury patients (Vocare System by NeuroControl) requires a high level of electrical current, which is applied in order to stimulate the nerves and create a direct response in the control and coordination system. Direct stimulation of the third sacral nerve is a widely-used method of treating total medullar injury at the upper motorneuron level; neuromodulation in cases of complete medullar injury has not been shown to be successful or achieve any results.

Where direct stimulation is not possible or applicable, modulation is used. There are a number of methods for bringing about neuromodulation of the lower urinary tract: chemical modulation uses substances such as capsaicin and resinaferatoxin (RTX) to modulate afferent neurons at the receptor level; electrical modulation uses a low level of electrical current, applied in pulses. Typically, the somatic component of the pudendum is electrically modulated, in order to evoke the recovery of the control and coordination systems.

Sacral neuromodulation

In 1988, Tanagho and Schmidt reported the positive results of sacral neuromodulation for the treatment of lower urinary tract dysfunction [1]. This method of electrostimulation involves continuous modulation of one or more of the sacral nerves by an implantable stimulator. In sacral neuromodulation, the applied electric current has an effect on the sensory component; this is known as the dominant effect.

Sacral neuromodulation is a proven method of treatment in the following types of cases:

1. Urinary incontinence as a result of detrusor hyperactivity;
2. Voiding dysfunction resulting from a lack of coordination between the reservoir and the closure mechanism;
3. Voiding dysfunction as a result of altered sensitivity of the bladder or the perineal region of the pelvis.

Development of a minimally-invasive lead implant technique
The development of a minimally-invasive technique for sacral nerve stimulation is based on experience gained in using a number of approaches. The following is a description of one such approach, namely Dr G. Mamo's surgical technique for lead implantation,

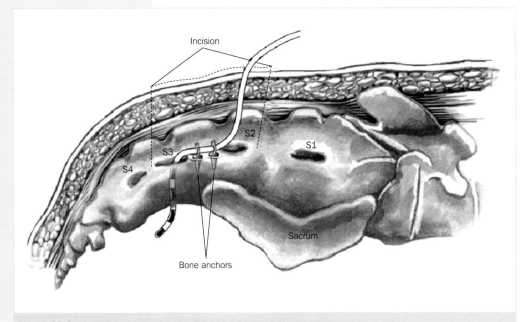

Figure 18.1 Lead implant technique: fixation of the lead with bone anchors.

which involves a paramedian incision and the use of bone anchors to fix the lead to the sacrum (Fig. 18.1).

The patient is placed in the a prone position, as during the test stimulation, and prepared. The procedure is performed under general anaesthesia without the use of any muscle relaxants. The landmarks for the S2, S3, and S4 foramina are identified and marked. The sacral nerve that elicits the best clinical response during test stimulation is then re-tested with the foramen needle and external test stimulator.

Once the appropriate motor response has been obtained, a paramedian incision measuring 2.5cm is made directly over the targeted foramen. The needle is removed and electrocautery is performed to reach the lumbrosacral fascia, which is incised longitudinally to expose the paraspinous muscle.

The muscle fibres are split and retracted laterally and medially to expose the periosteum. The test needle is placed in the foramen through the incision and the response is confirmed.

The chronic lead is placed next to the needle. The presence of dense fibrous tissue may require puncturing of the tissue using a 14-gauge angiocatheter needle prior to placement of the lead. An angio-catheter can be made into a sheath by shortening it to 2.5cm, slicing it longitudinally, and passing a suture through the proximal end (for removal). The sheath can be advanced over the needle to a location next to the nerve. Both the test and 14-gauge needles are removed, leaving the sheath in place. Once the chronic lead has been introduced, the sheath is removed, leaving the lead next to the nerve.

The lead is stimulated to confirm a good placement. If an appropriate response is obtained, the lead is fixed to the sacrum above the S3 foramen using two bone anchors (Fig. 18.1). The anchors are carefully advanced into the bone behind the lead and the anchor sutures are tied over the lead to fix it in place. Radiographs are used to confirm the position of the lead.

A subcutaneous pocket is created on the upper and lateral aspect of the buttock and the proximal end of the lead is then tunnelled subcutaneously and connected to the implantable neurostimulator with an extension.

Development of a staged implant procedure for sacral neuromodulation

The traditional procedure for sacral nerve stimulation involved the use of percutaneous test stimulation prior to implantation of a chronic system. The implantation procedure was performed after positive results had been obtained and the procedure was typically performed as a single-stage implant. The test stimulation sometimes gave inconclusive results, because test leads would migrate. The need for repeated test stimulations because of these inconclusive results often frustrated and discouraged patients. In January 1997, Janknegt and co-workers reported on a staged implant procedure using a chronic lead for the test stimulation [2].

The use of a chronic lead for screening was the first step in reducing the invasiveness of the sacral neuromodulation. A staged implant has specific advantages, including the following:

Key Points
- This technique involves a paramedian incision, and bone anchors to fix the lead to the sacrum.
- A chronic lead for screening reduces SNS invasiveness.

Key Points

• A staged implant has specific advantages.

• A percutaneous staged implant is described.

1. Shorter duration of the procedure, which uses an anaesthetic for the positioning of the quadripolar electrode with a lead to the external temporary stimulator;
2. The possibility of a longer testing period;
3. The absence of complications such as lead migration;
4. Effective monitoring of the stimulation efficacy (due to multiple stimulation sites and a long overall stimulation zone on the chronic lead);
5. Elimination of correlation complications (resulting from different lead placement) between the screening phase and the chronic lead.

In developing a minimally-invasive technique for implanting the neuromodulation lead, we considered the particular anatomy of the posterior side of the sacrum and drew on our experience in performing acute and chronic testing of sacral neuromodulation. We began by using materials and techniques normally associated with percutaneous positioning of kidney drainage at the pyelic level.

We gained a better understanding of the sacral anatomy through the experience of implanting extradural direct stimulators with sacral laminectomy on patients with complete spinal cord injury. As it is easy to identify the ideal position of the lead for a percutaneous test stimulation through a 'needle-lead' stimulation, we attempted to show the feasibility of a similar access for the positioning of the chronic lead using the same approach. This approach would eliminate the requirement for a surgical opening of the planes lying above the sacral foramen.

In December 1999, the first patient underwent the first staged, percutaneous implant, as follows.

Description of a percutaneous staged implant

The following technique was developed independently, but concurrently, by the authors (G. Mamo and M. Spinelli).

The patient is placed in a prone position, as in a test stimulation procedure. The bony landmarks are identified and drawn on the skin and a local anaesthetic is applied to anaesthetise the area where the stimulation lead will be implanted, such as posterior to the sacrum. By using local anaesthesia, the implanting clinician uses the patient's conscious sensory response to stimuli; this aids in placing the stimulation lead more accurately and reduces the potential for an inconclusive response. Other forms of anaesthetic, including general anaesthesia, can also be used during the procedure. Once the patient is anesthetised, and the operation field sterilised, the procedure can begin.

The foramen needle is inserted posterior to the sacrum. The needle is hand-guided into the foramen to a desired location. Electrical stimulation is applied to the needle to verify the correct positioning and motor and conscious sensory responses are tested. Fluoroscopy or radiography are used to confirm the position of the needle in the S3 foramen (Fig. 18.2a).

A guide-wire is then inserted through the needle (Fig. 18.2b). With the guide-wire in position, the needle is removed; the guide-wire will serve as a guide for the dilator (Fig. 18.2c).

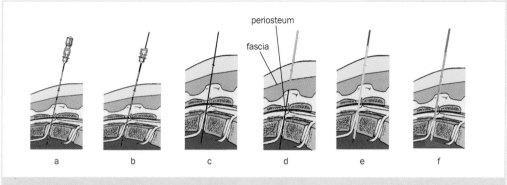

Figure 18.2 *Minimally-invasive procedure: the six steps.*

The insertion path is dilated using a metal dilator (8F) to a diameter sufficient for inserting a stimulation lead (Fig. 18.2d). Latero-lateral fluoroscopy is used to ensure that the tip of the dilator stops at the edge of the sacrum, at the level of the S3 foramen. The metal dilator is removed and a plastic dilator (8F) is positioned (Fig. 18.2e) using the guide-wire to guide the insertion. The guide-wire is then removed from the insertion path, at which stage care should be taken to avoid displacing the plastic dilator.

The stimulation lead is inserted through the plastic dilator to the desired location (Fig. 18.2f). To verify its position, an electrical signal is applied to the stimulation lead to evoke the patient's motor or sensory response; position and depth of the lead are adjusted to obtain the best responses. Typically, fluoroscopy is used to confirm and document the placement of the lead. Once good responses have been obtained, the plastic dilator is removed from the insertion path, at which stage, care should be taken to avoid displacing the stimulation lead. The stimulation lead position is re-verified by applying electrical stimulation.

Once the plastic dilator has been removed, the lead is fixed in place by creating an incision through the skin, anchoring the lead to the fascia layer, and closing the incision. Adjustable anchors such as the silicone anchor used with the Medtronic 3886 lead (or similar adjustable anchor) can be used (Figs. 18.3 and 18.4); care should be taken to avoid displacing the stimulation lead during anchoring.

Conclusions

Sacral neuromodulation continues to evolve. A less invasive approach to implantation has a number of benefits, as follows:

1. Our experience has shown that the staged, percutaneous approach with local anaesthesia is feasible and enables sub-chronic phase of the test stimulation to be eliminated;
2. The use of local anaesthesia enables the implanting physician to use the patient's conscious sensory responses to stimuli as an aid to accurate placement of the stimulation lead;

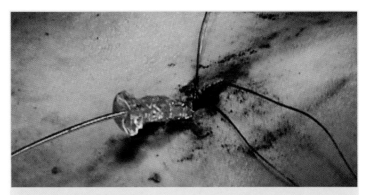

Figure 18.3 *Twist-lock inserted and anchoring suture attached to the fascia.*

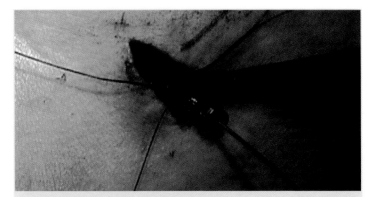

Figure 18.4 *Twist-lock ready to be fixed.*

3. The staged, percutaneous approach is quicker than the traditional implant procedure;
4. Patients are more willing to undergo the test stimulation;
5. Anchoring the lead mitigates its migration and reduces the likelihood of inconclusive results, thereby improving the success rate;
6. The percutaneous lead placement method may reduce adverse events associated with the surgical procedure required to implant the lead.

References

1. Tanagho EA, Schmidt RA. Electrical stimulation in the clinical management of the neurogenic bladder. *J Urol* 1988; 140: 1331–9.
2. Janknegt RA, Weil E, Eerdmans P. Improving neuromodulation technique for refractory voiding dysfunctions: two stage implant. *Urology* 1997; 49: 358–62.

19 Emerging indications for sacral nerve stimulation

General introduction

J.L.H.R. Bosch

Established indications for sacral nerve neuromodulation include refractory urge urinary incontinence, urinary urgency–frequency syndrome and urinary retention.

Urge incontinence in patients with or without an unstable bladder was the first indication to be studied extensively and systematically, and it appeared that those patients with urodynamic proof of an unstable detrusor were particularly good candidates for this treatment [1]. It also appeared that there are limits to the extent to which neuromodulation can suppress bladder instability; it is less effective if bladder capacity is very small and if the amplitude of unstable contractions is excessively high, as is sometimes the case in male patients with genuine incontinence due to an unstable bladder [2]. These men will have higher amplitudes of unstable contractions than female patients because of the much stronger outflow tract in men.

It seemed logical to test the value of this treatment in selected patients with a neurogenic cause of the detrusor instability. Proof of efficacy in these patients would be consistent with experimental evidence [3] and would also increase the credibility of this treatment, which has suffered from the fact that the exact mechanism of action is still elusive. The efficacy of neuromodulation was shown in patients with neurogenic bladder disease as a result of multiple sclerosis (MS) [4]; its application in detrusor hyperreflexia should, therefore, be termed an emerging rather than a future indication.

Empirically, it was recognised that several patients with chronic voiding dysfunction also suffered from pelvic pain syndromes (PPS). Some of these patients experienced a marked relief of pain during the subchronic test phase as well as after a permanent implant [5]; however, it was not clear why some patients did, whereas others did not, respond to this treatment. There are some indications that pain related to spastic behaviour of the pelvic floor musculature can be modulated by sacral nerve neuromodulation. It is, at present, unclear what proportion of so-called interstitial cystitis patients actually suffers from spasticity of the pelvic floor; furthermore, the aetiology of interstitial cystitis is still a matter of debate and research. Evaluation of the effects of neuromodulation in pain syndromes is particularly difficult because of the lack of objectively measurable parameters. Another problem seems to be the fact that a certain proportion of patients suffer from the late consequences of sexual abuse and/or incest [5]. Basic research in this field is hampered by the fact that there are no animal models

Key Points

- SNS poorly suppresses bladder instability when bladder capacity is small.
- It is also ineffective for high-amplitude, unstable, contractions.
- Effective in neurogenic bladder disease resulting from multiple sclerosis (MS), it is an 'emerging' indication.
- Some patients with chronic voiding dysfunction also have pelvic pain syndromes (PPS).
- In PPS patients without response to SNS, pelvic-floor muscle spasticity may be absent.
- Lack of objective parameters hampers evaluation of SNS in PPS.

Key Points

- SNS effectively treats faecal incontinence.
- SNS during voiding reduces urethral resistance (less spasticity of pelvic floor muscles).
- Upper motor-neuron lesions cause incontinence via detrusor hyperreflexia.
- This is attributable to formation of new reflex arc with afferent C fibres.
- Treatment: anticholinergic drugs/ clean intermittent catheterisation/other therapies affecting bladder smooth muscle.
- SNS inhibits detrusor by stimulation of afferent somatic sacral nerves.

of pelvic pain. The availability of newer functional imaging techniques of the central nervous system may soon be able to overcome some of these problems.

The application of sacral neuromodulation in the realm of colorectal surgery has been reported relatively early and seemed to work well in patients with faecal incontinence [6]. It was not surprising that chronic constipation due to spastic behaviour of the pelvic floor started to be explored as an indication when the treatment proved effective in patients with chronic urinary retention.

Using urodynamic methods, it has been shown that urethral resistance during voiding is lower with the stimulator in the on-mode than in the off-mode [7]. This counter-intuitive finding is consistent with the fact that neuromodulation can decrease spastic behaviour of the pelvic floor musculature.

In the following sections of this chapter, the above-mentioned emerging and future indications of sacral nerve neuromodulation are discussed by the pioneers of the study of its effects in these indications.

Neurogenic refractory urge incontinence

J.L.H.R. Bosch and E.J. Chartier-Kastler

Introduction

Incontinence in patients with an upper motor-neuron lesion is usually due to detrusor hyperreflexia. In the experimental cat model it has been demonstrated that, upon interruption of the spinobulbospinal pathways of the micturition reflex, a new sacral segmental reflex arc may become functional as a result of neuroplasticity [8]. This reflex arc with an afferent limb consisting of unmyelinated C fibres is responsible for detrusor hyperreflexia.

In incontinent patients with an upper motor-neuron lesion, the aim of treatment with anticholinergic drugs [9] is to reduce the overactivity of the bladder by a direct action on the bladder smooth muscle cells. If detrusor–sphincter dyssynergia leads to incomplete emptying of the bladder, clean intermittent (self)-catheterisation can be added to the treatment. In those who are refractory to conservative treatment with anticholinergic drugs with or without clean intermittent catheterisation, alternative therapies with variable success rates, such as intravesical instillations of capsaicin or resiniferatoxin [10], injections of botulinum toxin in the detrusor muscle [11], transvesical phenol injection of the pelvic plexus, augmentation ileocystoplasty, detrusor myectomy and even urinary diversion, have been advocated [12].

The aim of neuromodulation is to achieve detrusor inhibition by chronic electrical stimulation of afferent somatic sacral nerve fibres by means of an implanted electrode coupled to a subcutaneously-placed pulse generator.

How does neuromodulation work in patients with urinary incontinence associated with detrusor hyperreflexia?

The ratio of this treatment modality is based on the existence of spinal inhibitory systems which are capable of interrupting a detrusor contraction. In acute clinical tests, Vodušek *et al.* have shown that electrical stimulation of non-muscular sacral somatic nerve afferents in the pudendal nerve is most efficient in inducing bladder inhibition in patients with detrusor hyperreflexia due to traumatic spinal cord injury or MS [13]. These findings were recently confirmed by Shah *et al.* who stimulated the purely sensory dorsal nerve of the penis [14].

Most of these afferent somatic fibres reach the spinal cord via the sacral spinal nerves and dorsal roots of the sacral nerves. Of the sacral nerve roots, S3 is the most practical one for use in chronic electrical stimulation [15].

What results have been obtained in patients with urinary incontinence due to neurogenic bladder disease?

Peripheral nerve evaluation (PNE)

In a combined evaluation of 14 patients with detrusor hyperreflexia (mainly due to MS and complete and incomplete spinal cord lesions) that were reported in three papers, the percentage of successful test stimulations was 50% on average [4, 16, 17]. Hohenfellner *et al.* reported that none of four patients with a complete, or near-complete spinal cord lesion responded favourably to a test stimulation [16]. In a prospective study, Carone *et al.* performed a PNE in 24 patients with detrusor hyperreflexia due to a variety of neurological problems including suprasacral, suprapontine and cortical cerebral lesions [18]: in six and seven patients they found a more than 80% and a 50–80% improvement, respectively, for each of the parameters recorded in a voiding diary. These parameters included voided volume, voiding frequency and the number of leaking episodes. It seems that patients with an incomplete traumatic spinal cord lesion are better candidates for a PNE than those with a complete lesion [16].

Permanent implant: clinical results

The gender of permanently implanted patients has been reported in several studies [4, 17, 19, 20]: ten of 15 patients were female. This is not surprising as female patients with incontinence due to neurogenic bladder disease have more to gain from the treatment than men, because there are no acceptable urine collection devices for the female patient population. Sacral neuromodulation has been successfully employed in patients with detrusor hyperreflexia due to complete or incomplete traumatic spinal cord lesions. Combined data from three reports [17, 19, 20] indicate that, after a mean

Key Points

- SNS activates spinal inhibitory systems that interrupt detrusor contraction.
- S3 is the most practical nerve root for use in chronic stimulation.
- Good PNE candidates are patients with incomplete (*not* complete) spinal cord lesion.
- Good clinical SNS results are reported for spinal cord lesion, MS and myelitis.

follow-up of 19 months, four of eight implanted patients were cured; in two, the symptoms had improved significantly and the treatment had failed in another two patients.

Bosch and Groen first reported favourable results of sacral neuromodulation in patients with MS [4]. These results were subsequently confirmed after a longer follow-up (average 55 months) [20]. In these five women, the average number of leakages decreased from 5.1 to 0.5 per 24 hours; three women were able to stop using incontinence pads.

Additionally, Chartier-Kastler *et al.* reported on two women with neurogenic bladder disease due to myelitis [20]. The number of pads used decreased from 12.5 to 1 and from 8 to 0.5 per 24 hours after an average follow-up of 31 and 19 months, respectively.

Carone *et al.* performed permanent implants in six patients, including four with incomplete spinal cord lesions and one with MS patient [18]. A 3- and 6-month follow-up was reported in three patients and one patient, respectively: two of three patients were dry at 3 months.

Permanent implant: urodynamic results
Urodynamic studies with the stimulation on, at 6 months, revealed an improvement of maximal bladder capacity and volume at the first uninhibited contraction [1, 20]. The volume at the first unstable contraction increased in six of nine patients [20]. The average volume at first unstable contraction in the nine patients increased from 214– 340ml. Maximal detrusor pressure during unstable contractions decreased, remained the same, or increased in five, one and three patients, respectively. Hyperreflexia disappeared in one patient.

What are the future perspectives?

The results that have been obtained in a limited number of pilot studies are promising and warrant further exploration of the potential of sacral neuromodulation in patients with refractory urinary incontinence associated with neurogenic bladder disease. Because sacral neuromodulation is a non-destructive technique, it does not preclude the future use of other treatments. The long-term results will have to be studied carefully, recognising that the evolution of neurological disease can sometimes be unpredictable; this is particularly true for MS. To date, bladder augmentation has been avoided (or at least delayed) in patients with neurogenic bladder disease treated with neuromodulation. Formal multicentre studies in patients with incomplete traumatic spinal cord lesions and in patients with MS must be conducted to confirm the results that have been obtained in a limited number of centres. Neuromodulation will have to compete with other, newer treatment strategies, such as repeated bladder instillations with resiniferatoxin or repeated detrusorial microinjections with botulinum toxin. The cost-effectiveness of treatment with these agents must be compared with that of a permanent implant.

Interstitial cystitis

T.C. Chai

Introduction

Interstitial chronic cystitis (IC) is a diagnosis of exclusion. IC patients present with urinary frequency–urgency and chronic pelvic pain in absence of any identifiable aetiology such as urinary tract infection, bladder stones, bladder carcinoma or neurological disease. The National Institutes of Health (NIH) convened a panel in 1987 and 1988 [21] and proposed exclusionary and inclusionary criteria for IC to be used in NIH-sponsored studies. Although these criteria are not intended to comprise the definitive diagnostic tool for IC, they serve a useful purpose in helping clinicians to rule out other causes of lower urinary tract symptoms (LUTS).

It has been theorised that the glycosaminoglycan (GAG) layer of the apical (luminal) bladder urothelium is deficient in IC [22]. Furthermore, urinary potassium mediates all the IC symptoms because potassium can penetrate the GAG-deficient IC urothelium, depolarising suburothelial nerve endings. Therefore, if exogenous, high concentrations of potassium are infused into the bladder, those patients with IC will have an acute exacerbation of bladder pain, whereas those without IC will not [23]. Other workers are searching for a factor in the urine that can diagnose IC non-invasively and which can also shed light on pathophysiology. Various urinary substances have been studied and reported to differ significantly between IC and control urine specimens [24–28]. Growth factors such as heparin-binding, epidermal growth-factor-like growth factor (HB-EGF), epidermal growth factor (EGF), insulin-like growth factor 1 (IGF1), and insulin-like growth factor binding protein 3 (IGFBP3) were all significantly altered in urine from IC patients [29].

More interesting was the finding that the urine from IC subjects contained a low-molecular-weight protein, termed antiproliferative factor (APF), that significantly inhibited the normal uptake of ^{3}H-thymidine by cultured normal uroepithelium [30]; urine from normal subjects did not possess any inhibitory activity. The finding of APF activity suggests that alterations in the repair and regenerative ability of the urothelium may contribute to the pathogenesis of this disease. Other potential aetiologies include infectious, immunological, neurological and/or bladder-intrinsic (smooth muscle, extracellular matrix, urothelium) disruption; IC may be caused by several factors. It is beyond the scope of this section to present all proposed etiologies in detail; however, the alterations in urinary growth factors represent a unique opportunity to investigate whether these alterations 'normalise' after clinical treatment, thereby strengthening the mechanistic link between these urine growth factors and IC.

Because there is no known cause of IC, treatment of IC is highly empirical. Current treatments for IC include oral agents

Key Points
- Various criteria for interstitial cystitis (IC) diagnosis have been proposed by the National Institutes of Health.
- Urinary markers of IC are sought.
- These may include growth factors (e.g. HB-EGF) and antiproliferative factor (APF).
- IC treatment is empirical, as the cause is still unknown.

such as antimuscarinics (oxybutinin, tolterodine, imipramine), central neural agents (amitriptyline, gabapentin, benzodiazepines), and antihistamines (hydroxyzine). Intravesical agents such as dimethyl sulphoxide, heparin, steroids and silver nitrate are also used. These therapies have all been tried with varying success; however, without knowledge of the aetiologic mechanism(s), these treatments are geared towards symptom relief and not at reversing the pathophysiological deficit. Oral Elmiron® (sodium pentosanpolysulphate), which purportedly replenishes the urothelial apical GAG layer, can potentially reverse the pathophysiological deficit if IC is the result of a deficiency in that layer; however, there have been no studies to demonstrate either that GAG is replenished or that the permeability of the bladder in IC is decreased with Elmiron® treatment.

How does sacral neuromodulation work in interstitial cystitis?

Sacral neuromodulation is indicated in patients with idiopathic urinary urge incontinence, frequency–urgency syndrome, and urinary retention. Because the aetiology of these conditions is often uncertain, the manner by which sacral neuromodulation has been shown to be clinically effective is also uncertain. Certainly, a balance exists between bladder storage and emptying reflexes; theoretically, alterations in this balance may result in symptoms of urinary urge incontinence, frequency–urgency and urinary retention. However, until more precise diagnostic and/or aetiologic information is available, there will be an element of uncertainty regarding the mechanisms underlying the effectiveness of sacral neuromodulation.

Because IC has similar symptomatology to urinary frequency–urgency, the use of sacral neuromodulation should be contemplated. As detailed earlier, urinary growth factors are altered in IC. Measurements of these urinary factors during sacral

Table 19.1 Effect of 5 days' percutaneous S3 neuromodulation on signs and symptoms in six patients with interstitial cystitis

Assessment	Baseline	After 5 days of S3 neuromodulation	p-value
Pain scale (0-10)	7.0 ± 1.6	2.3 ± 3.2	0.05
Urgency scale (0-10)	6.0 ± 2.2	1.8 ± 1.7	0.02
Voiding frequency (per 24h)	23.3 ± 4.9	10.8 ± 4.4	0.001
Urine HB-EGF (ng/ml)	1.5 ± 2.1	11.0 ± 1.7	<0.0001
Urine APF activity (%)	-76.1 ± 31.0	-4.5 ± 8.8	<0.0001

neuromodulation may therefore provide information on the mechanistic link between sacral neuromodulation and improvement in IC symptoms.

What results have been obtained with neuromodulation in patients with interstitial cystitis?

Six patients with IC defined by NIH criteria and who underwent percutaneous S3 neuromodulation were studied recently [31]. The subjects underwent baseline assessment of voiding frequency, pain, and urinary urgency scores; additionally, urine HB-EGF and APF were measured. After 5 days of S3 neuromodulation, these same subjective and objective assessments were repeated. The results are shown in Table 19.1.

Both subjective and objective parameters improved during the neuromodulation, suggesting that sacral neuromodulation may be considered in the treatment of IC.

Future perspectives

The use of sacral neuromodulation for clinical conditions such as IC depends on the continued research into the aetiology(ies) of this enigmatic disease. In fact, the current clinical utility of sacral neuromodulation depends to a large degree on patients' subjective interpretation of their symptoms and of how these symptoms change with neuromodulation. Although voiding frequency diaries and pad usage may be considered to be objective tests, these still are within the realm of subjective reporting by the patients. Changes in objective tests (such as measurement of urine growth factors) during neuromodulation therefore represent an advance in the utilisation of sacral neuromodulation as a potential therapy for IC. Because the precise physiological mechanisms of the beneficial effects of sacral neuromodulation are still unclear, it is incumbent on all those interested in neuromodulation to continue mechanistic research. The combination of research into the aetiologies of voiding dysfunction (for example, IC, urinary urge incontinence and idiopathic retention) and into the mechanisms of neuromodulation will result in more precise and efficient clinical treatment for patients afflicted with these bladder conditions.

Pelvic pain

K. Everaert and F. Peeren

Introduction

The diagnosis of chronic pelvic pain syndrome (PPS) is made by exclusion in both men and women. After exclusion of endometriosis, chronic pelvic inflammatory disorders, uterine or ovarian

Key Points

- SNS currently relies on patients' (largely subjective) opinion of symptom improvement.
- Objective tests (e.g. growth-factor changes) therefore promote SNS use as IC therapy.
- Chronic PPS is diagnosed by exclusion (e.g. of IC).
- PPS is often related to pelvic floor dysfunction, through the pain cycle.

pathology in women, prostatitis in men, urological pathology (such as stone disease, cancer or carcinoma *in situ*), IC, or irritable bowel syndrome, a group of patients is left with the diagnosis of chronic PPS. At reproductive age, 15% of women appear to suffer from this disorder; in men, the incidence of pelvic pain is unknown but the condition is often referred to as abacterial prostatitis or prostatodynia (prevalence of 5–10%), and there is considerable confusion in terminology [32, 33]. Chronic pelvic pain is a diagnostic and therapeutic challenge and is often related to psychological and psychosomatic disorders [32,33].

The pathogenesis of pelvic syndromes remains unknown; however, in these patients, pelvic floor hyperactivity and pelvic congestion are common phenomena [34]. PPS is often related to dysfunction of the pelvic floor, with symptoms such as voiding dysfunction, urinary retention, constipation, dyschezia and dyspareunia. The pain cycle theory explains why pelvic floor spasms and pelvic pain are linked physiopathologically [35, 36]. Sustained physical trauma (pelvic surgery, heat), physiological impulses (for example, neurogenic inflammation due to nerve damage), and psychological impulses cause increasing muscle tension and spasms, diminishing the blood supply to the muscle. The tonic-muscle activity itself causes heat and accumulation of metabolites (such as potassium ions, lactic acid, histamine and bradykinin). The resultant ischaemia acidosis, and accumulation of metabolites produces increasing pain [37]. This mechanism is referred to as the pain cycle. Muscle spasms of the pelvic floor may be either the cause or the result of sustained pain.

Pelvic congestion is documented in 90% of women with pelvic pain syndromes and has been demonstrated by radiology, ultrasound and thermal techniques [38, 39]. Hypersensitivity to calcitonin gene-related peptide (CGRP) in women with pelvic pain suggests that a possible underlying neurovascular disorder is responsible for the pelvic congestion [40].

Both the pain cycle theory and the vascular hypothesis can easily be integrated in a disorder known as complex regional pain syndromes, which is a specific type of neuropathic pain accompanied by muscle spasm and vasodilatation and vasoconstriction [41]. The reported incidence varies from 1–35%, depending on the type of trauma (for example, fracture, nerve damage, infarction) following which the syndrome developed. Theoretically, primary neurogenic damage causes neurogenic inflammation, which is responsible for typical neurogenic pain (100%), muscle spasms (49%), vascular congestion (47% increase and 47% decrease in skin temperature) and dysfunctions (95%) [38]. Other examples of complex regional pain syndromes are Sudeck's atrophy and frozen shoulder or shoulder–hand syndrome. Clinicians must be careful in the diagnosis of complex regional pain syndromes as it is true that patients with psychogenic pseudoneuropathy, sustained by conversion–somatisation–malingering, not only lack physiological evidence of structural nerve fibre disease but display a characteristically atypical, semi-subjective, psychophysical sensorimotor profile [42]. No diagnostic tests for neuropathy are available for patients with chronic pelvic pain: sensory evoked potentials of the pudendal nerve or bladder neck have not been validated for this purpose.

How does sacral neuromodulation work in patients with pelvic pain?

Neuropathic pain and complex regional pain syndromes are successfully treated with dorsal column stimulation and peripheral nerve stimulation by pain clinicians and neurosurgeons [43]. Several neurophysiological mechanisms of action have been proposed: these include simple blocking of pain transmission by a direct effect in the spinothalamic tracts; activation of descending inhibitory pathways, effects on central sympathetic systems, segmental inhibition through coarse fibre activation and brain stem loops; inhibition by increasing GABA levels in the dorsal horn; and thalamocortical mechanisms masking the nociceptive input [43, 44].

Because chronic PPS can be seen as complex regional pain syndromes, SNS is an obvious therapeutic option.

What results have been obtained with sacral neuromodulation in pelvic pain syndromes?

We performed test SNS for 4–7 days in 26 patients with pelvic pain in whom conservative treatment had failed (unpublished results). When the subchronic test stimulation was successful, we implanted a neurostimulator (InterStim pulse generator) and a quadripolar electrode (model 3080) from Medtronic. Stimulation parameters were 0.8–3.4V, 14Hz, and a pulse width of 210θμs. A test SNS of the S3 root was effective in the treatment of pain in 16/26 patients: efficacy was noted if the patient scored less than 3 points on a visual analogue (VAS) 10-point pain scale and if there was a more than 50% reduction of the pain. Among the 16 responders, ten had a history suggesting underlying neurogenic disease such as failed back surgery (n=3), pelvic surgery (n=5), peripheral neuropathy (n=1) or brain injury (n=1). Of the ten patients who did not respond to the test stimulation, six had pain relief for 24–48 hours and one patient had pain relief for 4 days. A two-stage implant was performed in three patients and unnecessary insertion of a pulse generator was avoided in two patients. We implanted 11/16 patients; two failures occurred immediately after insertion of the implant and are to be considered false-positive test stimulation results. So far no late failures have been seen (follow-up of 36±8 months). In our opinion, SNS is a promising new treatment of therapy-resistant pelvic pain syndromes. The high incidence of initial false-positive tests may be attributable to the need for longer periods of test stimulation in patients with pelvic pain.

Key Points

- SNS was promising in therapy-resistant PPS but longer test periods may be needed.
- Confirmation (+selective nerve stimulation, sacral-nerve sensory-evoked potential evaluation, electromyography needed.

Future perspectives

Our preliminary results need confirmation in a prospective, placebo-controlled study to evaluate SNS for chronic PPS. Treatment of complex regional pain syndromes by neurostimulation demands optimal stimulation of all those nerves responsible for neurogenic inflammation. In some patients with chronic PPS who have several damaged sacral nerves, it is possible that we may need to stimulate more nerves than we actually do at present. One could suggest that patients with chronic PPS in whom SNS with one lead has failed would have had more relief if more sacral nerves had been stimulated. The development of more sensitive and specific diagnostic tests to determine which nerves cause neurogenic inflammation, and selective stimulation of these nerves, is needed. Sensory-evoked potentials of sacral nerves should be evaluated. Electromyography of sacral innervated muscles might also help us to determine which nerves are damaged and need to be stimulated.

Patients with chronic pelvic pain are suggested as having a complex regional pain syndrome; SNS is a promising new treatment modality for such patients.

Faecal incontinence

K.E. Matzel

Introduction

The concept of recruiting residual function of an organ by stimulating its nerve supply presents a novel approach in the field of colorectal surgery. Only a few reports have been published on the effect of the new treatment mode of SNS on anorectal function [6, 45–47]. Whereas the initial use of SNS in the field of urology was based on experimental work, its use in faecal incontinence has followed an entirely pragmatic approach.

How does neuromodulation work in faecal incontinence?

Clinical observations of the effect of SNS on anorectal function in urological patients have revealed two different, synergistic mechanisms of faecal continence: these are increased anorectal angulation and increased anal canal closure pressure [48]. Anatomical dissections have demonstrated a two-fold peripheral nerve supply to the striated pelvic floor muscles contributing these functions to anal continence. The sacral spinal nerve site is the most distal common location of this dual peripheral nerve supply to the striated pelvic floor and anal sphincter muscles; thus, by stimulating these nerves, both mechanisms can be elicited [48].

What results have been achieved with neuromodulation for the treatment of faecal incontinence?

Potential patients are screened for permanent SNS by means of a protocol consisting of two diagnostic and one therapeutic stage [48]. During the first phase, acute percutaneous nerve evaluation, the functional relevance of each sacral spinal nerve to striated anal sphincter function, is tested with the help of needle electrodes inserted bilaterally into the sacral foramina of S2, S3, and S4, and current is applied in a graduated fashion [49]. When the stimulation causes movement of the anal sphincter and/or pelvic floor (monitored visually or by anorectal manometry or electromyography; EMG) the therapeutic potential of SNS is assessed by temporary stimulation of the functionally most relevant sacral spinal nerve. The needle electrodes are replaced either by thin wire electrodes connected to an external impulse generator or by an operatively implanted foramen electrode that is exteriorised by an extension that can be connected to an external nerve stimulator [50, 51]. To document the functional benefit of low-frequency stimulation, its effect on bowel habits is monitored with the help of questionnaires (which are also used before and during participation in the protocol).

If symptoms have improved with temporary stimulation and if they recur after its discontinuation, the patient is considered a candidate for permanent electrode implantation. Two different techniques are applied: foramen electrodes are inserted through the sacral foramen, close to the site where the sacral spinal nerves enter the pelvic cavity [50], or cuff electrodes are placed around the sacral spinal nerves within the sacral canal after a dorsal laminectomy of the sacrum [52].

Because the initial treatment concept was to recruit residual function of the striated anal sphincter muscles, the initial application of SNS was confined to faecal incontinence due to reduced voluntary and reflexive striated anal sphincter function in patients with no detectable morphological defect, and in whom traditional conservative and surgical treatments had failed. The cause of faecal incontinence varied: it could be attributable to voluntary sphincter weakness occurring after operative anal and rectal procedures (for example, rectal resection for rectal prolapse) or secondary to lumbar spine fracture [6, 52].

The screening procedure also led to permanent implants in patients with functional or morphological deficits of the smooth-muscle internal anal sphincter (for example, those due to scleroderma, postoperative fragmentation or primary degeneration) and in patients with limited defects of the internal and external anal sphincters [45]. Symptomatic improvement was obtained in most patients for mid- and long-term follow-up, with success rates ranging from 85–100% [45, 52].

The physiological mode of action of SNS in the treatment of faecal incontinence is as yet undefined, but it does not seem to be attributable to a placebo effect [53]. Clinical findings are complex and partially contradictory; thus, the mechanism of action is likely

Key Points

- SNS affects nerves supplying both the striated pelvic floor and anal sphincter muscles.
- It thus activates two synergistic faecal continence mechanisms.
- Assess SNS potential by stimulation of functionally most relevant sacral spinal nerve.
- Effect of stimulation on bowel habit is monitored with questionnaires.

to be multifactorial. SNS can result in striated pelvic-floor muscle contraction or in facilitation of voluntary contraction in patients with abolished or limited residual striated anal sphincter function during temporary [6, 51] and chronic [52] stimulation, reflected in increased squeeze pressure, presumably mediated by α motor fibre stimulation. Despite the therapeutic benefit in some patients, the increase in squeeze pressure is limited to the phase of subchronic test stimulation [45].

During short-term stimulation, a reduction in rectal sensitivity and contractile activity, as well as in anal motility — potentially mediated by modulation of the sacral reflex arcs — was observed [51]. An increase in maximal tolerable volume [45] was reported during chronic stimulation, representing another effect of SNS on visceral function.

Despite the fact that the precise physiological mechanism of action of SNS on the continence function is not clearly defined as yet, reproducible clinical results can be achieved in patients identified by the three-step screening procedure and who present a wide range of causes of faecal incontinence. In a patient population in which conservative treatment fails and traditional surgical approaches are of limited success or are conceptually questionable, SNS thus offers a new treatment mode.

Future perspectives

To clearly define the spectrum of indications for SNS in faecal incontinence, it is necessary to classify patients not only by the extent of their symptoms but also by the relationship of the symptoms to aetiology and morphological and physiological findings. Not only will this help to explain the effect of SNS on deteriorated function but also it will teach us how to improve that effect — for instance, bilateral versus unilateral stimulation, stimulation of multiple sacral spinal nerves on different levels [54] and patient selection for optimal results.

Because faecal continence is governed by visceral and somatic functions that are less well understood than the function of the urinary tract, it is essential to investigate the interaction of autonomic and somatic nervous systems of the continence organ. A better understanding of this interaction will help us to explain the therapeutic effect of SNS in our field and will broaden the acceptance of this new therapy in colorectal surgery.

Chronic faecal constipation

E. Ganio

Introduction

Most physicians consider two or less evacuations per week as constipation. However, many patients are bothered by the subjective feeling of incomplete or difficult defecation and symptoms such as hard faeces, squeezing, the need for digital assistance or tenesmus. Pelvic causes of abnormal evacuation include rectal aganglionosis (Hirschsprung's disease), rectal intussusception or complete rectal prolapse, and anterior rectal wall hernia (rectocele); most of these can be cured by surgery. Many patients with rectal constipation suffer from a lack of coordinated activity of the rectum and the anal sphincters (outlet constipation) that is not amenable to simple surgical treatment. Biofeedback, stool softeners, and laxatives may help some patients, but often do not offer a satisfactory long-term solution. Sacral neuromodulation has been used experimentally in these patients to improve defecatory dysfunction by modifying the neural control of the sphincter and the proximal bowel [55].

How does neuromodulation work in patients with faecal constipation?

The physiological mechanism of SNS remains unclear, although it is likely to be multifactorial. SNS appears to have an effect on rectal motility, which could be of clinical importance [56,57]. The improvement in evacuation and the decrease in the number of unsuccessful attempts could be related to a change of rectal sensibility, leading to a better coordination between rectum and sphincter. Modulation of sacral reflex arcs regulating rectal tone and contractility may also have a potentially beneficial role in some patients [56].

What results have been obtained with sacral neuromodulation in patients with faecal constipation?

We submitted 25 patients with chronic outlet constipation to PNE. Inclusion criteria were as follows: difficulty (the need for digital assistance or squeezing) in emptying the rectum or a feeling of incomplete evacuation during more than 50% of the bowel movements in the previous year; failure of conventional drugs, diets or biofeedback therapy; and lack of relaxation or normal sphincter behaviour in constipated patients. Patients with inflammatory bowel diseases, with cardiac disease, or those who were pregnant, were excluded. The patients were referred to our institution for assessment of faecal disorders between January 1999 and December 2000 (unpublished results).

The results of the peripheral nerve evaluation (PNE) tests were evaluated with a defecation diary and with anorectal manovolumetry [56] before and on the last day of PNE. Patients completed a clinical diary of bowel movements, episodes of squeezing to empty the rectum, unsuccessful attempts to evacuate, and time necessary to evacuate in the 2 weeks preceding the PNE, during the PNE, and in the 2 weeks following PNE and at anorectal manometry before and on the last day of PNE.

The mean duration of the tests was 16 (range 7–28) days. During PNE we observed an improvement in bowel emptying, with a decrease in the Wexner's score [58] from 12 (range 8–15) before

Key Points
- SNS improves defecatory dysfunction by modifying neural bowel/sphincter control.
- SNS-induced pelvic-floor contraction improves perception of anal sphincter muscles.
- SNS appears to affect rectal motility, sensibility, tone and contractility.
- SNS is effective in cases of faecal incontinence and rectal constipation.

the test to 2.4 (range 0–6) during the test (p<0.01). The mean numbers of voluntary bowel movements per week (WBM) decreased during temporary SNS (prestimulation WBM 9.5, range 2–28; end of PNE WBM 6.4, range 2–14; p=0.2), as did the difficulty in emptying the rectum (prestimulation score 7, range 2–21; end of PNE score 2.1, range 0–6; p<0.01). The number of unsuccessful visits to the toilet fell from 29.2 (7–24) to 6.7 (0–28) per week; p=0.01. The time necessary to evacuate decreased from 12.5 (5–20) to 9.3 (5–30) minutes per bowel movement (p=0.4).

Nine of these patients (two male, seven female, mean age 53.4 years, range 31–72) underwent a definitive implant after a successful PNE test. The constipation was idiopathic (7) or secondary to myelitis (1) and to a herniated disc (1). All patients complained of outlet constipation with normal or prolonged left-colonic transit time (2) and without demonstrable anatomical alterations. The clinical diary was used to evaluate SNS results: Wexner's score decreased from 12.5 (range 9–16) before the SNS to 3.4 after 3 months (range 0–6; p<0.01) and to 2.9 at the last follow-up (4.9; range 3–15 months (p<0.01).

The most important manometric findings were (a) an increase in amplitude of maximal resting pressure (MRP): baseline 67±25 versus 69±14mmHg at the end of PNE and 78±10mmHg at 3 months' follow-up) and maximal squeeze pressure (MSP): 120±33mmHg baseline vs 140±52 at the end of PNE and 132±62 at 3 months' follow-up and (b) a reduction in the rectal volume for the feel (prestimulation 99±47ml to 81±37ml at last follow-up) and urge to defecate threshold (pre-stimulation 199±80ml, to 140±40ml at last follow-up). All the implanted patients showed an improvement in symptoms.

As in results reported by urologists, SNS seems to be effective with regard to both faecal incontinence and rectal constipation; it results more in a reduction of unsuccessful attempts and in a reduction of the difficulty to evacuate, rather than in a change in the number of daily evacuations. The increase in sphincter pressure, which could have a negative impact on evacuation, and the reduction in rectal volume for feel and urge threshold, suggest a possible influence of SNS on sensory fibres and this could lead to a better coordination between rectum and sphincter.

Our data confirm that SNS can benefit patients with symptoms of rectal outlet constipation.

Future perspectives

The evaluation of SNS continues. We need a better understanding of how the modulating effect of stimulation of sacral nerve afferent pathways affects the rectosphincteric and colonic complex. Attention must be given to colonic motility and to the basic functional mechanisms causing constipation, in order to characterise a subgroup of constipated patients that responds best to this therapy. In some patients (Figs. 19.1 and 19.2) we have observed a change of the left colon motility rhythm, which could suggest a possible extension of indications to the patients with constipation from colonic inertia.

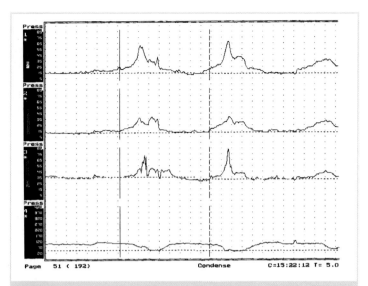

Figure 19.1 Left colonic manometry: trace 1,2, sigmoid colon; 3, rectum; 4, anal canal. Stimulation off: cyclic rhythmic activity every 40s.

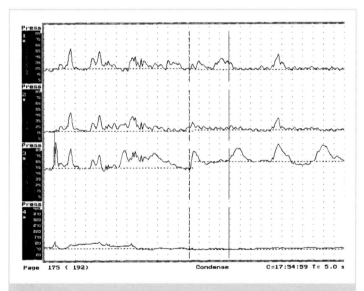

Figure 19.2 Left colonic manometry: trace 1,2, sigmoid colon; 3, rectum; 4, anal canal. Stimulation on: cyclic rhythmic activity every 20s.

Additionally, we have observed a marked improvement in the clinical, proctoscopic, and histological picture of a patient with solitary rectal ulcer syndrome, suggesting a neuroplastic effect of SNS on the rectal mucosa. Nevertheless, we are only now beginning exploration of the possible effects of SNS on intestinal function, and further long-term studies are needed.

237

References

1. Bosch JLHR, Groen J. Neuromodulation: urodynamic effects of sacral (S3) spinal nerve stimulation in patients with detrusor instability or detrusor hyperreflexia. *Behav Brain Res* 1998; 92: 141–50.
2. Bosch JLHR, Groen J. Disappointing results of neuromodulation in men with urge incontinence due to detrusor instability. *Neurourol Urodyn* 1997; 16: 347–9.
3. Shah N, Edhem I, Knight SL, Craggs MD. Acute suppression of detrusor hyperreflexia with detrusor-sphincter dyssynergia by electrical stimulation of the dorsal penile nerves in patients with a spinal injury. *Eur Urol* 1998; 33 (Suppl. 4): 60.
4. Bosch JLHR, Groen J. Treatment of refractory urge incontinence with sacral spinal nerve stimulation in multiple sclerosis patients. *Lancet* 1996; 348: 717–19.
5. Everaert K, Plancke H, Lefevre F, Oosterlinck W. The urodynamic evaluation of neuromodulation in patients with voiding dysfunction. *Br J Urol* 1997; 79: 702–7.
6. Matzel KE, Stadelmaier U, Hohenfellner M, Gall FP. Electrical stimulation of sacral spinal nerves for treatment of faecal incontinence. *Lancet* 1995; 346: 1124–7.
7. Groen J, Bosch JLHR. Relationship between detrusor instability and urethral resistance in patients treated with sacral neuromodulation. *Neurourol Urodyn* 2000; 19: 531–2.
8. de Groat WC, Kawatani T, Hisamitsu T *et al*. Mechanisms underlying the recovery of urinary bladder function following spinal cord injury. *J Auton Nerv Syst* 1990; 30: S71–8.
9. Urinary Incontinence Guideline Panel. Urinary incontinence in adults: clinical practice guidelines No. 92-0038. Rockville, MD: Agency for Health Care Policy and Research 1992, 38-43.
10. Chancellor MB, de Groat WC. Intravesical capsaicin and resiniferatoxin therapy: spicing up the ways to treat the overactive bladder. *J Urol* 1999; 162: 3–11.
11. Schurch B, Stöhrer M, Kramer G *et al*. Botulinum-A toxin for treating detrusor hyperreflexia in spinal cord injured patients: a new alternative to anticholinergic drugs? Preliminary results. *J Urol* 2000; 164: 692–7.
12. Mundy AR. The unstable bladder. *Urol Clin North Am* 1985; 12: 317–28.
13. Vodušek DB, Light JK, Libby JM. Detrusor inhibition induced by stimulation of pudendal nerve afferents. *Neurourol Urodyn* 1986; 5: 381–9.
14. Shah N, Edhem I, Knight SL, Craggs MD: Acute suppression of detrusor hyperreflexia with detrusor–sphincter dyssynergia by electrical stimulation of the dorsal penile nerves in patients with a spinal injury. *Eur Urol* 1998; 33 (Suppl. 4): 60.
15. Schmidt RA, Senn E, Tanagho EA. Functional evaluation of sacral root integrity. report of a technique. *Urology* 1990; 35: 388–92.
16. Hohenfellner M, Schultz-Lampel D, Matzel K *et al*. Functional rehabilitation of the neurogenic bladder by chronic sacral neuromodulation. *Aktual Urol* 1996; 27 (Suppl.): 89-91.
17. Ishigooka M, Suzuki Y, Hashimoto T *et al*. A new technique for sacral nerve stimulation: a percutaneous method for urinary incontinence caused by spinal cord injury. *Br J Urol* 1998; 81: 315–8.
18. Carone R, Bertapelle P, Zanollo A *et al*. Sacral neuromodulation in neurogenic lower urinary tract dysfunctions: results of a multicenter study group. *Urodynamica* 1999; 9: 177–82.
19. Schmidt RA. Treatment of unstable bladder. *Urology* 1991; 37: 28–32.
20. Chartier-Kastler EJ, Bosch JLHR, Perrigot M *et al*. Long-term results of sacral nerve stimulation (S3) for the treatment of neurogenic refractory urge incontinence related to detrusor hyperreflexia. *J Urol* 2000; 164: 1476–80.
21. Gillenwater JY, Wein AJ. Summary of the National Institute of Arthritis, Diabetes, Digestive and Kidney Diseases Workshop on Interstitial Cystitis, National Institutes of Health, Bethesda, Maryland, August 28–29, 1987. *J Urol* 1988; 140: 203–6.
22. Parsons CL, Lilly JD, Stein P. Epithelial dysfunction in nonbacterial cystitis (interstitial cystitis). *J Urol* 1991; 145: 732–5.
23. Parsons CL, Greenberger M, Gabal L *et al*. The role of urinary potassium in the pathogenesis and diagnosis of interstitial cystitis. *J Urol* 1998; 159: 1862–6.
24. Erickson DR, Mast S, Ordille S, Bhavanandan VP. Urinary epitectin (MUC-1 glycoprotein) in the menstrual cycle and interstitial cystitis. *J Urol* 1996; 156: 938–42.
25. Erickson DR, Sheykhnazari M, Ordille S, Bhavanandan VP. Increased urinary hyaluronic acid and interstitial cystitis. *J Urol* 1998; 160: 1282–4.
26. Okragly AJ, Niles AL, Saban R *et al*. Elevated tryptase, nerve growth factor, neurotrophin-3 and glial cell line-derived neurotrophic factor levels in the urine of interstitial cystitis and bladder cancer patients. *J Urol* 1999; 161: 438–41.

27. Rosamilia A, Clements JA, Dwyer PL *et al*. Activation of the kallikrein kinin system in interstitial cystitis. *J Urol* 1999; 162: 129–34.
28. Wei DC, Politano VA, Selzer MG, Lokeshwar VB. The association of elevated urinary total to sulfated glycosaminoglycan ratio and high molecular mass hyaluronic acid with interstitial cystitis. *J Urol* 2000; 163: 1577–83.
29. Keay S, Zhang CO, Kagen DI *et al*. Concentrations of specific epithelial growth factors in the urine of interstitial cystitis patients and controls. *J Urol* 1997; 158: 1983–8.
30. Keay S, Zhang CO, Trifillis AL *et al*. Decreased 3H-thymidine incorporation by human bladder epithelial cells following exposure to urine from interstitial cystitis patients. *J Urol* 1996; 156: 2073–78.
31. Chai TC, Zhang C, Warren JW, Keay S. Percutaneous sacral third nerve root neurostimulation improves symptoms and normalizes urinary HB-EGF levels and antiproliferative activity in patients with interstitial cystitis. *Urology* 2000; 55: 643–6.
32. Stones RW, Selfe SA, Fransman S, Horn SA. Psychosocial and economic impact of chronic pelvic pain. *Baillieres Best Pract Res Clin Obstet Gynaecol* 2000; 14: 415–31.
33. Nickel JC, Nigro M, Valiquette L *et al*. Diagnosis and treatment of prostatitis in Canada. *Urology* 1998; 52: 797–802.
34. Zermann DH, Ishigooka M, Doggweiler R, Schmidt RA. Neurourological insights into the etiology of genitourinary pain in men. *J Urol* 1999; 161: 903–08.
35. Mannheimer JF, Lampe GN. *Clinical Transcutaneous Electrical Nerve Stimulation*. 8th edition, F.A. Davis Company, 1988.
36. Everaert K, Stockman S, De Paepe H *et al*. The pain cycle, implications for the diagnosis and treatment of perineal pain. *Int Urogyn J*. 2001, 12:9–14.
37. Birklein F, Weber M, Ernst M *et al*. Experimental tissue acidosis leads to increasing pain in complex regional pain syndrome. *Pain* 2000; 87: 227–34.
38. Beard RW, Highman JH, Pearce S, Reginald PW. Diagnosis of pelvic varicosities in women with chronic pelvic pain. *Lancet* 1984; ii: 946–9.
39. Thomas DC, Stones RW, Farquhar CM, Beard RW. Measurement of pelvic blood flow changes in response to posture in normal subjects and in women with pelvic congestion by using a thermal technique. *Clin Sci* 1992; 83: 55–8.
40. Stones RW, Thomas DC, Beard RW. Suprasensitivity to calcitonin gene-related peptide but not vasoactive intestinal peptide in women with chronic pelvic pain. *Clin Auton Res* 1992; 2: 343–8.
41. Veldman PHJM, Reynen HM, Arntz IE, Goris RJA. Signs and symptoms of reflex sympathetic dystrophy: prospective study of 829 patients. *Lancet* 1993; 342: 1012–16.
42. Ochoa JL. Truths, errors and lies around 'reflex sympathetic dystrophy' and 'complex regional pain syndromes'. *J Neurol* 1999; 246: 875–9.
43. Kemler MA, Barendse GA, van Kleef M *et al*. Spinal cord stimulation in patients with chronic reflex sympathetic dystrophy. *N Engl J Med* 2000; 343: 618–24.
44. Kemler MA, Barendse GA, van Kleef M, Egbrink MG. Pain relief in complex regional pain syndrome due to spinal cord stimulation does not depend on vasodilatation. *Anesthesiology* 2000; 92: 1653–60.
45. Malouf AJ, Vaizey CJ, Nicholls RJ, Kamm MA. Permanent sacral nerve stimulation for faecal incontinence. *Ann Surg* 2000; 232: 143–8.
46. Rosen HR, Novi G, Urbarz C, Schiessel R. Sakrale nervenstimulation (SNS) als therapie der faekalen inkontinenz. *Z Gastroenterol* 1999; 37: 532.
47. Ganio E, Frascio M, Iboli B *et al*. Neuromodulation for faecal incontinence or anorectal dysfunction: outcome in eight patients with definitive implant. *Coloproctology* 1999; 5: 198.
48. Matzel KE, Schmidt RA, Tanagho EA. Neuroanatomy of the striated muscular anal continence mechanism: implications for the use of neurostimulation. *Dis Colon Rectum* 1990; 33: 666–73.
49. Hohenfellner M, Matzel KE, Schülz-Lampel D *et al*. Sacral neuromodulation for treatment of micturition disorders and faecal incontinence. In: R Hohenfellner, J Fichtner, A Novick (eds) *Innovation in Urologic Surgery*. Oxford: Isis Medical Media, 1997; 129–38.
50. Schmidt RA, Senn E, Tanagho EA. Functional evaluation of sacral nerve root integrity — report of a technique. *Urology* 1990; 15: 388–92.
51. Vaizey CJ, Kamm MA, Turner IC, Nicholls RJ, Woloszko J. Effects of short-term sacral nerve stimulation on anal and rectal function in patients with anal incontinence. *Gut* 1999; 44: 407–12.
52. Matzel KE, Stadelmaier U, Hohenfellner M, Hohenberger W. Chronic sacral spinal nerve stimulation for faecal incontinencel: long-term results with foramen and cuff electrode. *Dis Colon Rectum*; 44:59–66.

53. Vaizey CJ, Kamm M, Roy AJ, Nicholls RJ. Double-blind crossover study of sacral nerve stimulation for faecal incontinence. *Dis Col Rectum* 2000; 43: 298–302.

54. Matzel, KE, Stadelmaier U, Hohenfellner M. Asymmetry of pudendal motor function assessed during intraoperative monitoring. *Gastroenterology* 1999; 116: G4508.

55. Ganio E, Masin A *et al*. Short-term sacral nerve stimulation for functional anorectal and urinary disturbances. Results in 49 patients. *Dis Colon Rectum* 2000; 43: A17 [abstract].

56. Åkerval S, Fasth S, Nordgres S *et al*. Manovolumetry: a new method for investigation of anorectal function. *Gut* 1988; 29: 614–23.

57. Matzel KE, Sacral neurostimulation:principles and its role in the treatment of feacal incontinence. Proceedings of the 6th Biennial International Meeting of Coloproctology, April 2000; 101–3.

58. Agachan F, Chen T, Pfeifer J *et al*. A constipation scoring system to simplify evaluation and management of constipated patients. *Dis Colon Rectum* 1996; 39: 681–85.

20 Patient follow-up after sacral nerve stimulation system implantation for control of lower urinary tract dysfunction

J.L. Ruiz-Cerdá

Introduction

The follow-up schedule for monitoring patients after implantation of the sacral nerve stimulation (SNS) system for lower urinary tract (LUT) dysfunction is seldom referred to in the literature; in fact, no guidelines have yet been established. As in other conditions, a balance must be maintained between reasonable studies aimed at monitoring patients and detecting problems, and aggressive follow-up unlikely to make a difference other than increasing anxiety and expense. Basically, follow-up does not differ according to whether patients underwent surgery for urge urinary incontinence, voiding dysfunction, or urgency–frequency syndrome because it is governed by the fact that the effect of neuromodulation is temporary and, once the SNS system is removed or lost, the original symptoms return. As has been demonstrated in the results of therapy evaluation tests, once LUT dysfunction has been established it is permanent and patients will require lifelong SNS therapy [1–3]. For this reason, no matter what follow-up schedule has been implemented, as soon as the effect of neuromodulation decreases or becomes inadequate, the patient will immediately demand our help to rectify this situation. Follow-up is affected by factors such as loss of efficacy, undesirable response to stimulation, potential deterioration or damage of the implant, the risk of adverse events and complications and monitoring of electrical problems. Therefore, the issues involved in the follow-up of implanted patients can be addressed in terms not only of what, how and when this happens, but of how we are able to overcome problems when they arise.

Follow-up visit schedule and procedures

Follow-up is on an outpatient basis. The visits to the clinic should be scheduled as the physician deems necessary. Typically these are at 1 week, 1 month, 3 months, 6 months and as needed thereafter (probably at 6-monthly intervals). Patients must be systematically monitored at each visit according to the guidelines shown in Table 20.1.

> **Key Points**
> - No guidelines yet exist for patient follow-up after SNS implant for LUT dysfunction.
> - LUT dysfunction is permanent, so patients need lifelong SNS therapy.
> - Patients need help as problems arise.

Table 20.1 *Guidelines for follow-up visits: recommended procedures*

Procedure	Follow-up interval				
	1 week	1 month	3 months	6 months	Every 6 months
Physician assessment		X	X	X	X
3–7-day voiding diary		X	X	X	X
IPG site revision	X	X	X	X	X
Urine culture	X	X	X	X	X
IPG function: settings + battery life	X	X	X	X	X
Uroflowmetry + residual volume		X	X	X	X
Filling and voiding cystometry*				X	
Radiographs of lead position (AP-L) *	X			X	
Quality-of-life assessment				X	X

* After first year, one per year.

IPG, implanted pulse generator; AP, anteroposterior; L, lateral.

SNS therapy control team

An SNS therapy control team with specialised nursing expertise can help to support patients and provide any necessary information. The provision of information regarding SNS therapy continues after the implantation procedure. Questions constantly arise during the follow-up period. Patients voice concerns about issues such as how they will be monitored after the implantation procedure, whether the procedure will cure their condition, whether it will damage their nerves, whether it is reversible or whether they will need further surgery. Sometimes telephone contact is enough to make the patients feel that they are not alone with their implants; in addition, an SNS team may share the care of the demands of these patients.

First week after implantation

Hospitalisation after surgery typically lasts a few days but can extend to a longer period. Individuals can vary widely in their pain thresholds; thus, it is always appropriate to tailor the postoperative treatment to the individual. Stimulation is normally activated on the day after surgery. The patients must not only be aware of the stimulation as prominent but not painful but must also demonstrate a proper understanding of the operation of the SNS system. During the post-implantation period it is recommended that the team should verify the function of the implanted pulse generator (IPG), adjust the stimulation settings, observe the wound site and note any complications and adverse reactions. In addition, radiographs (AP and lateral) should be taken to document the position of the lead for future reference.

Follow-up visits

General status of the patient

Physician assessment at each visit is a basic requirement. The urologist must obtain the relevant physical and medical history, including work and activity status. Also necessary is any information about medication administered since the previous visit that may affect the patient's urological status, and about any LUT surgical procedures or interventions that might affect the patient's symptoms.

LUT symptoms

A voiding diary is the simplest tool by which to assess the effect of SNS on symptoms [1]. Prior to each visit, the patient must complete a voiding diary for a minimum of 3 days, although a week is preferable. A detailed voiding diary is recommended, whenever possible, recording such details as the times of voiding, the number of incontinence episodes and pads used, degree of leakage, residual and voided volume and the number of self-catheterisations. It is important to assess the individual fluid intake, remembering that this should include not only the fluids drunk but also the water content of food eaten. At each visit any changes in symptoms must be assessed, using a quantitative measure to gauge percentage improvement or deterioration.

IPG, lead and extension-sites revision

Physical examination of sites where the components were implanted and of their relation with bony structures is recommended. Erosion, seroma, haematoma and infection can occur during early follow-up. Pain at the IPG site is a frequent complication when the IPG has been implanted in a sensitive area or at the patient's beltline, when the pocket is too small, there is a loose electrical connection or there is an allergic response or rejection. Usually, surgical repositioning is necessary [1, 4].

Rule out urinary tract infection

The presence of urinary tract infection may cause stimulation to become inefficient. Urine culture must, therefore, be performed at each visit and at any time during the follow-up if the patient reports symptoms of infection.

IPG function

The primary goal of using an SNS system is to aid in the management of LUT dysfunction. In this sense, adequate programming of electrical settings is a basic requirement. Patients require their own, tailored, stimulation parameters to optimise the therapy, and their stimulation requirements may change over time. Efficacy directly depends on the contact between the lead and the nerve fibre. Even minor changes in the lead position (<1mm) or minimal fibrosis around the lead, can reduce the efficacy or create an undesirable degree of stimulation. Once the SNS system has been implanted, the only way to adapt to changes over time is by modifying the previous stimulation settings; thus, programmable

---

Key Points

- General status, LUT symptoms implanted pulse generator (IPG) lead, extension-site revision must be assessed.
- Urine culture is mandatory as urinary tract infection may impair SNS.
- IPG function must be individualised/monitored.

adjustment may be needed. A secondary goal of programming is to prolong the life of the battery. At each follow-up visit, IPG function must be revised systematically, checking the stimulation regimen within, responses and battery use.

Stimulation regimen with responses

The particular settings that provide the best therapeutic response vary from patient to patient. Table 20.2 details standard initial settings. Every time the IPG is reprogrammed it is mandatory to document all stimulation parameters that may have altered since the previous follow-up visit. Communication between the programmer and the IPG is achieved telemetrically and the console programmer is used to adjust stimulation parameters. Responses should be evaluated in conjunction with clear communication with the patient.

Electrode polarity

The IPG is activated initially by selecting the appropriate electrode (the one giving the best response) as the cathode and the outer casing as the anode. For further modifications, it is necessary to visualise the shape of the electrical field set following the changes in sensory and motor responses (Figs. 20.1 and 20.2). At each follow-up visit, the values of the threshold voltage and impedance should be determined for each electrode's contacts. It should be noted that patients' sensory and motor responses can vary, not only in relation to threshold but also regarding the degree of discomfort and the therapeutic responses that are obtained.

Electrode impedance

Measurement of the impedance provides information about the integrity of the leads and extensions over time. To monitoring purposes, the casing must be programmed as positive and the electrodes

Table 20.2 Standard initial settings for SNS

Parameter	Initial setting	Range	Do not exceed
Amplitude (V)	0.10	0–10.5	One setting below discomfort
Pulse width (µs)	180–210	60–450	270
Rate (Hz)	10–14	2–130	19
Electrode polarity	Unipolar/bipolar	Each electrode = off, (+) or (-); casing = off or (+)	
Mode	Continuous (20s) or cycling (8s)	Cycle on: 0.1s–24h; Cycle off: 0.1s–24h	Mode used depends on patient's tolerance to stimulation
Softstart/stop (s)	4	1–8	
Magnet function	On	On–off	

negative, one at a time. As a general rule, the most effective electrode for long-term stimulation is the contact that exhibits the lowest voltage threshold and the lowest impedance.

Amplitude

The long-term results show that the voltage needed for an optimal response increases slightly during the initial 6–12 months postoperatively but remains relatively constant thereafter [5]. In some patients it may be necessary to adjust the stimulation parameters

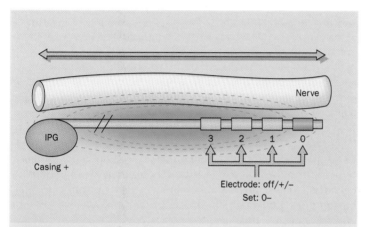

Figure 20.1 *Electrical field with a monopolar configuration. The casing is set to positive (+) and at least one contact negative (-). Monopolar stimulation creates a broad and flat electrical field.*

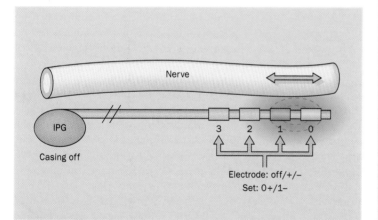

Figure 20.2 *Electrical field with a bipolar configuration in which the current flows between two or more electrodes of the lead. The casing is set to off and at least one electrode must be positive and one negative. Bipolar stimulation shapes a narrow and deep electrical field; it focuses the flow of current over a smaller area than unipolar stimulation.*

to maintain an optimal response or to regain it after temporary deterioration. It is best to adjust the amplitude by gradual increase of the settings (with the IPG on) in order to avoid uncomfortable increases in stimulation. The amplitude should be slowly increased, by increments of 0.1V, until the subject senses stimulation and/or muscle responses are obtained. An ideal response is obtained with a current of 0.5V: a lesser current denotes that the electrode is very close to the nerve; a greater current indicates that the electrode is too far away. After the appropriate responses have been obtained, the amplitude should be decreased by approximately 1V; fine-amplitude resolution then allows increments of 0.05V, which can be useful in sensitive patients or in those in whom the sensory and motor threshold responses are very close. Setting of the correct limits for the patient must always be the final stage of programming. The physician can set limits for the amplitude so that the patient cannot exceed these limits when using the patient programmer; this method reduces the potential for uncomfortably high settings, limits the parameters that the patient can adjust (thus ensuring optimal therapy) and facilitates patient compliance.

Pulse rate and width

Pulse rate and width are closely related to efficacy. Even minor changes in pulse rate can significantly improve efficacy, particularly in patients with voiding dysfunction, who, as a rule, respond better to low frequencies in the range of 10–12pps. Patients with urge incontinence and urgency–frequency syndrome respond better to high frequencies in the range of 15–18pps or even higher, although it is recommended not to exceed 20pps.

Mode

The IPG output can be set in continuous or cycling mode. In the latter, stimulation is cycled on and off automatically, improving both the life of the IPG battery and also the patient's comfort. In very sensitive patients the 'softstart' mode is useful; this is characterised by a gradual increase in amplitude as stimulation starts and gradual decrease in amplitude as stimulation ceases.

Optimisation of battery life

The IPG battery life depends on the period of use, the amplitude, rate and pulse width, the number of active electrodes and the output mode. An additional factor is fibrosis around the electrode, which necessitates an increase for effective modulation. The life expectancy is between 7–10 years. Correct settings can maximise battery longevity. For example, if two negative electrodes and one positive electrode are activated, the resulting IPG battery life is only 77% of that of a bipolar combination. For a given set of parameters, a unipolar setting will require approximately 35% more power from the IPG than a bipolar setting. Merely cycling one 'cycle-off' period for every two 'cycle-on' periods adds approximately 12 months (or 35%) to the life of the IPG.

Some of the steps that can be taken to optimise battery life are shown in Table 20.3. They extend longevity and decrease the

Table 20.3 *Preferential electrical setting to optimise battery life*

Preference	Procedure
Unipolar vs multipolar stimulation	Set only 1 (+) and 1 (-) whenever possible
Low vs high settings	Set amplitude, pulse width and rate as low as possible
Single vs multiple configuration	Change the electrode settings and combinations over time
Bipolar vs unipolar	Use bipolar stimulation whenever possible
Cycling vs continuous mode	Instruct the patient to turn off the IPG when it is not needed
To estimate vs not estimate battery life	Use the longevity estimate chart
IPG, implanted pulse generator.	

Key Points
- Baseline LUT function must be evaluated.
- No correlation between symptoms and urodynamic test results has been found.
- Urodynamic studies are useful only as indicators during follow-up.

probability of accommodation to the stimulation. Once settings are stable during the course of the follow-up, it is important to estimate battery life expectancy using the longevity estimate chart, so that both patient and physician may have realistic expectations about the life of the battery. It is useful to calculate for how many hours on average in each 24-hour period the subject currently uses stimulation. Normally, incontinent patients use stimulation 24 hours per day to control episodes of leakage. In such subjects, the two voltage levels that can be set are used to control symptoms during the day and at night; however, the level of stimulation necessary during the day is often uncomfortable when the patient is trying to sleep, when a lower setting is appropriate for comfort. Those patients with voiding dysfunction should be instructed to use stimulation for only as long as necessary.

Evaluation of LUT function

Urodynamic evaluation is a baseline assessment tool necessary to describe the behaviour of the bladder, urethra and pelvic floor muscles during the filling and voiding phases [6,7]; however, it is not useful in evaluating the primary efficacy of SNS therapy. It has been shown that urodynamic improvement occurs as a result of SNS therapy and that urodynamic effects are associated with clinical results [5]; however, no complete correlation has been found between the urodynamic findings and patient symptomatology. Thus, urodynamic studies should be used only as indicators during follow-up of LUT function.

For patients with urge incontinence, filling cystometry 6 months after implantation and for each year thereafter is recommended to measure any improvement in the ability to store urine. However, it must be borne in mind that the loss of urodynamically demonstrable bladder overactivity does not appear to be mandatory for an excellent symptomatic result. About one half of the patients with persistent bladder overactivity are cured; on the other hand, about one quarter of those who have no bladder overactivity at follow-up are not cured. This is true in idiopathic as well as neurogenic cases [5]. Uroflowmetry and measurement of post-void residual volume are easy to perform and can be scheduled for each visit; however, not many changes in these parameters are shown in these patients because SNS does not compromise detrusor contractility.

For patients with voiding dysfunction, uroflowmetry and post-void residual volume measurements must be performed at each visit. At 6 months after implantation, filling cystometry with pressure/flow measurement can be studied for comparison with baseline data. However, bladder contractility and urethral resistance data are not always available, owing to the inability of most of these patients to void preoperatively. Nevertheless, the data indicate that the origin of the problem is not the bladder but the pelvic floor musculature [8]. For this reason, sphincter electromyiography recorded during the filling and voiding phases seems to be a more appropriate method of evaluation of any improvement in pelvic floor muscle relaxation.

Quality-of-life assessment

Quality of life may be constantly changing. A validated quality-of-life questionnaire is recommended to measure the direct impact on quality of life of the alleviation of patients' symptoms.

Stimulation problems

The first indication that a subject may not be receiving appropriate levels of stimulation, or that a problem has developed with the implanted device (lead migration, wire breakage), is a change in the degree of stimulation perceived. A knowledge of the basic concepts of electricity is essential in order to investigate these problems; in addition, troubleshooting guidelines can help their management.

Basic concepts of electricity

Current is the flow of electrons from one point to another. The amount of current that flows between two points in an electrical circuit depends on two factors — voltage and resistance. Resistance represents any hindrance to current flow. In the body, resistance is termed impedance, which takes into account the tissue's ability to store electrical charge, as well as its resistive opposition to the movement of electrons. The relationship between voltage, current, and resistance is expressed by Ohm's law (Fig. 20.3). During electrical stimulation, the amount of charge flowing between two points is the critical therapeutic specification; therefore, the control of charge flow is of primary importance. SNS therapy is based on a voltage-controlled source; therefore, when a short or open circuit occurs, the flow of current delivered by the SNS system will vary, as will the perception of stimulation by the patient (Figs. 20.4 and 20.5).

Troubleshooting guidelines

Stimulation problems during the early stages of follow-up are associated with incorrect use of the programmer, telemetry or patient programmer. As the duration of follow-up increases, so does the risk of deterioration of the implanted system.

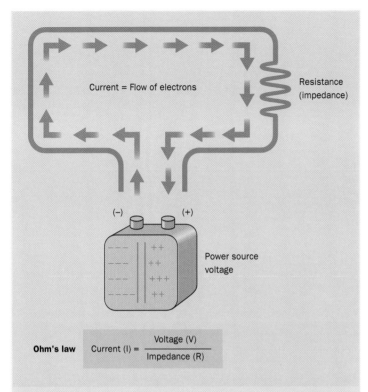

Figure 20.3 *Diagram showing an electrical circuit. The circuit is derived from an electrically charged power source. The electrical current (flow of electrons) occurs between the negative (-) and positive (+) poles. Resistance represents any hindrance to the flow of current. The relationship between voltage, current and resistance is expressed by Ohm's law. When resistance is constant, current is directly proportional to the voltage: the greater the voltage the greater the current. When voltage is constant, Ohm's law also means that current is inversely related to the resistance: the greater the resistance, the less the current.*

Lack of stimulation and intermittent stimulation

Normally, when stimulation is not perceived by the patient, this means that there has been physical damage to the system. Rupture of a wire produces an open circuit; this can occur as a result of severe stretching or twisting. Sometimes, the patient himself provokes the rupture, as in the so-called 'twiddler's syndrome', in which repeated manipulation of the IPG inside the pocket breaks the wire. Excessive tightening of the set screws may also cause physical damage leading to a short circuit. Sometimes, seepage of fluid into connections or junctions produces leakage of current. Intermittent stimulation can be caused by lead fracture or by a loose connection at the junction of an extension and the IPG or of the lead and an extension (Fig. 20.6).

Inadequate or undesirable stimulation pattern

The displacement of the lead from its original position can produce inadequate stimulation of an inappropriate nerve [9]. Usually,

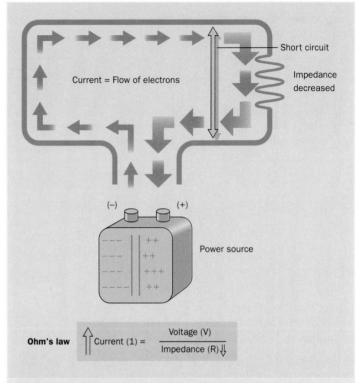

Figure 20.4 *Electrical short-circuit situation. The resistance is suddenly decreased (as happens when two bare wires touch) and the flow of current attempts to become infinite as the voltage remains constant.*

radiography resolution is unable to show minimal migrations; however, movements of less than 1mm can alter the stimulation pattern. In some cases the stimulation has undesirable effects, such as burning sensation, pain and stimulation of the bowel or genital regions. In this situation, it is necessary to investigate whether the sensation is induced by the current, by turning off the IPG. Electrically-induced undesirable stimulation is caused by leakage of current, which occurs when body fluids touch active electrodes, thus causing the stimulation of adjacent tissues. The burning sensation is confined to the site of the leakage, and calls for surgical revision (Fig. 20.7).

Long-lasting effects

Those studies that have reported on follow-up investigations have generally recorded long-lasting success [10–13]. However, a recent study by Bosch and Groen has shown that, after 5 years, there was some deterioration in the success rate of neuromodulation in some of their patients [11]. No explanation was given for this loss of

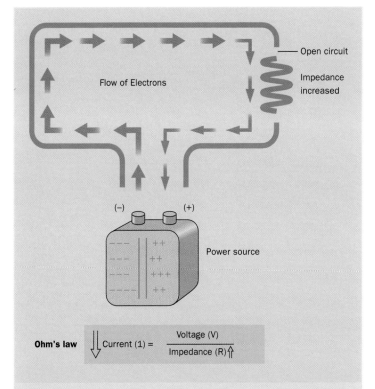

Open circuit

Impedance increased

Flow of Electrons

(−)   (+)

Power source

Ohm's law   Current (1) = $\dfrac{\text{Voltage (V)}}{\text{Impedance (R)}\Uparrow}$

Figure 20.5 *Electrical open circuit occurs. The resistance is suddenly increased (as happens when a wire ruptures); the flow of current attempts to become zero as the voltage remains constant.*

Key Points

- Effect of SNS may decline in some patients after 5 years.
- This may be due to electrical, mechanical or physiological causes.
- Electrical stimulation is contraindicated in pregnancy.
- Pregnancy termination is not necessary on inadvertent stimulation.
- IPG should be inactivated in pregnancy if return of voiding dysfunction can be tolerated.

effect, but its cause may have been related to mechanical problems such as displacement of the electrode, increasing impedance due to fibrosis or electrode erosion. For some patients there may even have been a physiological reason for the declining effectiveness.

What to do in pregnancy

Electrical stimulation has been considered to be a contraindication in pregnant women because of its potential to cause teratogenicity or abortion. A recent study has evaluated whether electrical stimulation has any adverse effects on pregnant rats and fetuses. All pregnant rats were healthy during the gestation period and no abortions were noted; no adverse effects were found in pregnant rats and their fetuses after electrical stimulation of the sacral dorsal roots. In clinical practice, termination of pregnancy is not necessary for prospective mothers when electrical stimulation is performed inadvertently during early pregnancy. It is advisable to turn off the IPG during pregnancy if the patient can tolerate the return of voiding dysfunction [14].

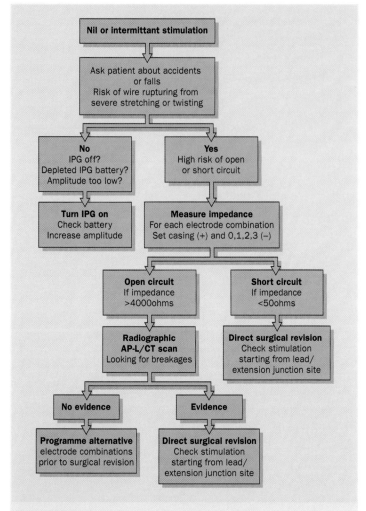

Figure 20.6 *Troubleshooting algorithm for when stimulation is either not perceived or is intermittent.*

Conclusions

Physicians must be committed to long-term follow-up of these patients. It is important that such patients are seen regularly for a long period after surgery. Successful results are due to management of all aspects of the patient's care, not just the technical aspects of surgery and follow-up procedures.

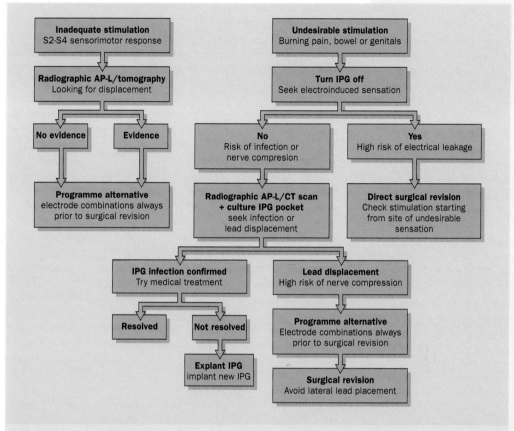

Figure 20.7 Troubleshooting algorithm for when stimulation is inadequate or undesirable.

References

1. Schmidt R, Jonas U, Oleson K et al. Sacral nerve stimulation for the treatment of refractory urinary urge incontinence. *J Urol* 1999; 162: 352–7.
2. Bemelmans B, Mundy A, Craggs M. Neuromodulation by implant for treating lower urinary tract symptoms and dysfunction. *Eur Urol* 1999; 36: 81–91.
3. van Kerrebroeck P. The role of electrical stimulation in voiding dysfunction. *Eur Urol* 1998; 34(Suppl 1): 27–30.
4. Weil EH, Ruiz-Cerdá JL, Eerdmans PH et al. Clinical results of sacral neuromodulation for chronic voiding dysfunction using unilateral sacral foramen electrodes. *World J Urol* 1998; 16: 313–21.
5. Bosch JLHR, Groen J. Sacral nerve neuromodulation in the treatment of patients with refractory motor urge incontinence: long-term results of prospective longitudinal study. *J Urol* 2000; 163: 1219–22.
6. Hassouna MM, Siegel S, Lycklama à Nijeholt AAB et al. Sacral neurostimulation in the treatment of urgency–frequency symptoms: a multicenter study on efficacy and safety. *J Urol* 2000; 163: 1849–54.
7. Janknegt RA, Hassouna MM, Siegel S et al. Long-term effectiveness of sacral nerve stimulation for refractory urge incontinence. *Eur Urol* 2001; 39: 101–6.
8. Shaker H, Hassouna MM. Sacral root neuromodulation in the treatment of various voiding and storage problems. *Int Urogynecol J* 1999; 10: 336–43.
9. Fowler CJ, Swinn MJ, Goodwin RJ et al. Studies of the latency of pelvic floor contraction during peripheral nerve evaluation show that the muscle response is reflexly mediated. *J Urol* 2000; 163: 881–3.

10. Chartier-Kastler EJ, Bosch JLHR, Perrigot M *et al*. Long-term results of sacral nerve stimulation (S3) for the treatment of neurogenic refractory urge incontinence related to detrusor hyperreflexia. *J Urol* 2000; 164: 1476–80.

11. Bosch JLHR, Groen J. Seven years of experience with sacral (S3) segmental nerve stimulation in patients with urge incontinence due to detrusor instability or hyperreflexia. *Neurourol Urodyn* 1997; 16: 426–7.

12. Grünewald V, Jonas U, the MDT-103 Multicenter Study Group. Sacral electrical nerve stimulation for treatment of severe voiding dysfunction. *J Urol* 1999; 275 (abstr. 1064).

13. Jonas U, Grünewald V, the MDT-103 Multicenter Study Group. Sacral electrical nerve stimulation for treatment of severe voiding dysfunction, *Eur Urol* 1999; 35 (Supll): 17.

14. Wang Y, Hassouna MM. Electrical stimulation has no adverse effect on pregnant rats and fetuses. *J Urol* 162: 1785–7.

Index

Abbreviations: LUT, lower urinary tract; PNE, peripheral nerve evaluation; SNS, sacral nerve stimulation; UT, urinary tract.

L

laboratory tests, 74–5
laminectomy, sacral, 204–14
    cuff electrode placement via, 204–7
    tailored, 208–14
leads and cables
    implantable, 85, 87
    in follow-up, 243
    migration/repositioning, 191, 195
    minimally-invasive technique, 218–19, 221
    routing, 30, 31
    in test stimulation, 82, 83, 101, 105, 118–19, 122, 184–5
        adverse events related to, 187
        fixed to skin, 119, 122, 123
leg response to stimulation, 12, 103, 104, 118
lignocaine (lidocaine)
    fos-immunoreactivity and effects of, 61–2
    PNE, 102
    pudendal block, 44
local anaesthetic
    fos-immunoreactivity and effects of, 61–2
    PNE, 102
    pudendal block, 44
lower urinary tract, see urinary tract
lumbodorsal fascia, see thoracolumbar fascia
lumbosacral fascia in minimally-invasive surgery, 219

M

magnet, control, 86, 127
males, see men
Mamo technique, minimally-invasive lead implantation, 218–19
materials, implant, 86–8
mechanical nerve injury, 29–33, 38
medical history, 72
Medtronic, 81
    MDT-103 (randomised prospective study), 183–96
    permanent implants
        model 3023 neurostimulator/pulse generator, 84, 126
        model 3031 patient programmer, 127
        model 3080 quad lead, see Quad electrodes
        model 3886 lead, 221
        model 7432 console programmer, 85, 127
        quadripolar extension, see quadripolar design
    test stimulation equipment, 100
        model 3057 test lead, 82, 118
        model 3625 test stimulator, 82, 83
men
    clinical examination specific to, 74
    pelvic pain syndrome, 230
    sacral shape, 10
micturating (voiding) cystourethrography (VCUG), 75, 76
micturition reflexes (voiding reflexes), 18–21
    afferent input and, 21–3, 23–5, 26
    bladder outlet obstruction and, 64
    cystitis and, 58
    urinary retention and, 157
    see also voiding
minimally-invasive SNS, 217–22
Minnesota Multiphase Personality Inventory, SNS candidates
        with urinary retention, 174–6, 177
motor effects of neuromodulation, 51
motor neuron lesions, upper, 224
motor system in brain, emotional, 91
muscle action potentials, compound (CMAPs), recording,
        107–8, 109, 113, 114
myogenic bladder, 92

N

needle (foramen), test stimulation, 82, 117, 121
    insertion, 117, 120
    stylet removal, 118, 121
nerve(s)
    electrodes, see electrodes
    injury, potential for/prevention of, 29–41
    stimulation, see electrical stimulation
    see also specific (types of) nerves
nerve growth factor (NGF), 55–6
    distribution, 62–4
    normal, 62–3
    pathological conditions, 63–4
nerve root, see sacral nerve root
NeuroControl Vocare System, 217
neurogenic bladder, 92, 224–7
neurogenic urge incontinence, 224–7
neurological examination, 74
neuromodulation, sacral, see sacral nerve stimulation
neuropathic pain, 230–1
neuropeptides, 55–67
    distribution, 56–60, 62–4
    normal, 56–8, 62–3
    pathological conditions, 58–60, 63–4
NGF, see nerve growth factor
nociception, visceral, 62
    see also pain

O

older persons, see elderly

P

pacemakers, heart, 2
paediatric urological conditions, 90
pain
    neuropathic, 230–1
    pelvic, syndromes of, 223, 229–32
    persistent, NGF and, 63
    test stimulation-related, 187–8
    visceral, urgency–frequency and, 167
    see also nociception
parasympathetic nucleus, 6
patient programmer (stimulator)
    chronic stimulator, 84, 85–6, 88, 127, 140
    test stimulator, 119
patient screener, 105
pelvic congestion, 230
pelvic floor muscles
    neuromodulation and patient rediscovery of, 51
    urethral external sphincter overactivity and, 95
pelvic floor response, PNE, 103, 104
pelvic floor stimulation, 3–4
    afferent pathways in, 23
pelvic nerve stimulation, 4
pelvic pain syndromes, 223, 229–32
percutaneous extension hardware, 83–4
percutaneous neurostimulation testing, see peripheral nerve
        evaluation
percutaneous staged implants, see staged implants
perineum-to-bladder reflex, 22–3
perineurium, breaching, 32
peripheral nerve evaluation (PNE; percutaneous neurostimula-
        tion testing; test stimulation), 76, 77–8, 99–106, 184–9
    acute responses, 103–5
    documentation, 105–6
    adverse event study, 184–9
    atlas of, 117–23
    clinical examples, 44, 45, 47
    electrophysiological monitoring during, 112, 113–14
    in faecal constipation, 235–6
    future applications, 88, 106
    hardware, see hardware
    location for, 100
    patient preparation, 99–100
    in pelvic pain syndromes, 231
    positioning of patient, 100
    predictive value, 96, 105–6
    preparation of patient, 99–100, 100
    staged implants and, 219
    in urge incontinence, 141–2, 225